Complete Self Assessment
for Medical Finals

Complete Self Assessment for Medical Finals

KINESH PATEL BA (HONS) MB BS
Senior House Officer
Department of Medicine
Hammersmith Hospital
London, UK

NEIL PATEL MB BS
Foundation Year 2
St Peter's Hospital
Chertsey
Surrey, UK

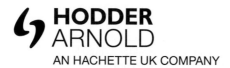
HODDER
ARNOLD
AN HACHETTE UK COMPANY

First published in Great Britain in 2007 by
Hodder Education, a member of the Hodder Headline Group,
338 Euston Road, London NW1 3BH

http://www.hoddereducation.com

Distributed in the United States of America by
Oxford University Press Inc.,
198 Madison Avenue, New York, NY10016
Oxford is a registered trademark of Oxford University Press

Hodder Headline's policy is to use papers that are natural, renewable and
recyclable products and made from wood grown in sustainable forests.
The logging and manufacturing processes are expected to conform to the
environmental regulations of the country of origin.

Whilst the advice and information in this book are believed to be true and
accurate at the date of going to press, neither the authors nor the publisher
can accept any legal responsibility or liability for any errors or omissions
that may be made. In particular, (but without limiting the generality of the
preceding disclaimer) every effort has been made to check drug dosages;
however it is still possible that errors have been missed. Furthermore,
dosage schedules are constantly being revised and new side-effects
recognized. For these reasons the reader is strongly urged to consult the
drug companies' printed instructions before administering any of the drugs
recommended in this book.

British Library Cataloguing in Publication Data
A catalogue record for this book is available from the British Library

Library of Congress Cataloging-in-Publication Data
A catalog record for this book is available from the Library of Congress

ISBN 978 0 340 88944 2

1 2 3 4 5 6 7 8 9 10

Commissioning Editor: Georgina Bentliff and Sara Purdy
Project Editor: Jane Tod
Production Controller: Lindsay Smith
Cover Design: Nichola Smith
Cover Image: © Alfred Pasieka/Science Photo Library
Indexer: Laurence Errington

Typeset in 10 on 13pt Minion by Phoenix Photosetting, Chatham, Kent
Printed and bound in India

What do you think about this book? Or any other Hodder Arnold
title? Please visit our website at www.hoddereducation.com

Contents

To our parents

Preface

The rise of multiple choice questions (MCQs) and extended matching questions (EMQs) as examination tools in medical school finals has meant that it is not only knowledge that students are tested on, but also exam technique. To this end, it is essential that students attempt large numbers of questions before their exams, to gain the confidence and speed that are necessary to ensure success.

This book provides 500 MCQs, 150 EMQs and 50 X-ray questions, divided into 16 sections covering the breadth of the medical curriculum. We suggest that students attempt the questions in each section after revising that particular topic: this will both consolidate knowledge and highlight deficiencies in learning.

The questions have been specifically written to include topics that regularly recur in finals. Student sitting their exams will undoubtedly recognize themes from this book; despite often seeming otherwise, there are only a finite number of facts undergraduates are expected to know! As with any exam, there is a considerable variety in difficulty: some questions are easier, while others are more challenging. Students should aim to attain a mark of 60 per cent of attempted questions scored correct; knowledgeable undergraduates may perform significantly better.

We wish you luck in your studies.

Kinesh Patel
Neil Patel

Acknowledgements

We would like to thank all the staff at Hodder, especially Georgina Bentliff and Jane Tod for their help with this project.

We are also grateful to Dr Kate Tatham and Dr Lucy Dolman for their invaluable comments and corrections to the manuscript.

Abbreviations

AAA	abdominal aortic aneurysm
ACE	angiotensin-converting enzyme
ACTH	adrenocorticotrophic hormone
ADH	antidiuretic hormone
ADP	adenosine diphosphate
ADPKD	autosomal dominant polycystic kidney disease
AFB	acid-fast bacilli
ALL	acute lymphoblastic leukaemia
ALP	alkaline phosphatase
ALT	alanine transaminase
AMA	antimitochondrial antibody
AML	acute myeloid leukaemia
ANA	antinuclear antibody
ANCA	antineutrophil cytoplasmic antibody
AP	anteroposterior
APTT	activated partial thromboplastin time
ARDS	adult respiratory distress syndrome
5-ASA	5-aminosalicylic acid
AST	aspartate transaminase
AV	atrioventricular
BiPAP	bilevel positive airways pressure
CK	creatine kinase
CLL	chronic lymphocytic leukaemia
CML	chronic myeloid leukaemia
CMV	cytomegalovirus
CNS	central nervous system
COPD	chronic obstructive pulmonary disease
COX-2	cyclo-oxygenase-2
CPAP	continuous positive airway pressure
CRH	corticotrophin-releasing hormone
CRP	C-reactive protein
CSF	cerebrospinal fluid
CT	computed tomography
DDH	developmental dysplasia of the hip

DIC	disseminated intravascular coagulation
DMARD	disease-modifying antirheumatic drug
DMSA	dimercaptosuccinic acid
DTPA	diethylenetriamine penta-acetic acid
DVT	deep vein thrombosis
ECG	electrocardiogram
ENT	ear, nose and throat
ERCP	endoscopic retrograde cholangiopancreatography
ESR	erythrocyte sedimentation rate
ETS	endoscopic transthoracic sympathectomy
FAP	familial adenomatous polyposis
FEV_1	forced expiratory volume in 1 s
FSH	follicle-stimulating hormone
FVC	forced vital capacity
GBM	glomerular basement membrane
GCS	Glasgow Coma Scale
G-CSF	granulocyte colony-stimulating factor
GGT	gamma-glutamyl transferase
GHB	gamma hydroxybutyric acid
GI	gastrointestinal
GnRH	gonadotrophin-releasing hormone
GORD	gastro-oesophageal reflux disease
GP	general practitioner
G6PD	glucose-6-phosphate dehydrogenase
γ-GT	gamma-glutamyl transferase
GTN	glyceryl trinitrate
Hb	haemoglobin
HBeAg	hepatitis B e antigen
HCG	human chorionic gonadotrophin
HIT	heparin-induced thrombocytopenia
HLA	human leucocyte antigen
HNPCC	hereditary non-polyposis colorectal cancer
HOCM	hypertrophic obstructive cardiomyopathy
HPOA	hypertrophic pulmonary osteoarthropathy
HPV	human papillomavirus
HRT	hormone replacement therapy
5-HT	5-hydroxytryptamine
i.v.	intravenous
IgA	immunoglobulin A
IgE	immunoglobulin E
INR	international normalized ratio
ITP	idiopathic thrombocytopenic purpura
ITU	intensive therapy unit
IVF	*in vitro* fertilization
IVU	intravenous urogram/urography
JVP	jugular venous pressure/pulse
LBBB	left bundle branch block

LDH	lactate dehydrogenase
LMWH	low-molecular weight heparin
MAHA	microangiopathic haemolytic anaemia
MAO	monoamine oxidase
MCV	mean corpuscular volume
MEN	multiple endocrine neoplasia
metHb	methaemoglobin
MPO	myeloperoxidase
MRCP	magnetic resonance cholangiopancreatography
MRI	magnetic resonance imaging
MRSA	meticillin-resistant *Staphylococcus aureus*
NASH	non-alcoholic steatohepatitis
NICE	National Institute for Clinical Excellence
NSAID	non-steroidal anti-inflammatory drug
OGD	oesophagogastroduodenoscopy
PA	postero-anterior
pANCA	perinuclear antineutrophil cytoplasmic antibody
Pco_2	partial pressure of carbon dioxide
PE	pulmonary embolism
Po_2	partial pressure of oxygen
PPI	proton pump inhibitor
PSA	prostate-specific antigen
PT	prothrombin time
PTH	parathyroid hormone
PTHrP	parathyroid hormone-related peptide
Sao_2	arterial oxygen saturation
SIADH	syndrome of inappropriate antidiuretic hormone secretion
SLE	systemic lupus erythematosus
TB	tuberculosis
TIA	transient ischaemic attack
TIPS	transjugular intrahepatic portosystemic shunting
TNF	tumour necrosis factor
TRH	thyrotrophin-releasing hormone
TSH	thyroid-stimulating hormone
TURP	trans-urethral resection of the prostate
UDP	uridine diphospho
VIP	vasoactive intestinal peptide
$\dot{V}/\dot{Q}$	ventilation–perfusion
WCC	white cell count

CHAPTER 1

The cardiovascular system

MULTIPLE CHOICE QUESTIONS

1 Rheumatic fever is:
   a) Caused by group A staphylococcus
   b) Common in the developed world
   c) A cause of mitral regurgitation
   d) Treated with intravenous flucloxacillin
   e) Associated with movement disorders

2 Aortic stenosis is commonly associated with:
   a) A slow rising pulse
   b) Corrigan's sign
   c) de Musset's sign
   d) Atrial fibrillation
   e) Syncope

3 Regarding arterial ulceration of the peripheries:
   a) It is painless
   b) The commonest site is above the medial malleolus
   c) Tissue reperfusion does not aid healing
   d) The edge is usually rolled
   e) Venous stripping is a useful treatment

4 The chest X-ray is of use in the diagnosis of the following conditions:
   a) Pericardial effusion
   b) Acute pericarditis
   c) Heart failure
   d) Coarctation of the aorta
   e) Bacterial endocarditis

5 Regarding abdominal aortic aneurysms:
   a) A computed tomography (CT) scan is an essential pre-operative investigation if rupture is suspected
   b) They affect males and females equally
   c) Repair is generally considered once the diameter has exceeded 3.5 cm
   d) Trash foot is a complication of surgery
   e) Repair is not possible if the patient is unable to tolerate a laparotomy

6   Hypertension:
   a) Is usually idiopathic
   b) Is usually secondary to other causes in those aged under 40 years
   c) Can be caused by Conn's syndrome
   d) Is associated with microaneurysm formation in the retina
   e) Can be caused by the use of heroin

7   Regarding the electrocardiogram (ECG):
   a) It is taken with 12 leads
   b) The normal axis is from 0° to 120°
   c) ST segment elevation in all leads usually indicates a myocardial infarct
   d) The PR interval is prolonged in Mobitz type II heart block
   e) The first change in acute myocardial infarction is the appearance of Q waves

8   The following drugs decrease the mortality of heart failure:
   a) Digoxin
   b) Dobutamine
   c) Verapamil
   d) Carvedilol
   e) Enalapril

9   The following statements are true of intermittent claudication:
   a) It usually starts in the foot
   b) Management involves strict alcohol abstinence
   c) The pain is not relieved by rest
   d) Exercise encourages collateral artery development
   e) Beta-blockers may help alleviate the symptoms

10 Options for management of critical limb ischaemia include:
   a) Vascular stenting
   b) Amlodipine
   c) Lumbar sympathectomy
   d) Limb amputation
   e) Compression stockings

11 Atrial fibrillation:
   a) Is more common in the elderly
   b) Is associated with hypothyroidism
   c) Is usually treated with amiodarone
   d) Is correlated with haemorrhagic stroke
   e) Always causes an irregularly irregular pulse

12 The following are characteristic features of angina:
   a) Retrosternal chest pain
   b) Pain that is worse with arm movement
   c) A split second heart sound
   d) ST segment depression on the resting ECG
   e) A tender chest wall

13 Regarding heart sounds:
   a) The aortic valve is heard closing before the pulmonary valve
   b) The third heart sound occurs in early systole
   c) A fourth heart sound indicates ventricular stiffness
   d) A third heart sound is a sign of heart failure
   e) Reversed splitting of the second heart sound is found in left bundle branch block

14 Regarding peripheral vascular rest pain:
   a) It is untreatable
   b) The pain is relieved at night
   c) It starts in the calf
   d) Elevation of the legs relieves the pain
   e) It is usually relieved by paracetamol

15 Cardiovascular causes of clubbing include:
   a) Pericarditis
   b) Atrial myxoma
   c) Malignant hypertension
   d) Infective endocarditis
   e) Rheumatic fever

16 The following arrhythmias are associated with a regular heart rate:
   a) Atrial fibrillation
   b) Atrial flutter
   c) First-degree heart block
   d) Mobitz I block
   e) Mobitz II block

17 The murmur of mitral regurgitation is best heard:
   a) With the patient sitting forward
   b) In systole
   c) On inspiration
   d) At the apex of the heart
   e) Radiating to the carotids

18 Causes of a raised jugular venous pressure include:
   a) Postural hypotension
   b) Congestive cardiac failure
   c) Atrial fibrillation
   d) Constrictive pericarditis
   e) Superior vena cava obstruction

19 Coarctation of the aorta leads to:
   a) Transient ischaemic attacks
   b) Radio-femoral delay
   c) Notching of the ribs on chest X-ray
   d) Hypertension
   e) Cardiomegaly

20   The following are recognized risk factors for ischaemic heart disease:
   a) Smoking
   b) Diabetes mellitus
   c) Stress
   d) Cystinuria
   e) Hypothyroidism

21   Recognized complications of carotid endarterectomy include:
   a) Stroke
   b) Hypoglossal nerve damage
   c) Tracheal perforation
   d) Thyroid dysfunction
   e) Foster Kennedy syndrome

22   Cardinal features of critical limb ischaemia include:
   a) Absence of hairs
   b) Gangrene
   c) Impaired capillary refill
   d) Rest pain
   e) Ankle pressure <100 mmHg

23   ST elevation on ECG in leads II, III and aVF alone:
   a) Indicates anterior myocardial infarction
   b) Indicates inferior myocardial infarction
   c) Could indicate acute pericarditis
   d) Could be a trivial finding
   e) Is normal in children

24   Consequences of lower limb venous insufficiency include:
   a) Ankle oedema
   b) Haemosiderin pigmentation
   c) Necrobiosis lipoidica
   d) Eczema
   e) Neuropathic ulceration

25   Subacute bacterial endocarditis is:
   a) Associated with systolic murmurs
   b) Commoner in intravenous drug users
   c) Treated with at least six weeks of oral penicillin
   d) Commoner in diabetics
   e) Associated with splinter lesions

26   The following are risk factors for varicose veins:
   a) Deep vein thrombosis (DVT)
   b) Uterine cancer
   c) Intermittent claudication
   d) Bed rest
   e) Pregnancy

27 Causes of arterial aneurysms include:
  a) Polycythaemia
  b) Trauma
  c) Marfan's syndrome
  d) Syphilis
  e) Vasculitis

28 The following are causes of heart failure:
  a) Hyperthyroidism
  b) Ischaemic heart disease
  c) Atrial myxoma
  d) Hypertension
  e) Atrial fibrillation

29 The following treatments are used in angina:
  a) Isosorbide mononitrate
  b) Glyceryl trinitrate
  c) Enalapril
  d) Fentanyl patches
  e) Metoprolol

30 Systolic murmurs are found in:
  a) Mitral stenosis
  b) Aortic stenosis
  c) Ventricular septal defect
  d) Pulmonary regurgitation
  e) Pregnancy

31 Bradyarrhythmias include:
  a) Wolff–Parkinson White syndrome
  b) Mobitz type II
  c) Atrial flutter
  d) Sick sinus syndrome
  e) The Wenckebach phenomenon

32 The jugular venous pulse (JVP):
  a) Shows cannon waves in tricuspid stenosis
  b) Is elevated in congestive heart failure
  c) Shows cannon waves in heart block
  d) Can be palpated in the anterior triangle of the neck
  e) Paradoxically falls on inspiration in constrictive pericarditis

33 Treatment options for atrial fibrillation include:
  a) Anticoagulation with warfarin for 6 months
  b) Cardioversion
  c) 1 per cent lidocaine intravenously
  d) Digoxin
  e) Ablation of an aberrant conduction pathway

34 Causes of sudden cardiac death include:
   a) Acute mitral stenosis
   b) Aortic stenosis
   c) Hypertrophic obstructive cardiomyopathy
   d) Aortic regurgitation
   e) Acute pericarditis

35 The following drugs improve the outcome of acute myocardial infarction:
   a) Aspirin
   b) ACE inhibitors
   c) Calcium channel blockers
   d) Beta-blockers
   e) Thrombolytics

36 Symptoms of cardiac failure include:
   a) Dyspnoea
   b) Orthopnoea
   c) Cheyne–Stokes respiration
   d) Chest pain
   e) Palpitations

37 Complications of myocardial infarction include:
   a) Severe chest pain
   b) Cardiogenic shock
   c) Sinus bradycardia
   d) Pericarditis
   e) Spontaneous aortic rupture

38 Primary causes of cardiomyopathy include:
   a) Schistosomiasis
   b) Alcohol
   c) Smoking
   d) Genetics
   e) Hypertension

39 Causes of high-output heart failure include:
   a) Pellagra
   b) Thyrotoxicosis
   c) Anaemia
   d) Paget's disease
   e) Scleroderma

40 A general practitioner might use the following to treat hypertension:
   a) Losartan
   b) Doxazosin
   c) Amlodipine
   d) Isosorbide mononitrate
   e) Bendroflumethiazide

Answers: see pages 16–21

EXTENDED MATCHING QUESTIONS

1 CHEST PAIN

Match the case histories below with the most likely cause of chest pain

A   Inferior myocardial infarction
B   Angina
C   Dissecting aortic aneurysm
D   Acute pericarditis
E   Oesophageal reflux

F   Anterior myocardial infarction
G   Pulmonary embolism
H   Costochondritis
I   Herpes zoster
J   Spontaneous pneumothorax

1   A 32-year-old librarian goes to the emergency department with chest pain. He is also feeling short of breath, but looks comfortable at rest. His pulse is 88 beats/min and respiratory rate 18 breaths/min. Examination reveals decreased expansion on the right side of his chest with a hyper-resonant percussion note.

2   A 31-year-old pharmacist presents to the emergency department with a 2-day history of central chest pain and associated shortness of breath. He says that the pain is worse on inspiration and movement. Examination reveals a muscular man with normal heart and breath sounds. He is tender over the lower sternum.

3   A 27-year-old student presents to his general practitioner (GP) with a 3-day history of central chest pain, which he describes as sharp and stabbing in character. The pain radiates to the neck and left arm, and is relieved by sitting upright. The GP immediately performs an ECG which shows ST elevation in all leads.

4   A 78-year-old former miner collapses while in the garden. The ambulance crew bring him in saying that he was complaining of central, crushing chest pain at the scene. He is now pale and sweaty, and keeps saying that he thinks he is going to die. An ECG shows ST elevation in leads II, III and aVF, with ST depression in I, aVL and aVR.

5   A 69-year-old journalist is brought to the emergency department via ambulance. He complains of severe central chest pain radiating through to his back. He looks pale and clammy and is sweating. An ECG is performed in resus which shows a sinus tachycardia. His pulse is 110 beats/min, blood pressure 170/100 mmHg in his right arm and 130/70 mmHg in the left.

2 ST CHANGES ON ECG

Match the description of the ST segment abnormalities with the most likely diagnosis

A   Pericarditis
B   Anterior myocardial infarction
C   Inferior myocardial infarction
D   Lateral myocardial infarction
E   Posterior myocardial infarction

F   Prolonged QT interval
G   Angina
H   Digoxin
I   Hypokalaemia
J   High take off

1   Convex upwards ST elevation in leads II, III, aVF, ST depression in I, aVL
2   Concave downwards ST depression in all leads with T wave inversion.
3   Concave upwards ST elevation in all leads except aVR
4   Leads V_1–V_3 show prominent R waves, ST depression and large inverted T waves
5   Convex upwards ST elevation in leads I, aVL, V5, V6

3 SECONDARY HYPERTENSION

All of the patients below present with hypertension. Match the most likely cause of their hypertension to each case history

A	Conn's syndrome	F	Renal artery stenosis
B	Cushing's syndrome	G	Polycystic kidney disease
C	Acromegaly	H	Coarctation of the aorta
D	Phaeochromocytoma	I	Congenital adrenal hyperplasia
E	Hyperthyroidism	J	Iatrogenic

1 A 43-year-old vet is found to have a blood pressure of 170/110 mmHg. A routine set of blood tests is normal apart from Na^+ 148 mmol/L, K^+ 3.1mmol/L. Further testing reveals a low plasma renin and elevated aldosterone.

2 A 79-year-old diabetic woman has a blood pressure incidentally found to be 162/103 mmHg. Her GP starts her on some enalapril to try to bring it under control. Three days later, she is admitted to hospital with a 1-day history of oliguria. Her urea is 15 mmol/L and creatinine 400 μmol/L.

3 A 32-year-old decorator goes to see his GP complaining that he suffers from hot flushes and episodic headaches. He is generally fit and well but has been seeing a psychologist for panic attacks and palpitations. Examination reveals a fine tremor, a blood pressure of 200/130 mmHg, and a tachycardia of 110 beats/min. While the GP is examining his abdomen, he has another panic attack.

4 A 22-year-old chef presents with blood pressure of 180/70 mmHg. Examination reveals the presence of a delay between the radial and femoral pulses.

5 A 27-year-old waitress goes to her GP for a repeat prescription of the oral contraceptive pill. He measures her blood pressure and finds it to be 170/105mmHg – previously it had been 130/75 mmHg. Examination is otherwise unremarkable.

4 ARRHYTHMIAS

Match the electrocardiographic abnormalities with the arrhythmias below

A	Wenckebach phenomenon	F	Atrial flutter
B	Ventricular fibrillation	G	Sick sinus syndrome
C	Wolff–Parkinson–White syndrome	H	Atrial fibrillation
D	Ventricular tachycardia	I	Third-degree heart block
E	First-degree heart block	J	Asystole

1 P waves are present but there is a broad complex regular bradycardia at a rate of 30 beats/min

2 A slurred upstroke to the QRS complex

3 No visible atrial activity with morphologically normal QRS complexes

4 Completely irregular electrical activity, with no coordination visible

5 Progressive lengthening of the PR interval until there is not a ventricular response

5 DRUGS USED IN CARDIOLOGY TO TREAT HYPERTENSION

Match the drugs below to the class to which they belong

A Enalapril
B Verapamil
C Bendroflumethiazide
D Metoprolol
E Losartan

F Clonidine
G Hydralazine
H Doxazosin
I Spironolactone
J Sodium nitroprusside

1 β-blocker
2 Angiotensin receptor antagonist
3 α_1-blocker
4 α_2-stimulant
5 Calcium channel blocker

6 SIDE-EFFECTS OF DRUGS USED IN CARDIOLOGY TO TREAT HYPERTENSION

Match the side-effects listed below with the most likely pharmacological cause. Each option may be used once, more than once, or not at all

A Enalapril
B Verapamil
C Bendroflumethiazide
D Metoprolol
E Losartan

F Clonidine
G Hydralazine
H Doxazosin
I Spironolactone
J Sodium nitroprusside

1 Systemic lupus erythematosus
2 Chronic cough
3 Gynaecomastia
4 Bronchospasm
5 Gout

7 HEART SOUNDS

Match the most likely cardiac lesion with the findings below

A Aortic regurgitation
B Aortic stenosis
C Atrial septal defect
D Mitral regurgitation
E Mitral stenosis

F Tricuspid regurgitation
G Pulmonary stenosis
H Ventricular septal defect
I Hypertrophic obstructive cardiomyopathy
J Pulmonary regurgitation

1 Ejection systolic murmur, heard best in expiration at the right second intercostal space close to the sternum, radiating into the neck.
2 Wide fixed splitting of the second heart sound.
3 Early diastolic murmur, heard best at the lower left sternal edge with the patient leaning forward in expiration.
4 Late systolic murmur with third and fourth heart sounds, double apical impulse, jerky carotid pulse.
5 Mid-diastolic murmur, heard best at the apex in expiration.

8 FEATURES OF INFECTIVE ENDOCARDITIS

A patient arrives in the UK from overseas, and gives a 6-month history of untreated infective endocarditis. Match the signs below with the clinical findings

A   Clubbing
B   Janeway lesions
C   Cerebral emboli
D   Conjunctival haemorrhage
E   Roth spots

F   Splinter haemorrhages
G   Haematuria
H   Osler's nodes
I   Splenomegaly
J   Petechiae

1   Tender subcutaneous nodules found on the distal pads of the digits
2   Small linear lines under the nails
3   Small non-blanching spots under the skin
4   Fundoscopy reveals small retinal haemorrhages
5   Non-tender macules on the palms and soles of the feet

9 INVESTIGATIONS IN CARDIOLOGY

The tests used below are all used in cardiology. Match the most useful investigation from this list for the patients below

A   Chest X-ray
B   Echocardiography
C   ECG
D   Pericardiocentesis
E   Exercise electrocardiography

F   Thallium scan
G   Cardiac magnetic resonance imaging
H   Coronary angiography
I   Holter monitoring
J   Tilt-table testing

1   A 36-year-old butcher tells her GP that she is having palpitations at home. She suddenly feels her heart start beating quickly for about 2 min, and then the palpitations suddenly disappear. She says that she never experiences any chest pain. An ECG is entirely normal.
2   A 69-year-old retired postman goes to hospital with central crushing chest pain. An ECG is performed which shows ST elevation in leads V_3–V_6.
3   A 43-year-old soldier cannot perform his sentry duties as he collapses after about 30 min of standing upright. The doctor suspects neurocardiogenic syncope.
4   A 23-year-old tree surgeon comes to the emergency department and gives a history of collapsing after playing football. He has had two similar previous occurrences. Examination reveals a double apical pulsation and a late systolic murmur. A chest X-ray shows an enlarged heart.
5   A 73-year-old attends his local cardiology department with exertional chest pain. The cardiologist is unsure whether the patient has angina. The resting ECG is normal, and the doctor therefore asks for an exercise stress test. Unfortunately the treadmill test is abandoned after 22 s, as the patient complains of severe pain in his arthritic left knee.

10 AORTIC REGURGITATION

Match the signs of aortic regurgitation below with their descriptions

A   de Musset's sign
B   Early diastolic murmur
C   Quincke's sign
D   Pistol-shot femorals
E   Austin Flint murmur

F   Corrigan's sign
G   Waterhammer pulse
H   Duroziez's sign
I   Displaced apex beat
J   Widened pulse pressure

1   Nailbed capillary pulsation
2   A blood pressure of 180/80 mmHg
3   Head nodding in time with the pulse
4   Visible carotid pulsations
5   A double murmur heard over the femoral artery when it is compressed distally and then released.

11 SIDE-EFFECTS OF DRUGS USED TO TREAT ARRHYTHMIAS

Match the case histories below with the drug most likely to cause the side-effects described.
Each option may be used once, more than once, or not at all

A   Adenosine
B   Flecainide
C   Lidocaine
D   Amiodarone
E   Digoxin

F   Verapamil
G   Propafenone
H   Disopyramide
I   Sotalol
J   Isoprenaline

1   A 68-year-old man who is started on an antiarrhythmic drug to control his atrial fibrillation presents to his GP 6 months later with weight loss, tremor, weakness, palpitations and heat intolerance.
2   A junior doctor tries to control a supraventricular tachycardia in a patient in resus. He does not realize that the patient has also taken metoprolol that evening. Unfortunately the patient develops asystole and dies.
3   A 73-year old woman goes to her GP 2 years after being started on a drug for three episodes of ventricular tachycardia. She is having difficulty breathing, and has fine crackles throughout both lungs. The GP orders chest X-ray which is reported as 'honeycomb lung'.
4   A 67-year-old man attends the emergency department with a productive cough and fever. The only medication he takes is for his atrial fibrillation. A routine ECG is performed which shows widespread T wave inversion with downwards-sloping ST segments.
5   A 52-year-old man goes to his GP complaining that while the new medicine he has been started on for his palpitations has cured his heart troubles, he is now impotent.

12 VAUGHAN WILLIAMS' CLASSIFICATION OF DRUGS USED TO TREAT ARRHYTHMIAS

Classify each antiarrhythmic drug by using one of the options below

A   Ia
B   Ib
C   Ic
D   II
E   III

F   IV
G   Active in all four classes
H   Active in none of the classes
I   Active in classes I and II
J   Active in classes III and IV

1   Digoxin
2   Amiodarone
3   Verapamil
4   Flecainide
5   Lidocaine

13 SIGNS OF CARDIAC DISEASE

Choose the diagnosis from the list below which best correlates with the examination findings

A   Rheumatic fever
B   Tricuspid regurgitation
C   Aortic stenosis
D   Atrial septal defect
E   Heart failure

F   Infective endocarditis
G   Hypertrophic cardiomyopathy
H   Complete heart block
I   Mitral stenosis
J   Aortic regurgitation

1   An 80-year-old woman goes to her GP for some laxatives. He notes that both her cheeks have a flushed appearance, and that she has a cardiac murmur.
2   A 29-year-old bricklayer goes for a routine health check-up. His doctor is intrigued when he finds that his patient has an ejection systolic murmur and a fourth heart sound.
3   A 73-year-old man goes to the emergency department feeling very unwell. The doctor examining him documents that his JVP demonstrates 'cannon' a waves, and asks for some further investigations.
4   An 83-year-old man, who has smoked all his life, is well known to the local cardiologist. He has not been well recently. When feeling his radial pulse, the consultant notes that alternate pulsations are strong and weak.
5   A 71-year-old woman goes to the emergency department having collapsed. The doctor finds that she has a slow rising pulse.

14 SYMPTOMS AND SIGNS OF CARDIAC DISEASE

Match the symptoms of cardiac disease with their descriptions

A   Cheyne–Stokes respiration
B   Pulsus alternans
C   Paroxysmal nocturnal dyspnoea
D   Xanthomata
E   Arcus senilis

F   Erythema marginatum
G   Orthopnoea
H   Xanthelasma
I   Pulsus paradoxus
J   Clubbing

1   An 89-year-old man says that he cannot sleep with fewer than three pillows.
2   A 28-year-old journalist goes to his GP after being discharged from hospital, where he has been an inpatient for two weeks having had a myocardial infarction. The GP notices nodules on the backs of the patient's hands and elbows.
3   A 92-year-old woman calls her GP to her nursing home as she is feeling short of breath. He notices that she has a respiratory rate of 25 breaths/min initially but then becomes apnoeic for 15 s before returning to a rate of 25 breaths/min.
4   A 61-year-old man goes to his GP for an insurance health check. Before she performs fundoscopy, she notices a whitish discoloration around the iris.
5   A 47-year-old artist is admitted to hospital with severe asthma. Written on the observations chart are blood pressures of 130/70 mmHg in expiration and 105/58 mmHg in inspiration.

15 CARDIAC SYNCOPE

All of the patients below have collapsed. Match the case scenarios with the most likely diagnosis from the list below

A   Neurocardiogenic syncope
B   Cardiac tamponade
C   Sick sinus syndrome
D   Pacemaker failure
E   Myxoma

F   Pulmonary stenosis
G   Aortic stenosis
H   Hypertrophic cardiomyopathy
I   Ventricular tachycardia
J   Myocardial infarction

1   A 59-year-old insurance salesman collapses on the train and is taken to the local emergency department. His pulse is irregular with some long pauses. An ECG shows irregularly spaced QRS complexes with each preceded by a normal P wave.
2   A 45-year-old firefighter goes to his GP after having collapsed several times. Physical examination reveals a diastolic murmur, with an added sound in early diastole, which his GP tells him sounds like a plop. An ECG is unremarkable.
3   A 21-year-old supermarket assistant goes to her doctor complaining that she collapses after about 2 h behind the fish counter. She denies incontinence of urine or tongue biting.
4   A 74-year-old man goes to his GP, having apparently fainted while playing football with his grandson. The GP examines him, but apologizes that he has forgotten his stethoscope. He finds a slow rising pulse and a thrill over the praecordium. An ECG shows left ventricular hypertrophy.
5   A 37-year-old film producer goes to the emergency department with some left-sided chest pain. He has been up all night celebrating the release of his latest picture. On examination, he has dilated pupils and is tachycardic. The ECG shows ST elevation in leads V_3–V_6.

Answers: see pages 21–26

X-RAY QUESTIONS

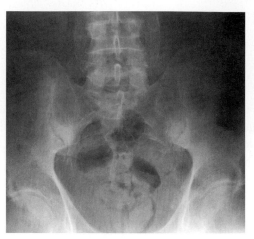

1

1   A 63-year-old man presents to Accident & Emergency complaining of severe abdominal pain. His blood pressure is 90/50 mmHg. A plain abdominal X-ray is requested. What is the most likely cause of this patient's abdominal pain?

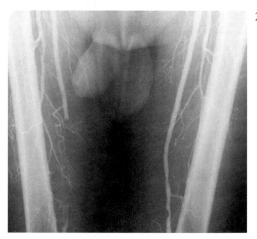

2

2   An 82-year-old man calls an ambulance as he notices that his leg has gone cold. On arrival in the emergency department, the doctor notes that he is in atrial fibrillation and cannot feel his right leg.
   a) What investigation has been performed?
   b) What is the cause of this patient's cold leg?

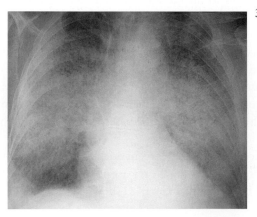

3

3   An 83-year-old woman calls an ambulance at 3 am, having just woken up acutely short of breath. On auscultation, she has crackles to both mid-zones.
   a) Explain why this patient is feeling short of breath.
   b) Outline initial treatment for this condition.

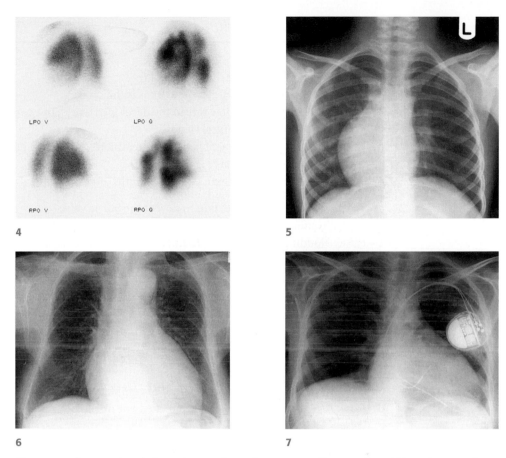

4

5

6

7

To answer the questions below, please refer to the corresponding numbered X-ray images above.

4   A 29-year-old woman goes to see her doctor 3 days after the birth of her first child, saying that she has noticed that she has started coughing up blood, and feels a little short of breath. He sends her straight to hospital.
   a) What investigation has been performed?
   b) What is the cause of this patient's symptoms?

5   A GP sees a child whose mother complains that he has a chronic cough. On examination, the heart sounds are indistinct. He requests a chest X-ray.
   a) What abnormality is shown on the chest X-ray?
   b) Why may this child have a chronic cough?

6   A 74-year-old man goes to see his GP, saying that he feels tired all the time and cannot walk as far as he used to be able to, due to shortness of breath. What abnormality is shown on the chest X-ray that may explain this patient's symptoms?

7   The surgical house officer on call is asked to check a chest X-ray requested from the orthopaedic pre-assessment clinic.
   a) What is the foreign body shown on the chest X-ray?
   b) Where do the wires terminate?

Answers: see pages 26–27

ANSWERS

MCQ ANSWERS

1. a) False. Group A β-haemolytic streptococcus is the cause.
   b) False. Rheumatic fever is now rare in the developed world, but common worldwide.
   c) True. It is also a cause of mitral stenosis.
   d) False. Intravenous benzylpenicillin is the treatment of choice. Flucloxacillin is used for staphylococcal infections.
   e) True. Sydenham's chorea occurs up to 6 months after the original disease.

2. a) True. It is caused by obstruction to flow at the aortic valve.
   b) False. Prominent carotid pulses are seen in aortic regurgitation.
   c) False. Nodding of the head in time with the pulse is a sign of severe aortic regurgitation.
   d) False. Sinus rhythm is usual – atrial fibrillation is more associated with mitral disease.
   e) True. Severe limitation of cardiac output can lead to syncopal episodes.

3. a) False. Arterial ulcers are intensely painful.
   b) False. This is the classic site for venous ulceration. Arterial ulcers are located over the pressure areas of the foot, heel and toes.
   c) False. Reversing the ischaemia can lead to complete healing of the ulcer.
   d) False. Arterial ulcers are normally punched out due to poor healing.
   e) False.

4. a) True. A rapid increase in heart size and a globular shadow are features.
   b) False. It is often a clinical diagnosis.
   c) True. Enlargement in heart size is almost universal.
   d) True. Rib notching on the underside is characteristic.
   e) False. Bacterial endocarditis is not seen on chest X-ray.

5. a) False. Urgent laparotomy is mandatory to avoid unnecessary delay, if there is a high clinical suspicion of rupture.
   b) False. They are more common in males.
   c) False. 5.5 cm is the commonly quoted threshold.
   d) True. Embolization of the aneurysm can occlude the small vessels of the feet, leading to areas of necrosis.
   e) False. Endovascular repair is another option.

6. a) True. This is so-called essential hypertension.
   b) False. Even in young people, essential hypertension is more common than secondary causes.
   c) True. Hyperaldosteronism is a cause of secondary hypertension.
   d) False. This is a hallmark of diabetic eye disease. Early hypertensive changes include narrowing of the retinal arteries.
   e) False. Heroin, unlike cocaine, does not cause hypertension.

7 a) False. The ECG is taken with 9 leads which are resolved into 12 leads.
   b) False. The normal axis is from −30° to 90°.
   c) False. This is more likely to be acute pericarditis.
   d) False. The PR interval is normal but the occasional QRS complex is dropped.
   e) False. ST segment elevation is usually the first sign of infarction.

8 a) False. Digoxin has no effect on mortality.
   b) False. Positive inotropes increase mortality in heart failure.
   c) False. Calcium channel blockers do not affect mortality.
   d) True. Beta-blockers have been counterintuitively shown to decrease mortality.
   e) True. Angiotensin-converting enzyme (ACE) inhibitors all decrease mortality and morbidity.

9 a) False. It normally affects the calf or the buttock.
   b) False.
   c) False. Resting reduces the work performed by the muscles, reducing ischaemic pain.
   d) True.
   e) False. Beta-blockers tend to exacerbate intermittent claudication by decreasing blood flow to the limb.

10 a) True.
   b) False. There is no role for calcium channel antagonists.
   c) True. This increases skin perfusion and may promote healing of arterial ulcers.
   d) True. While undesirable, it is often the best option to avoid the spread of gangrene.
   e) False. These are contraindicated in severe peripheral vascular disease.

11 a) True. The incidence increases with age.
   b) False. Thyrotoxicosis is a well-recognized cause.
   c) False. Digoxin is first-line therapy for rate control.
   d) False. Patients have a higher chance of ischaemic stroke.
   e) True. It is a hallmark of atrial fibrillation.

12 a) True.
   b) False. This is more consistent with a strained muscle.
   c) False. This is a normal examination finding.
   d) False. Resting ECG is normal in up to 80 per cent of cases.
   e) False. This is more suspicious of costochondritis.

13 a) True. This is the normal second heart sound and is responsible for audible splitting on inspiration.
   b) False. The third heart sound is normally heard soon after the second sound in early diastole.
   c) True.
   d) True.
   e) True. The pulmonary valve closes before the aortic valve in left bundle branch block (LBBB), leading to a split heart sound on expiration.

14 a) False. Analgesia and/or reperfusion procedures may alleviate the pain.
   b) False. It occurs continuously at rest.
   c) False. The pain starts by affecting the superficial tissues of the toes and forefoot.
   d) False. For relief, patients often dangle their legs out of the bed at night, increasing peripheral perfusion.
   e) False. Only strong analgesics, such as opioid derivatives, relieve the pain.

15 a) False.
   b) True. This is a primary cardiac tumour, usually in the left atrium.
   c) False.
   d) True. Cardiac causes are atrial myxoma, infective endocarditis and congenital cyanotic cardiac disease.
   e) False.

16 a) False. Atrial fibrillation is characteristically irregularly irregular.
   b) True. The heart rate is usually a factor of 300 (i.e. 150, 75, 60, 50) depending on the degree of atrioventricular (AV) block.
   c) True.
   d) False. Mobitz heart block types I and II have occasional missed beats.
   e) False.

17 a) False. This accentuates aortic regurgitation.
   b) True. It is a pan-systolic murmur.
   c) False. Left-sided murmurs are best heard in expiration.
   d) True. This is the best place for mitral murmurs.
   e) False. Aortic stenosis radiates towards the carotids.

18 a) False.
   b) True. There is increased right ventricular filling pressure.
   c) False.
   d) True. There is restricted right ventricular filling.
   e) True. The distended jugular veins do not have a pulsation in superior vena cava obstruction.

19 a) False.
   b) True. The narrowing leads to blood reaching the radial pulses before the femoral pulses.
   c) True. The characteristic notching occurs on the underside of the ribs where the intercostal vessels run.
   d) True. Hypertension occurs predominantly in the upper limbs.
   e) True. Untreated coarctation leads to heart failure.

20 a) True. They are strongly correlated.
   b) True. Diabetes mellitus is another important risk factor.
   c) True.
   d) False. Elevated homocysteine levels are a minor risk factor.
   e) True.

21 a) True. Possibly up to 5 per cent of patients suffer a stroke.
   b) True. Due to the close proximity of the nerve to the incision site.
   c) False.
   d) False.
   e) False. Foster Kennedy syndrome is papilloedema in one eye and optic atrophy in the other, caused by a meningioma of the optic nerve.

22 a) False. While the absence of hairs can be a sign of chronic ischaemia, it is not a cardinal feature of critical ischaemia.
   b) True.
   c) False. It is a reflection of poor peripheral perfusion, but not a cardinal feature of critical ischaemia.
   d) True. Critical ischaemia requires an ankle pressure less than 50 mmHg, with persistent rest pain requiring analgesia for over two weeks, or arterial ulceration or gangrene.
   e) False. See d) above.

23 a) False.
   b) True.
   c) False. This presents with ST elevation in all leads.
   d) False. ST elevation in multiple leads is always significant.
   e) False.

24 a) True. Fluid oozes from the capillaries into the surrounding tissue.
   b) True. Brown in colour, it is a by-product of haemoglobin degradation.
   c) False. A dermatological condition associated with diabetes mellitus, it may be mistaken for venous insufficiency. Lipodermatosclerosis, however, is associated with venous insufficiency.
   d) True. It causes pruritus, commonly over the medial malleolus.
   e) False. It occurs in diabetes mellitus as a consequence of peripheral neuropathy. Venous ulcers occur in venous insufficiency.

25 a) True. Vegetations on cardiac valves cause flow murmurs.
   b) True. Dirty needles are a well-recognized cause.
   c) False. Intravenous antibiotics are always indicated in the first instance.
   d) False. Diabetes mellitus is not a risk factor.
   e) True. Small haemorrhages under the nails are also seen in trauma.

26 a) True. Venous valves are damaged by previous DVT, predisposing to valvular incompetence.
   b) True. Pelvic tumours can block venous return, causing venous hypertension.
   c) False.
   d) False. Prolonged standing can lead to venous hypertension.
   e) True. This is for the same reason as for pelvic tumours.

27 a) False.
   b) True. Penetrating or iatrogenic trauma may give rise to an arterial aneurysm.
   c) True. This is an autosomal dominant condition, one of whose features is ascending aortic dissection and aneurysm.
   d) True. It affects the ascending aorta and arch.
   e) True. For example, Takayasu's arteritis, which causes aneurysms of the aortic arch.

28 a) True. Hyperthyroidism is a cause of high-output heart failure.
    b) True. This is an important cause in the Western world.
    c) True.
    d) True. This is the most common cause.
    e) True. Most arrhythmias can lead to heart failure.

29 a) True. This is a long-acting nitrate which vasodilates coronary vasculature.
    b) True. This is a short-acting vasodilator, usually an oral spray.
    c) False. This is an ACE inhibitor used in hypertension.
    d) False. This is an opiate and not appropriate for anginal pain.
    e) True. Beta-blockers reduce myocardial oxygen demand.

30 a) False. A mid-diastolic murmur is characteristic.
    b) True. An ejection systolic heart murmur is best heard at the upper right sternal edge.
    c) True. A pan-systolic murmur.
    d) False.
    e) True. The hyperdynamic circulation can lead to an innocent murmur.

31 a) False. Pre-excitation of the ventricles causes runs of tachycardia.
    b) True. This is a form of second-degree heart block.
    c) False. It is generally associated with rates of 300 or 150 per minute.
    d) True. Sino-atrial node disease leads to bradycardia.
    e) True. This is also known as Mobitz type I second-degree heart block.

32 a) False. Cannon waves are seen in complete heart block when the right atrium contracts against a closed tricuspid valve.
    b) True. This is a useful clinical sign indicating elevated right heart pressure.
    c) True.
    d) False. The JVP cannot be palpated.
    e) False. The JVP paradoxically rises on inspiration in constrictive pericarditis.

33 a) False. If anticoagulation is appropriate, it should be instituted for life.
    b) True. This is appropriate for new-onset atrial fibrillation.
    c) False. Lidocaine is used in ventricular arrhythmias.
    d) True. Digoxin is used for rate control.
    e) False. This is used in atrial flutter.

34 a) False.
    b) True. Severe aortic stenosis leads to syncope and can cause sudden death.
    c) True. This is a cause of sudden death particularly in young people.
    d) False.
    e) False.

35 a) True.
    b) True.
    c) False.
    d) True.
    e) True.

36 a) True.
   b) True.
   c) True. This is a sign of severe disease. Redistribution of blood leads to increased pulmonary blood volume.
   d) False. This would be more in keeping with ischaemia.
   e) False. Arrhythmias are a cause of heart failure but not usually a symptom.

37 a) False. This is a presenting feature.
   b) True. This is a poor prognostic sign.
   c) True. A variety of arrhythmias is possible post-infarct.
   d) True. This occurs immediately post-myocardial infarction or classically after 6 weeks (Dressler's syndrome).
   e) False.

38 a) False.
   b) True. It is a well-recognized complication of chronic alcohol use.
   c) False. This causes ischaemic heart disease.
   d) True. Hypertrophic obstructive cardiomyopathy (HOCM) is the commonest genetic cardiac disease.
   e) True. This predominantly causes dilated cardiomyopathy.

39 a) False. Beri beri (vitamin B_1 deficiency) is however a cause.
   b) True.
   c) True.
   d) True. Increased vasculature to bone can lead to heart failure.
   e) False. It is not associated.

40 a) True. This is an angiotensin II receptor blocker.
   b) True. This is an alpha-blocker; not a first-line agent.
   c) True. This is a calcium channel blocker.
   d) False. Nitrates are not used to treat hypertension.
   e) True. This is a thiazide diuretic.

EMQ ANSWERS

1 CHEST PAIN

1 J **Spontaneous pneumothorax.** A hyper-resonant percussion note and decreased expansion indicate air within the thorax: there is no lung tissue to inflate and cause movement of the chest wall.

2 H Musculoskeletal chest pain or **costochondritis** is common: it is typically worse on inspiration as the muscles contract. A history of cough or strenuous physical activity can often be elicited.

3 D **Acute pericarditis** is suggested by the young patient with chest pain relieved by sitting upright. The ST elevation not corresponding to any particular cardiac territory is also typical.

4 A This unfortunate gentleman has had an **inferior myocardial infarction**. There is ST elevation in the inferior chest leads corresponding to the territory supplied by the right coronary artery.

5 C This is a typical history for a **dissecting aortic aneurysm**. The central chest pain radiating to the back is caused when blood from the lumen of the aorta tracks between the intima and the media.

2 ST CHANGES ON ECG

1 C **Inferior myocardial infarction.** Leads II, III and aVF correspond to the inferior portion of the heart: the area supplied by the right coronary artery. Reciprocal ST depression is common in leads looking at the heart from the opposite direction.

2 H This 'reverse tick' pattern of widespread concave ST depression is associated with **digoxin**.

3 A Widespread concave upwards ST segment elevation indicates acute **pericarditis**; contrast this with the convex ST elevation in a few leads of cardiac ischaemia.

4 E **Posterior myocardial infarction** is an important diagnosis. As the ECG leads are traditionally placed on the anterior surface of the heart, reciprocal changes are noted, with prominent R waves and ST depression in the septal leads.

5 D **Lateral myocardial infarction.** These leads correspond to the lateral surface of the heart; it is this region that has suffered coronary occlusion most probably as a result of a blocked circumflex artery.

3 SECONDARY HYPERTENSION

1 A **Conn's syndrome** (primary hyperaldosteronism) is suggested by the elevated aldosterone levels, which cause retention of sodium and loss of potassium. A significantly elevated aldosterone:renin ratio is usually diagnostic.

2 F This patient has developed acute renal failure secondary to the administration of an ACE inhibitor. ACE inhibitors are contraindicated in bilateral **renal artery stenosis** due to their ability to significantly diminish glomerular filtration rate.

3 D This gentleman has the characteristic features of a **phaeochromocytoma**: headaches, hot flushes, panic attacks, palpitations and hypertension. The GP has caused the release of catecholamines into the systemic circulation by compressing the adrenal tumour while examining the patient.

4 H Radio-femoral delay is a sign of **coarctation of the aorta**, a condition that typically affects young men. If long-standing, a chest X-ray may show notching of the inferior borders of the ribs due to collateral vessel formation.

5 J **Iatrogenic.** Monitoring of blood pressure is important for patients on the oral contraceptive pill. This patient has quite marked hypertension, most likely as a result of her medication. In these circumstances, the pill should be stopped immediately.

4 ARRHYTHMIAS

1 I **Third-degree heart block** is diagnosed by the presence of complete atrioventricular dissociation. P waves are present but have no bearing on ventricular activity. The broad complex bradycardia is the result of a spontaneous escape rhythm.

2 C This is the characteristic feature of **Wolff–Parkinson–White syndrome**. An abnormal piece of tissue links the atria and the ventricles resulting in pre-excitation: on the ECG this is manifested as a short PR interval and a slurred upstroke to the QRS complex.

3 H The normal QRS complexes indicate that ventricular depolarization is being appropriately triggered from above the atrioventricular node. The lack of P waves suggests **atrial fibrillation**.

4 B **Ventricular fibrillation** is diagnosed by completely haphazard electrical activity, with no recognizable complexes. Urgent treatment is indicated!

5 A Progressive PR interval prolongation until a QRS complex is missed occurs in Mobitz type 1 second-degree heart block, which is also known as the **Wenckebach phenomenon**.

5 DRUGS USED IN CARDIOLOGY TO TREAT HYPERTENSION

1 D **Metoprolol** is the only beta-blocker listed. These drugs end in the suffix -olol.

2 E **Losartan**. Angiotensin II RecepTor ANtagonists end in the suffix -artan.

3 H **Doxazosin** is an α_1-blocker used as a second/third-line agent in the management of hypertension. It has a particular use in hypertensive men with symptoms of prostatic disease, where it can increase urinary flow rates.

4 F **Clonidine** is a centrally acting α_2-stimulant. It is not commonly used nowadays to treat hypertension, as withdrawal of the agent may lead to a rebound hypertensive crisis.

5 B **Verapamil** is a calcium channel blocker used both in the treatment of hypertension and as an antiarrhythmic.

6 SIDE-EFFECTS OF DRUGS USED IN CARDIOLOGY TO TREAT HYPERTENSION

1 G **Hydralazine** is most associated with a lupus-like syndrome. This is usually reversible upon stopping the drug.

2 A **Enalapril**, an ACE inhibitor, prevents the breakdown of bradykinin and thereby causes a subgroup of patients to have a chronic cough. Angiotensin II receptor antagonists do not suffer from this same problem.

3 I A well recognized side-effect of **spironolactone** is gynaecomastia; other drugs causing this adverse reaction include digoxin, cimetidine and some antipsychotics.

4 D **Metoprolol** can cause bronchospasm, particularly in those with asthma, as it antagonizes the β_2-receptor (which causes bronchodilatation).

5 C **Bendroflumethiazide**, a thiazide diuretic, causes hyperuricaemia and may precipitate gout.

7 HEART SOUNDS

1 B **Aortic stenosis** is responsible for this murmur; characteristically it is louder in expiration, heard best at the upper right sternal edge, and radiates into the neck. In severe cases, reversed splitting of the second sound may occur.

2 C **Atrial septal defect**. Usually the second heart sound is split on inspiration, with a single sound in expiration. Fixed splitting occurs when respiration makes no difference to the interval between the aortic and pulmonary components of the second sound.

3 A **Aortic regurgitation**. Note that this murmur is heard best at the lower left sternal edge, not in the 'aortic area' at the upper right sternal edge.

4 I A variety of murmurs may be heard in **hypertrophic obstructive cardiomyopathy (HOCM)**. A jerky pulse, double apical impulse, third and fourth heart sounds (due to left ventricular hypertrophy), and a late systolic murmur due to outflow tract obstruction can all be clinical features.

5 E **Mitral stenosis** is associated with a low-pitched mid diastolic murmur, which is best heard with the bell of the stethoscope.

8 FEATURES OF INFECTIVE ENDOCARDITIS

1 H **Osler's nodes** may be found on either the tips of the fingers or the toes. They are painful; contrast this with Janeway lesions.

2 F In infective endocarditis, **splinter haemorrhages** are the result of immune complex deposition. However they are more commonly found in healthy individuals in association with trauma.

3 J **Petechiae** are the most common cutaneous manifestation of infective endocarditis; they may occur on the skin or mucosal surfaces such as the conjunctivae and palate.

4 E **Roth spots** refer to retinal haemorrhages. These are rarely found in modern medicine as endocarditis is usually diagnosed before immunological phenomena such as this have a chance to develop.

5 B **Janeway lesions** are blanching macules, which are characteristically non-tender.

9 INVESTIGATIONS IN CARDIOLOGY

1 I This is a good history for a paroxysmal supraventricular tachycardia, with sudden onset and abatement of symptoms. To confirm the diagnosis, **Holter monitoring** (a 24 h ECG) is required.

2 H This gentleman is having an acute myocardial infarction. Out of the options given, the best answer is **coronary angiography**, which, as well as confirming the diagnosis, offers the possibility of treatment.

3 J Neurocardiogenic or vasovagal syncope is a common cause of loss of consciousness. Typically it occurs after a period of standing, when blood accumulates in the lower limbs due to venous pooling. The diagnosis is made by **tilt-table testing**.

4 B The diagnosis here is hypertrophic obstructive cardiomyopathy. The best investigation to evaluate cardiac chamber size and wall thickness is transthoracic **echocardiography**.

5 F Non-invasive cardiac evaluation of a patient who cannot exercise can be done with either **thallium scanning** (where uptake of radioactive isotope is measured) or stress echocardiography (where dobutamine is used to stimulate the heart and ultrasound used to look for wall motion abnormalities).

10 AORTIC REGURGITATION

1 C Quincke's sign
2 J Widened pulse pressure
3 A de Musset's sign
4 F Corrigan's sign
5 H Duroziez's sign

The signs of aortic regurgitation are caused by a hyperdynamic circulation, which causes flow murmurs, bounding pulses and a widened pulse pressure. Some of the signs listed here are rarely seen in clinical practice as patients undergo valve replacement before they can develop.

11 SIDE-EFFECTS OF DRUGS USED TO TREAT ARRHYTHMIAS

1 D The clinical syndrome described is hyperthyroidism. This is a well recognized side-effect of **amiodarone**, which can cause both hyper- and hypothyroidism.

2 F An important drug reaction occurs between **verapamil** and beta-blockers. These two drugs must not be given together because of the risk of hypotension and asystole.

3 D Honeycomb lung is the term used to describe severe pulmonary fibrosis. **Amiodarone**-induced lung disease is a common side-effect, and occurs in about 1 in 10 patients.

4 E The 'reverse tick' ECG with downwards sloping ST segments and T wave inversion is characteristic of **digoxin**.

5 I Beta-blockers such as **sotalol** can cause sexual dysfunction, as can thiazide diuretics such as bendroflumethiazide.

12 VAUGHAN WILLIAMS' CLASSIFICATION OF DRUGS USED TO TREAT ARRHYTHMIAS

1 H Digoxin is **active in none of the classes** above. It works by reducing conductivity in the AV node, and is therefore useful in supraventricular tachycardias such as atrial fibrillation.

2 G Amiodarone is a predominantly class III antiarrhythmic: as such, it prolongs the duration of the action potential and the refractory period. However, it does have **activity in all four classes**, though its exact mechanism of action is still unclear.

3 F Verapamil, a calcium channel blocker, is a **class IV** agent. It is used for the control of supraventricular tachycardias; it must not be administered with beta-blockers because of the risk of asystole.

4 C Class I agents inhibit the influx of sodium into the cardiac myocyte. Flecainide is a **class Ic** drug – it has no effect on the duration of the action potential. Class Ia drugs cause prolongation of the action potential, whereas class Ib result in shortening.

5 B Lidocaine is a **class Ib** drug, sometimes used in the management of ventricular arrhythmias.

13 SIGNS OF CARDIAC DISEASE

1 I The presence of a malar flush indicates that the diagnosis is **mitral stenosis**.

2 G A fourth heart sound indicates a non compliant ventricle. The most common cause of an ejection systolic murmur and an abnormal ventricle in a patient of this age is **hypertrophic cardiomyopathy**

3 H When the right atrium contracts against a closed tricuspid valve, as occurs in **complete heart block**, huge cannon waves are seen in the jugular venous pulse.

4 E **Pulsus alternans** is a sign of severe heart failure – most probably due to ischaemic heart disease in this patient.

5 C Syncope is a classic presentation of **aortic stenosis**. A slow rising pulse is also consistent with this diagnosis.

14 SYMPTOMS AND SIGNS OF CARDIAC DISEASE

1 G **Orthopnoea**, the inability to lie flat, is a sign of heart failure, typically manifested by patients using multiple pillows at night. It is caused by the redistribution of blood resulting in pulmonary venous congestion.

2 D The history of early myocardial infarction suggests the possibility of familial hypercholesterolaemia. The lesions on the backs of the hands are **xanthomata**, depositions of lipids that occur over tendons.

3 A Alternating hyper- and hypoventilation is referred to as **Cheyne–Stokes respiration**, and is a sign of severe heart failure, or brainstem lesions.

4 E **Arcus senilis,** or corneal arcus, is a common clinical finding in the middle-aged or elderly population. However, it may point to a familial hyperlipidaemia in younger patients.
5 I **Pulsus paradoxus** is an exaggeration of the normal pattern of a fall in arterial pressure on inspiration (up to 10 mmHg). This sign can be elicited in cardiac tamponade and sometimes in severe asthma.

15 CARDIAC SYNCOPE

1 C **Sick sinus syndrome** occurs when the cardiac conduction system is normal, but the sinoatrial node does not produce regular P waves. This results in an irregular pulse, often with pauses. Treatment is by pacemaker insertion.
2 E This astute doctor has heard the characteristic sound of an atrial **myxoma.** The diastolic tumour plop occurs when the tumour moves inferiorly on its peduncle.
3 A The most common cause of collapse is **neurocardiogenic syncope.** This typically occurs after a prolonged period of standing, as blood pools in the lower limbs. Consciousness is rapidly regained upon falling to the ground.
4 G This patient has signs of **aortic stenosis:** syncope, a slow rising pulse, and left ventricular hypertrophy. The risk of sudden death in these circumstances is high, and a presentation such as this warrants urgent treatment.
5 J The history of left-sided chest pain and ST elevation on the ECG is highly suggestive of an anterior **myocardial infarction.** The likely cause in this gentleman is cocaine-induced vasospasm, which would explain the tachycardia and dilated pupils.

X-RAY ANSWERS

1 The X-ray shows a large calcified abdominal aortic aneurysm. There is an exponential risk of rupture as these increase in size; this patient's pain may well be due to blood dissecting through the vessel wall.

2 a) Radiological contrast has been injected to show the vessels of the lower limbs: an angiogram.
   b) There is a filling defect in the right femoral artery, indicating arterial occlusion. An embolus is more likely than thrombosis given the history of atrial fibrillation.

3 a) The clinical finding of bilateral crackles and chest X-ray showing bilateral ill-defined mid-zone shadowing and cardiomegaly suggests pulmonary oedema as the cause of this patient's dyspnoea.
   b) Pulmonary oedema is initially treated with:
   - high-flow oxygen
   - intravenous furosemide
   - intravenous glyceryl trinitrate (GTN)
   - intravenous diamorphine.

4 a) A ventilation–perfusion ($\dot{V}/\dot{Q}$) scan.
   b) The scans show normal homogenous lung ventilation (the two left images), but multiple filling defects in the perfusion scans (right images). These findings are typical of multiple pulmonary emboli. Pregnant women, and those who have recently delivered, are thrombophilic and are at a higher chance of developing deep vein thrombosis (DVT)/pulmonary embolism (PE).

5 a) The chest X-ray shows dextrocardia, a right-sided heart. This explains why the heart sounds were difficult to auscultate.

   b) Situs inversus, where the organs are situated in the opposite side of the body, is associated with Kartagener's syndrome. Dysfunction of cilia in this condition leads to chronic lung infections and bronchiectasis.

6 The heart is grossly enlarged on this postero-anterior chest X-ray: the width of the heart should be no greater than half the width of the thorax in a healthy person. The symptoms described by this patient and the X-ray findings together suggest a diagnosis of heart failure.

7 a) The metallic device is a permanent pacemaker, used to treat cardiac arrhythmias. They are usually implanted on the left side of the chest, as in this case.

   b) The superior lead is situated in the right atrium; the inferior lead is in the right ventricle.

CHAPTER 2

The respiratory system

MULTIPLE CHOICE QUESTIONS

1 Causes of bronchiectasis include:
   a) Kartagener's syndrome
   b) Asthma
   c) Pulmonary embolism
   d) Cystic fibrosis
   e) Asbestosis

2 Cystic fibrosis is:
   a) Inherited as an autosomal dominant condition
   b) Common worldwide
   c) Associated with cirrhosis
   d) Diagnosed by DNA analysis
   e) Associated with a median life expectancy of 20 years

3 Regarding chest drains:
   a) They are not always indicated for tension pneumothorax
   b) They should be kept clamped overnight
   c) Diaphragmatic penetration is a complication
   d) They are usually inserted under general anaesthetic
   e) The normal insertion site is the second intercostal space in the mid-clavicular line

4 Examination of the chest in lung consolidation reveals:
   a) Reduced chest wall movement
   b) Mediastinal displacement towards the affected side
   c) Mediastinal displacement away from the affected side
   d) Decreased vocal resonance
   e) A dull percussion note

5 Cavity formation on chest X-ray occurs in:
   a) Tuberculosis
   b) Streptococcal pneumonia
   c) Staphylococcal pneumonia
   d) Wegener's granulomatosis
   e) Bronchial carcinoma

6   The following associations regarding respiratory failure are true:
   a) Type I: partial pressure of oxygen (P_{O_2}) normal, partial pressure of carbon dioxide (P_{CO_2}) low
   b) Type I: P_{O_2} low, P_{CO_2} high
   c) Type I: P_{O_2} low, P_{CO_2} normal
   d) Type II: P_{O_2} normal, P_{CO_2} low
   e) Type II: P_{O_2} low, P_{CO_2} high

7   Exudative pleural effusions:
   a) Have a protein content >30 g/L
   b) Have a lactate dehydrogenase (LDH) <200 IU/L
   c) Can be caused by pneumonia
   d) Should never be drained
   e) Occur in bronchial carcinoma

8   Causes of haemoptysis include:
   a) Goodpasture's syndrome
   b) Extrinsic allergic alveolitis
   c) Pulmonary embolism
   d) Mitral stenosis
   e) Spontaneous pneumothorax

9   Pulmonary embolism:
   a) Causes a type I respiratory failure
   b) Causes a type II respiratory failure
   c) Can produce characteristic electrocardiogram (ECG) changes
   d) Is often diagnosed by percutaneous pulmonary angiography.
   e) Is associated with a loud second heart sound

10 Clubbing is a feature of the following respiratory conditions:
   a) Severe chronic obstructive pulmonary disease (COPD)
   b) Chronic bronchitis
   c) Asthma
   d) Bronchiectasis
   e) Emphysema

11 A tension pneumothorax:
   a) Should be diagnosed by a postero-anterior (PA) chest X-ray
   b) Leads to tracheal deviation towards the affected side
   c) Is common in young, tall, slim men
   d) Is treated by aspiration of air from the second intercostal space in the mid-clavicular line
   e) Is more common than simple pneumothorax

12 Well-recognized features of life-threatening asthma include:
   a) Rapidly falling P_{CO_2}
   b) Bradycardia
   c) Pulsus alternans
   d) Development of alkalosis
   e) Silent chest

13 Obstructive sleep apnoea:
   a) Occurs more often in men
   b) Leads to daytime somnolence
   c) Can be diagnosed by formal sleep studies
   d) Is treated with home bilevel positive airways pressure (BiPAP)
   e) Can be treated conservatively

14 The following organisms are causes of community-acquired pneumonia:
   a) *Mycoplasma pneumoniae*
   b) *Chlamydia pneumoniae*
   c) *Klebsiella pneumoniae*
   d) *Escherichia coli*
   e) *Staphylococcus aureus*

15 The following drugs are commonly used in the treatment of asthma:
   a) Terbutaline
   b) Montelukast
   c) Salmeterol
   d) Chlorphenamine
   e) Doxazosin

16 Pulmonary tuberculosis:
   a) Predominantly affects the lung bases
   b) Can cause erythema nodosum
   c) Is treated with at least 6 months of dual antibiotic therapy
   d) Classically forms cavities on chest X-ray
   e) Is rising in incidence in the UK

17 The following cancers are common causes of lung metastases:
   a) Breast
   b) Colon
   c) Lymphoma
   d) Liver
   e) Pancreas

18 Bronchial carcinoma is associated with:
   a) Radiation exposure
   b) Low social class
   c) Asbestos exposure
   d) Pipe smoking
   e) Passive smoking

19 The following are recognized causes of transudative pleural effusion:
   a) Hyperthyroidism
   b) Cardiac failure
   c) Nephrotic syndrome
   d) Liver failure
   e) Tuberculosis

20 Features consistent with a diagnosis of bronchial carcinoma include:
   a) Clubbing
   b) Haemoptysis
   c) Erythema nodosum
   d) Hoarse voice
   e) An elevated jugular venous pulse (JVP)

21 Sarcoidosis is associated with:
   a) Typical presentation in the first decade of life
   b) Bilateral hilar lymphadenopathy
   c) Erythema multiforme
   d) Hypocalcaemia
   e) An elevated serum angiotensin-converting enzyme

22 Causes of lung fibrosis include:
   a) Asbestosis
   b) Pneumoconiosis
   c) Severe asthma
   d) Propranolol
   e) Amiodarone

23 Features of bronchiectasis include:
   a) Clubbing
   b) Cerebral abscesses
   c) Haemoptysis
   d) Hyperexpanded chest
   e) Purulent sputum production

24 Lung transplantation is an effective treatment for:
   a) Asthma
   b) Emphysema
   c) Cryptogenic fibrosing alveolitis
   d) Cystic fibrosis
   e) Bronchial carcinoma

25 The following agents are used as first-line therapy for tuberculosis:
   a) Ciprofloxacin
   b) Ethambutol
   c) Pyrazinamide
   d) Imipenem
   e) Clarithromycin

26 Bronchial carcinoma is associated with:
   a) Hypothyroidism
   b) Syndrome of inappropriate antidiuretic hormone secretion (SIADH)
   c) Cushing's syndrome
   d) A myasthenia-like syndrome
   e) Hypertrophic pulmonary osteoarthropathy

Answers: see pages 44–47

EXTENDED MATCHING QUESTIONS

1 COMMUNITY-ACQUIRED PNEUMONIA

Choose the most likely organism for each case below

A   *Klebsiella pneumoniae*
B   *Escherichia coli*
C   *Streptococcus pneumoniae*
D   *Staphylococcus aureus*
E   *Mycoplasma pneumoniae*

F   *Chlamydia pneumoniae*
G   *Chlamydia psittaci*
H   *Haemophilus influenzae*
I   *Legionella pneumophila*
J   *Pseudomonas aeruginosa*

1   A previously healthy 22-year-old student returns from a holiday at a hotel in Ibiza and presents to the emergency department 2 days later with a fever of 39°C, a dry cough and diarrhoea. A chest X-ray shows a lobar pneumonia.

2   An 85-year-old is brought by ambulance to hospital, with a fever and cough productive of rusty-coloured sputum. A full blood count shows a white cell count of 17×10^9/L.

3   A 76-year-old who has just recovered from influenza becomes very unwell with a fever and cough. Chest radiography shows patchy bronchopneumonia throughout the lung fields, with bilateral pleural effusions.

4   A 32-year-old intravenous drug user with multiple skin abscesses develops dyspnoea and cough. Chest X-ray shows widespread bronchopneumonia.

5   An 18-year-old student is brought to hospital by a friend from his halls of residence. He has been unwell for 3 days with headache, cough, fever and an unusual rash which looks like little bull's eyes.

2 INVESTIGATION OF RESPIRATORY DISEASE 1

Match the clinically most useful investigation to each case below

A   Chest X-ray
B   High-resolution computed tomography (CT) of the thorax
C   CT pulmonary angiogram
D   Spirometry
E   Magnetic resonance imaging (MRI) of the thorax

F   Pulmonary angiogram
G   CT of the thorax
H   Peak flow
I   Skin prick testing
J   Bronchoscopy

1   A previously healthy 24-year-old pregnant woman collapses suddenly and is brought to hospital by ambulance. On arrival, she is saturating at 83 per cent on air. Blood gas analysis on oxygen shows a P_{O_2} of 6 kPa and P_{CO_2} of 4 kPa.

2   A 58-year-old builder presents with a 3-month history of shortness of breath. He has smoked 20 cigarettes a day for the past 40 years. Chest X-ray reveals a 3 cm central mass in the right hilum.

3   A 68-year-old bus driver presents to his general practitioner (GP) complaining of a 6-month history of gradually worsening shortness of breath. He has smoked for 50 years. A chest X-ray shows hyperexpanded lung fields but no focal lesions.

4   A 28-year-old student with known asthma presents to the emergency department with a 1 h history of wheezing. Examination reveals a respiratory rate of 27 breaths/min and widespread expiratory wheeze.

5   An elderly woman is admitted from her nursing home with a fever and productive cough. Chest examination reveals crackles in the right upper zone with increased vocal resonance.

3 DRUGS USED IN ASTHMA

Each of the drugs below is used in asthma. Choose the drug that best fits each of the statements below

A Terbutaline
B Salmeterol
C Montelukast
D Magnesium sulphate
E Theophylline
F Omalizumab
G Aminophylline
H Sodium cromoglicate
I Prednisolone
J Fluticasone

1 A leukotriene antagonist.
2 An inhaled drug used as a reliever by patients with symptomatic asthma.
3 The best drug to add to the regimen of a man who is using his reliever once every day.
4 The final pharmacological intervention in the management of chronic asthma.
5 A monoclonal antibody that binds to immunoglobulin E (IgE), used in patients refractory to conventional treatment.

4 SHORTNESS OF BREATH

Match the most likely cause of shortness of breath with the cases below

A Asthma
B Anaemia
C Pulmonary embolism
D COPD
E Bronchial carcinoma
F Pulmonary fibrosis
G Pneumothorax
H Tuberculosis
I Pulmonary oedema
J Foreign body

1 A 57-year-old miner is brought to his GP by his wife who is concerned as he has been becoming increasingly short of breath. He is clubbed and has bibasal fine inspiratory crackles.
2 A 74-year-old retired secretary with severe osteoarthritis presents to her GP with a 6 month history of increasing shortness of breath. Examination reveals a respiratory rate of 22 breaths/min, pulse of 94 beats/min and pale conjunctivae.
3 A 22-year-old basketball player presents to hospital having experienced the sudden onset of severe shortness of breath. His respiratory rate is 28 breaths/min, but is saturating normally at 98 per cent on room air.
4 A 35-year-old who has only ever been in hospital for the miscarriages of her two pregnancies is brought in by ambulance in extreme respiratory distress, with a respiratory rate of 45 breaths/min. The chest X-ray is unremarkable. Despite the best efforts of the medical team, she dies 1 h later.
5 A 2-year-old is brought in to hospital by her mother, who left her unattended for a moment. Chest examination reveals reduced expansion and no air entry into the right lung.

5 CAUSES OF CLUBBING

Match the most likely cause of clubbing with the cases below

A   Bronchial carcinoma
B   Idiopathic pulmonary fibrosis
C   Empyema
D   Cirrhosis
E   Inflammatory bowel disease

F   Subacute bacterial endocarditis
G   Bronchiectasis
H   Cyanotic heart disease
I   Congenital
J   Mesothelioma

1   A 74-year-old woman who smokes 20 cigarettes per day presents with a 4-month history of gradually increasing shortness of breath and haemoptysis. On further questioning, she admits that she has lost 5 kg in weight. Examination reveals a thin, clubbed patient with no signs in the chest.

2   A 29-year-old homeless intravenous drug addict presents to the emergency department with a long history of fever and malaise. Positive examination findings include pyrexia at 39°C, small retinal haemorrhages and microscopic haematuria.

3   A previously healthy 26-year-old accountant attends his GP with a 3-day history of cough, cold, fever and muscle pain. The GP cannot find any abnormality on clinical examination apart from clubbing.

4   A 64-year-old non-smoking builder presents to his GP with a 6 month history of shortness of breath, pleuritic pain and weight loss of 10 kg. Examination reveals clubbing and bibasal pleural effusions.

5   A 20-year-old with cystic fibrosis has a routine appointment with his GP. Her GP notices that her fingers and toes are all clubbed and that she has coarse crackles heard throughout the lungs.

6 COMPLICATIONS OF ANTITUBERCULOUS THERAPY

Match the drug side-effects below with the most likely pharmacological cause

A   Erythromycin
B   Isoniazid
C   Ciprofloxacin
D   Capreomycin
E   Streptomycin

F   Pyrazinamide
G   Clarithromycin
H   Rifampicin
I   Ethambutol
J   Trimethoprim

1   A 32-year-old being treated for tuberculosis complains that his urine has turned pink.

2   A 61-year-old with pulmonary tuberculosis presents to his physician saying that he cannot distinguish colours as well as he could before.

3   A 78-year-old with resistant tuberculosis complains that he has noticed hearing loss since starting his new medication.

4   A 19-year-old immigrant who only takes some of her medication for tuberculosis notices that the sensation in her hands and feet is not as sharp as it once was.

5   A 43-year-old is admitted to hospital having taken his antituberculous therapy for 2 months. He is profoundly jaundiced.

7 COMPLICATIONS OF SMOKING

Match the complications of smoking to the case scenarios below

A   Ischaemic heart disease
B   Peripheral vascular disease
C   Bladder cancer
D   Oesophageal carcinoma
E   COPD

F   Bronchial carcinoma
G   Polycythaemia
H   Oral cancer
I   Premature delivery
J   Subfertility

1   A 60-year-old man is taken to hospital by ambulance complaining of central chest pain and sweating. He has smoked 25 cigarettes a day for the past 40 years.
2   A 63-year-old with a 50 pack year history of smoking is referred to hospital after complaining of blood in her urine, but no dysuria. She has never experienced any similar episodes in the past.
3   A 58-year-old taxi driver with an 80 pack year history of smoking goes to his GP complaining of tiredness and headache. His GP notices he is plethoric but can find no other abnormality on clinical examination.
4   A 74-year-old retired waiter, who has smoked 10 cigarettes a day for 60 years, makes an appointment with his doctor as he has become impotent. As he enters the doctor's surgery, he clasps both buttocks saying that they hurt when he walks.
5   A 58-year-old smoker presents to his doctor with tiredness. She notices that his right eye is drooping, and that the pupil is smaller than the other one.

8 EXAMINATION FINDINGS IN RESPIRATORY DISEASE

Match the examination findings in the right chest of a 50-year-old male with the most likely underlying pathological process

A   Asthma
B   Pleural effusion
C   Fibrosis
D   Consolidation

E   Pneumothorax
F   Lobar collapse
G   Obstructive lung disease

1   Chest wall movement is diminished, with a dull percussion note. Auscultation reveals bronchial breathing and increased vocal resonance.
2   Chest wall movement is markedly reduced, with a hyper resonant percussion note. Breath sounds are absent.
3   Percussion is normal, but auscultation reveals fine inspiratory crackles. There is reduced chest wall movement. Vocal resonance is increased.
4   There is a wheeze, with a prolonged expiratory phase. Chest wall movement is generally reduced; percussion is normal. Vocal resonance is normal.
5   There is reduced chest wall movement with a stony dull percussion note. Vocal resonance is absent.

9 INVESTIGATION OF RESPIRATORY DISEASE 2

For each case below, select the most appropriate investigation

A	CT pulmonary angiogram	E	CT of the thorax
B	Forced expiratory volume in 1 s/forced vital capacity (FEV$_1$/ FVC) ratio	F	Sputum analysis
		G	Arterial blood gas analysis
C	Bronchoscopy	H	Pleural biopsy
D	Anti-glomerular basement membrane (GBM) antibody	I	Skin prick testing
		J	Pleural aspiration

1   A 78-year-old man is admitted with severe bronchopneumonia, with a respiratory rate of 42 breaths/min and oxygen saturation on air of 87 per cent. The medical registrar asks you to see if he is in type I or type II respiratory failure.
2   A previously healthy 55-year-old woman is admitted with shortness of breath. Chest X-ray shows a large right pleural effusion of unknown aetiology.
3   A 23-year-old medical student becomes short of breath after returning from his elective in Antigua. On hospital admission, his saturations are 92 per cent on air, chest X-ray is normal.
4   An 18-year-old cleaner presents to the emergency department with haemoptysis. A chest X-ray shows blotchy shadowing; blood tests show haemoglobin (Hb) 10.7 g/dL, urea 22 mmol/L and creatinine 300 µmol/L.
5   A 24-year-old Somalian presents to his GP with cough, shortness of breath, weight loss and night sweats. The GP orders a chest X-ray which shows shadowing in the right upper zone.

10 HAEMOPTYSIS

Match the causes of haemoptysis with each case history below

A	Pulmonary embolism	F	Mesothelioma
B	Goodpasture's syndrome	G	Bronchial carcinoma
C	Pneumonia	H	Wegener's granulomatosis
D	Mitral stenosis	I	Bronchiectasis
E	Tuberculosis	J	Pulmonary metastases

1   A 28-year-old biochemist presents to respiratory outpatients with a 2-month history of haemoptysis and malaise. She is currently waiting for an outpatient appointment for the ear, nose and throat (ENT) clinic as she has also recently developed recurrent epistaxis. A chest X-ray performed by her GP has a 3 cm round nodule in the left upper lobe.
2   An 82-year-old woman is referred to chest clinic with a 3-month history of haemoptysis. She also admits that she has felt increasingly short of breath over the same period. Examination reveals a thin woman with red cheeks, with a tapping apex beat. There is a mid-diastolic murmur heard best at the apex, and some crackles at the lung bases.
3   A 68-year-old with pancreatic cancer presents to the emergency department with a 5-h history of haemoptysis and shortness of breath. He is saturating at 92 per cent on air, with a respiratory rate of 32 breaths/min. A chest X-ray shows a small triangular area of increased density in the right lung field.
4   A 42-year-old civil engineer presents to his GP with haemoptysis. He is a non-smoker who has only ever been to see his doctor in the past for subfertility. Clinical examination reveals widespread coarse crackles throughout both lungs; the GP cannot feel his apex beat despite the patient being slim.
5   A 71-year-old vicar is admitted to hospital with a 2-day history of fever and cough productive of rusty-coloured sputum. Chest examination reveals a dull percussion note in the left base, with bronchial breathing.

11 PLEURAL EFFUSION

Match the causes of pleural effusion with the case histories below

A Hypothyroidism
B Systemic lupus erythematosus
C Nephrotic syndrome
D Bronchial carcinoma
E Cirrhosis

F Tuberculosis
G Cardiac failure
H Pneumonia
I Acute pancreatitis
J Pulmonary embolism

1 A 47-year-old homeless man presents to the emergency department with vague abdominal pain. He is unkempt and smells strongly of alcohol. Examination reveals a respiratory rate of 28 breaths/min, with some abdominal tenderness and multiple spider naevi. A chest X-ray shows a left-sided pleural effusion.

2 A 74-year-old with inoperable bowel cancer goes to see his GP having become short of breath earlier that day. He is tachycardic at 110 beats/min; an ECG reveals sinus tachycardia with an axis of +110°.

3 An 89-year-old calls an ambulance from her sheltered accommodation because she has become increasingly short of breath over the course of the day. On examination, she is apyrexial, her jugular venous pulse is 8 cm, and she has bilateral crackles bibasally.

4 A 29-year-old nurse presents to hospital with symptoms of malaise, fatigue, shortness of breath and ankle swelling. A chest X-ray reveals bilateral pleural effusions. Her blood tests show Hb 9.0 g/dL, white cell count (WCC) 5.3×10^9/L, albumin 27 g/L, and cholesterol 8.3 mmol/L. A urine dipstick is positive for protein ++++.

5 A 31-year-old Algerian teacher presents to his GP with a 3-month history of fever, and night sweats. He has lost 5 kg in weight over the past month. A chest X-ray shows right upper lobe shadowing and a right-sided pleural effusion.

12 COMPLICATIONS OF DRUGS USED IN RESPIRATORY MEDICINE

Match the case histories below with the drug most likely to cause the complication

A Salbutamol inhaler
B Ipratropium bromide inhaler
C Montelukast
D Sodium cromoglicate
E Theophylline

F Amoxicillin
G Oxygen
H Beclometasone inhaler
I Doxapram
J Prednisolone

1 A poorly controlled asthmatic visits his GP and is prescribed a new medication. He returns 4 weeks later complaining of white patches on his tongue and pharynx.

2 A 60-year-old woman with severe COPD presents to her GP with severe back pain. A thoracic spine X-ray shows collapse of T6, T8 and T9. Her GP says that her medication may be to blame.

3 A 21-year-old artist returns to her GP saying that the medication that he gave her means that she can no longer paint with such precision due to tremor.

4 A 73-year-old woman, with a long history of smoking, is given an inhaler for her respiratory disease. At her next visit, she mentions that her mouth is constantly dry.

5 An 82-year-old man takes an entire packet of his tablets in an attempt to kill himself. He later calls an ambulance, which rushes him to hospital. On arrival, he has a broad complex tachycardia, which soon degenerates into ventricular fibrillation. No treatment is successful, and half an hour later he is pronounced dead.

13 RESPIRATORY FAILURE

Match the case histories to the diagnoses given

A   Myasthenia gravis
B   Guillain–Barré syndrome
C   Asthma
D   Pneumonia
E   Drug reaction

F   COPD
G   Pulmonary embolism
H   Pulmonary oedema
I   Extrinsic allergic alveolitis
J   Motor neurone disease

1   A 26-year-old cleaner presents to her emergency department with fatigue, wheeze, and shortness of breath. The doctor notices that both her eyelids are droopy, and her respirations are shallow, and performs some blood tests and a chest X-ray. Blood gases show a P_{O_2} of 8.9 kPa and a P_{CO_2} of 3.8 kPa. The chest X-ray shows a mass above the heart in the superior mediastinum.

2   A 72-year-old man is brought to hospital by ambulance with difficulty breathing. His breathing has been getting worse over the past few months. Blood gases show P_{O_2} of 7.4 kPa, P_{CO_2} of 6.2 kPa and pH 7.38. On examination, his entire body is wasted and his tongue is fasciculating.

3   An 80-year-old man is admitted to the orthopaedic ward having tripped on an uneven pavement and broken the neck of his femur. He has been in considerable pain. Around 6 am, the nurses notice that his respiratory rate is 7 breaths per minute, his arterial oxygen saturation (S_aO_2) has dropped to 91 per cent, and his pupils are 2 mm.

4   A 32-year-old baker comes to hospital with shortness of breath and numbness and weakness in his feet. He is usually well but has just got over a bout of food poisoning after he ate a cold chicken salad. He says the weakness is getting worse: he now has difficulty bending his knees. He is admitted, but three days later is transferred to the intensive therapy unit (ITU) for ventilation.

5   A 64-year-old farmer has been seen in the respiratory clinic for many years for his chronic lung disease. He has never smoked. Examination reveals coarse crackles throughout the lungs. A blood gas analysis shows P_{O_2} of 7.6 kPa and a P_{CO_2} of 5.4 kPa. Precipitins to *Micropolyspora faeni* are positive.

14 PULMONARY OEDEMA

Match the most likely cause of pulmonary oedema with the information given below

A   Mitral stenosis
B   Congestive cardiac failure
C   Intracranial haemorrhage
D   Renal artery stenosis
E   Constrictive pericarditis

F   Adult respiratory distress syndrome (ARDS)
G   Nephrotic syndrome
H   Myocardial infarction
I   Iatrogenic
J   Cardiomyopathy

1   A 73-year-old woman comes to hospital with difficulty breathing. Examination reveals a mid-diastolic murmur heard best at the apex, and crackles to both mid-zones.

2   A 35-year-old diver is brought to the emergency department after nearly drowning. He is brought to the emergency department in respiratory distress and is ventilated and taken to ITU. The chest X-ray the next day shows bilateral diffuse infiltrates in both lungs.

3   An 86-year-old man is brought in to hospital in the evening as his wife is concerned about his black, tarry stools. He is usually fit and well, but has had three heart attacks in the past. His Hb is found to be 6.7 g/dL and the medical registrar asks for him to be given 4 units of blood. The next morning his Hb is 10.4 g/dL, but he is extremely short of breath. An X-ray confirms pulmonary oedema.

4   A 47-year-old Bengali man is admitted to hospital with central chest pain. An ECG shows ST elevation which continues despite medical therapy. He becomes hypotensive, blood pressure of 90/55 mmHg, and short of breath. A chest X-ray shows pulmonary oedema.

5   A 79-year-old retired gardener comes to hospital as he is short of breath, but denies any chest pain. He has been a lifelong smoker, and is known to be hypertensive. His GP recently started him on some new medication to help control his blood pressure. His chest X-ray shows bilateral pulmonary oedema.

15 COMPLICATIONS OF LUNG CANCER

The patients below all have bronchial carcinoma. Match the complications of lung cancer with the case histories

A   Liver metastases
B   Hypertrophic pulmonary osteoarthropathy
C   Hypercalcaemia
D   Superior vena cava obstruction
E   Horner's syndrome

F   Bone metastases
G   Eaton–Lambert syndrome
H   Cachexia
I   Syndrome of inappropriate antidiuretic hormone
J   Peripheral neuropathy

1   A 62-year-old man tells his oncologist that in the past 2 weeks his face has become increasingly swollen. On examination, he is plethoric with dilated veins over his thorax.

2   A 74-year-old patient goes to her GP complaining of lethargy, constipation, abdominal pain and nocturia. She also says her mood has been low recently and she does not enjoy the activities she once did.

3   A 54-year-old banker goes to his GP because of weakness in his right hand. The GP notices that he also has a small right pupil and a drooping right eyelid.

4   An 81-year-old man has a routine appointment with his GP for a medication review. During the consultation he tells her that his wrists are both painful. When the wrists are X-rayed the ends of the bones look like onion skin.

5   A GP notices that his 85-year-old patient has drooping eyelids. However, after repeated attempts to make her open her eyes fully, the droopiness disappears.

Answers: see pages 48–53

X-RAY QUESTIONS

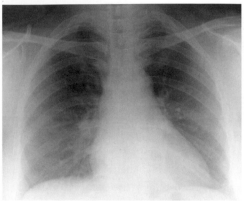

1 Film A

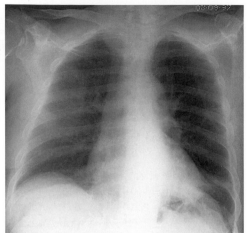

1 Film B

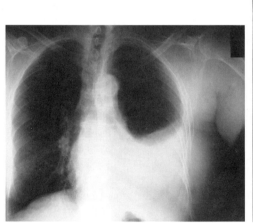

2

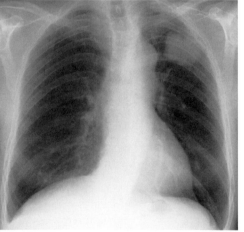

3

To answer the questions below, please refer to the corresponding numbered X-ray images above.

1   Some medical students are shown two chest X-rays of the same patient taken a day apart. They wonder why they look so different. What is the difference between the two films?

2   A 49-year-old woman presents to her GP with increasing shortness of breath. The past medical history is unremarkable apart from a mastectomy for breast carcinoma 4 years ago. What is the cause of her shortness of breath?

3   A 66-year-old man presents to his GP, saying that in addition to his usual cough, he has now noticed that there are streaks of blood in his sputum. What is the most likely cause of this patient's haemoptysis?

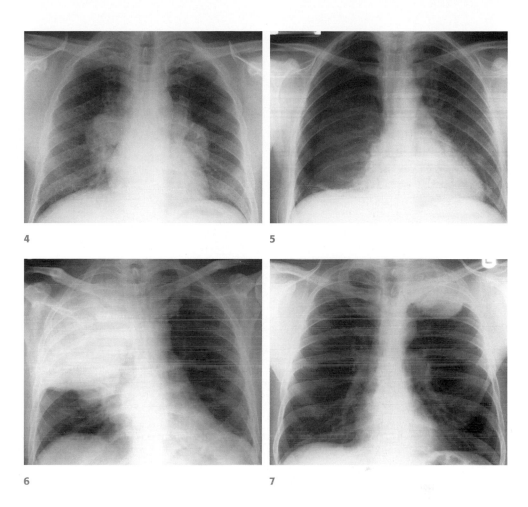

To answer the questions below, please refer to the corresponding numbered X-ray images above.

4 A 31-year-old woman seeks medical attention as she has noticed a rash on her legs. Her GP finds tender nodules over her shins. He also asks that she go to the local hospital for a chest X-ray. What is the cause of this patient's symptoms?

5 A 32-year-old man goes to the emergency department as he is feeling short of breath. He says he has never been in hospital before. The junior doctor asks one of the nurses to arrange a chest X-ray before he sees the patient.
   a) Why is this patient feeling short of breath?
   b) What is the most appropriate treatment?

6 A 39-year-old homeless man goes to the emergency department with fever and cough. A junior doctor requests a chest X-ray.
   a) What is the cause of this patient's symptoms?
   b) What is the most likely responsible organism?

7 A 73-year-old man goes to see his GP as he has noticed that his left eye is drooping. The GP also finds that the left pupil is 2 mm and the right pupil 4 mm. He requests a chest X-ray.
   a) Which clinical syndrome has the GP found?
   b) What is the underlying cause of this patient's problems?

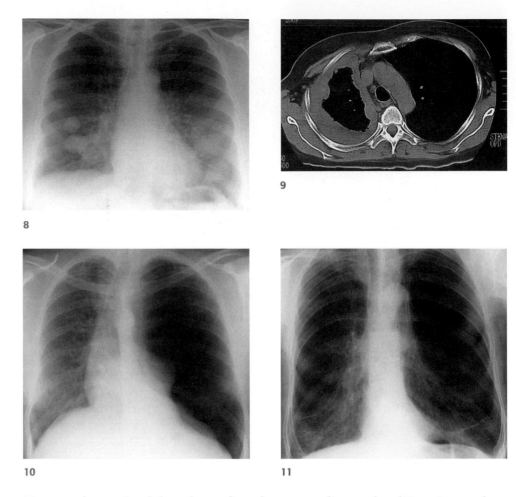

8

9

10

11

To answer the questions below, please refer to the corresponding numbered X-ray images above.

8   A 63-year-old man goes to see his doctor complaining of a chronic cough and weight loss.
    a) What is the cause of this patient's cough?
    b) Which underlying conditions predispose to the development of these lesions?

9   A 59-year-old dockworker sees his doctor complaining of shortness of breath. The chest
    X-ray is reported as being highly abnormal, and a CT scan of the thorax is requested.
    a) What is the cause of this patient's shortness of breath?
    b) Why has this patient contracted this disease?

10 The medical house officer is called to the wards urgently as one of her patients is acutely
    short of breath. The nurse says that he is saturating at 84 per cent on high-flow oxygen.
    She feels his pulse: it is weak and thready. The doctor asks the nurse to call the radio-
    grapher to perform a chest X-ray.
    a) Why is this patient feeling short of breath?
    b) What is the appropriate treatment?

11 A 71-year-old man, with an 80 pack per year history of smoking, goes to see his GP as he
    has noticed that he has become short of breath over the past 6 months. The GP requests
    a chest X-ray. Why is this patient feeling short of breath?

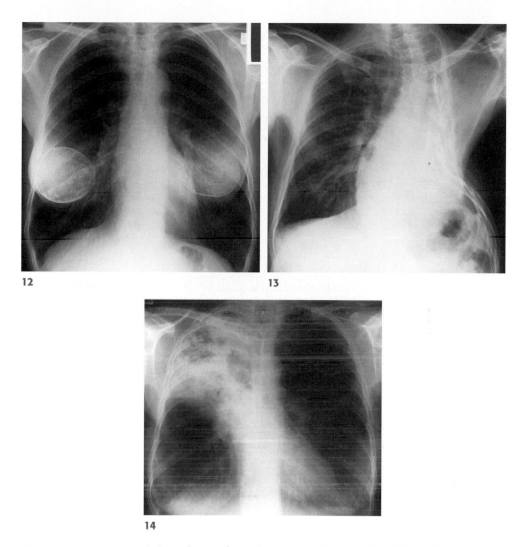

12

13

14

To answer the questions below, please refer to the corresponding numbered X-ray images above.

12 A 28-year-old woman is admitted to hospital electively for the removal of a small mole. The house officer clerking her in notes that she has had a cough for the past week, and requests a chest X-ray. He is quite surprised by the result. Why is this chest X-ray abnormal?

13 An 83-year-old man is admitted for a cholecystectomy. He has a preoperative chest X-ray, as he mentions that he had some surgery, just before the war.
   a) Which operative procedure has this patient undergone?
   b) What was the underlying condition that led to this operation?

14 A 41-year-old homeless man seeks medical attention as he has noticed that he has lost 7 kg in weight over the past 4 months. On examination, he has some peculiar red tender lesions on his lower limbs. What is the cause of this man's symptoms?

Answers: see pages 53–54

ANSWERS

MCQ ANSWERS

1   a) True. This syndrome, comprising ciliary dysfunction and situs inversus is a rare cause of bronchiectasis.
    b) False.
    c) False.
    d) True. Cystic fibrosis is a common cause of bronchiectasis.
    e) False.

2   a) False. Cystic fibrosis is autosomal recessive.
    b) False. Cystic fibrosis affects predominantly a Caucasian population; its incidence is high in Western Europe but low in Africa.
    c) True. About 5 per cent of sufferers develop liver cirrhosis.
    d) True. The ΔF508 mutation is the most common in Britain.
    e) False. Patients can expect to live until 40 years with modern treatments.

3   a) False.
    b) False. Clamping can lead to tension pneumothorax.
    c) True. 'There is no organ in the thoracic or abdominal cavity that has not been pierced by a chest drain.'
    d) False. Local anaesthetic is sufficient.
    e) False. This is the recommended site for emergency aspiration of a tension pneumothorax.

4   a) True.
    b) False. There is no mediastinal shift with consolidated lung; the volume of lung remains unaffected. Expansion of the lung is limited by the affected tissue.
    c) False.
    d) False. Vocal resonance is increased as sound travels better through denser material.
    e) True. This is an important clinical sign.

5   a) True. It occurs typically in the upper zones on the chest X-ray.
    b) False.
    c) True. *Staphylococcus aureus* can cause lung abscesses.
    d) True. The cavities are noted to move through the lung fields on serial chest X-rays.
    e) True.

6   a) False. A low P_{O_2} has to accompany respiratory failure. A P_{O_2} of less than 8 kPa is often used in clinical practice.
    b) False. This is type II respiratory failure.
    c) True. The P_{O_2} is low and the P_{CO_2} is normal or low in type I respiratory failure.
    d) False. Respiratory failure is unlikely when the P_{O_2} is normal.
    e) True. This is characteristic of type II failure.

7 a) True. This is a defining characteristic. Transudates typically have protein contents
       <30 g/L.
   b) False. Exudates have a lactate dehydrogenase level of over 200 IU/L.
   c) True. This is a common cause.
   d) False.
   e) True.

8 a) True. This is a vasculitic disorder featuring proliferative glomerulonephritis and
       pulmonary haemorrhage. Anti-glomerular basement membrane antibodies are
       characteristic.
   b) False.
   c) True.
   d) True. Other important causes include tuberculosis, lung cancer, pneumococcal
       pneumonia, bronchitis, anticoagulants.
   e) False. Haemoptysis may be a feature in a traumatic pneumothorax.

9 a) True. Pulmonary emboli commonly lead to hypoxia and a normal or low P_{CO_2} –
       hallmarks of type I respiratory failure.
   b) False. Hypoventilation is not a usual feature of pulmonary emboli, so CO_2 levels are
       not raised.
   c) True. The $S_1Q_3T_3$ (S wave in I, Q wave in III and inverted T wave in III) is well-
       recognized but uncommon.
   d) False. CT pulmonary angiography and ventilation–perfusion ($\dot{V}/\dot{Q}$) scanning
       diagnose a large majority of emboli. Pulmonary angiography is rarely indicated.
   e) True. The pulmonary component of the second heart sound may be loud due to
       right heart strain.

10 a) False. The respiratory causes of clubbing include suppurative lung disease such as
       bronchiectasis and empyema, pulmonary fibrosis, bronchial carcinoma and
       mesothelioma.
   b) False.
   c) False.
   d) True.
   e) False.

11 a) False. A tension pneumothorax is a clinical diagnosis.
   b) False. Deviation occurs away from the affected side.
   c) False. Spontaneous pneumothorax is common in this population.
   d) True. This emergency treatment is then followed by chest drain insertion.
   e) False. Simple pneumothoraces are much more common.

12 a) False. Rising P_{CO_2} is a late feature of severe asthma.
   b) True.
   c) False. This is a sign of severe cardiac failure.
   d) False.
   e) True. Poor respiratory effort indicates a poor prognosis without rapid intervention.

13 a) True.
    b) True.
    c) True.
    d) False. Continuous positive airway pressure (or CPAP) is used to keep the airway open.
    e) True. Weight loss can result in spontaneous resolution of symptoms.

14 a) True. It usually affects young people, often living in shared accommodation.
    b) True.
    c) False. This is a nosocomial infection.
    d) False.
    e) True. This typically affects the debilitated and causes a severe pneumonia.

15 a) True. This is a β_2-agonist in the same class as salbutamol – a short-acting broncho-dilator.
    b) True. This is a leukotriene antagonist which blocks interleukins thought to be involved in the pathogenesis of asthma.
    c) True. This is a long-acting β_2-agonist.
    d) False. Antihistamines are not effective in asthma.
    e) False. This is an α_1-blocker which is used for hypertension and benign prostatic hyperplasia.

16 a) False. TB is usually found in the apices of the lungs.
    b) True. TB is an important cause.
    c) False. Triple or even quadruple agent therapy is mandatory in the initial stage of treatment to avoid resistance.
    d) True.
    e) True. Increased immigration and HIV-associated tuberculosis has meant that the incidence is now increasing.

17 a) True. The breast, colon, kidney and lung are the most common tumours that meta-stasize to the lung.
    b) True.
    c) False.
    d) False.
    e) False.

18 a) True. This is an uncommon cause.
    b) True. Poorer sections of society are more likely to smoke.
    c) True. This increases the risk of bronchial carcinoma and pleural mesothelioma.
    d) True.
    e) True.

19 a) False. Hypothyroidism is a rare cause.
    b) True.
    c) True. Hypoalbuminaemia leads to a decrease in hydrostatic pressure.
    d) True. Hypoalbuminaemia is responsible.
    e) False. Tuberculosis is a cause of exudative effusion.

20 a) True.
   b) True.
   c) False.
   d) True. Laryngeal nerve palsy can cause a hoarse voice and characteristic bovine cough.
   e) True. Superior vena caval obstruction leads to an elevated JVP and swollen face.

21 a) False. The third and fourth decades are the most common times when patients present.
   b) True. The combination of hilar lymphadenopathy and erythema nodosum is pathognomonic of sarcoidosis.
   c) False.
   d) False. Hypercalcaemia is often found due to increased activation of vitamin D in the lung.
   e) True. This can also be elevated in a wide range of conditions.

22 a) True.
   b) True.
   c) False.
   d) False.
   e) True. This is an idiosyncratic or type B reaction.

23 a) True. This is almost universal.
   b) True. This is a rare complication.
   c) True. This can be massive.
   d) False.
   e) True. It is often produced in large quantities.

24 a) False.
   b) True. Those particularly amenable to transplantation are patients who develop the disease at an early age.
   c) True.
   d) True.
   e) False.

25 a) False. The commonly used first-line agents are rifampicin, isoniazid, pyrazinamide and ethambutol.
   b) True.
   c) True.
   d) False.
   e) False.

26 a) False.
   b) True. Ectopic hormone secretion can lead to a variety of endocrine disorders.
   c) True. From adrenocorticotrophic hormone (ACTH) secretion.
   d) True. The Lambert–Eaton myasthenic syndrome.
   e) True. Bony overgrowth is well-recognized but the mechanisms remain unclear.

EMQ ANSWERS

1 COMMUNITY-ACQUIRED PNEUMONIA

1 I This student has *Legionella pneumophila* infection from a water-cooled air condition-ing system, giving pneumonia with gastrointestinal upset.

2 C *Streptococcus pneumoniae* is the most likely cause of pneumonia in adults, classically causing the production of rusty-coloured sputum.

3 D This is a classic history for pneumonia caused by *Staphylococcus aureus*, which usually causes pneumonia after a preceding infection with influenza.

4 D Intravenous drug users are susceptible to pneumonia caused by *Staphylococcus aureus* due to the introduction of bacteria within the bloodstream from dirty needles.

5 E *Mycoplasma pneumoniae* commonly affects young people living in close proximity. Erythema multiforme is a well recognized feature of *Mycoplasma* infection.

2 INVESTIGATION OF RESPIRATORY DISEASE 1

1 C This woman has had a pulmonary embolus; her pregnancy makes her blood hyper-coagulable. A **CT pulmonary angiogram** is the investigation of choice; conventional pulmonary angiography is not routinely carried out nowadays.

2 J Bronchial carcinoma is the most likely diagnosis. A **bronchoscopy** will provide valuable histology which will both confirm the diagnosis and help guide treatment. The patient will also need a CT of the chest and abdomen to look for metastases.

3 D This history is compatible with COPD in a long term smoker. **Spirometry** is mandatory to confirm the diagnosis, and helps quantify the level of damage to the lungs.

4 H The most useful test in acute asthma is the **peak flow**: this helps stratify patients into mild, moderate, severe or life-threatening. Imaging is not generally helpful.

5 A **Chest X-ray** is useful in this setting to confirm the diagnosis of pneumonia and the examination findings of consolidation.

3 DRUGS USED IN ASTHMA

1 C **Montelukast** is a leukotriene antagonist, and offers benefit to a minority of patients. It is usually tried in patients whose asthma is not controlled on inhaled steroids and long-acting β_2 agonists.

2 A **Terbutaline** is a short-acting β_2 agonist that is used to relieve acute exacerbations of asthma such as wheezing or coughing. Salbutamol is also in this class.

3 J By far the best choice for patients with symptomatic asthma (using salbutamol/terbutaline inhalers more than three times per week) while on intermittent short-acting β_2 agonists is the addition of a regular inhaled corticosteroid such as **fluticasone** or beclometasone.

4 I Oral corticosteroid should be the last therapy to be tried in patients with asthma. Weaning should be attempted as soon as the asthma is brought under control to avoid side-effects. However, some patients do remain on long term **prednisolone**.

5 F **Omalizumab** is an expensive new therapy for asthma, licensed for hospital use only. It can be used in patients with symptoms even on high-dose inhaled corticosteroids and β_2 agonists.

4 SHORTNESS OF BREATH

1 F While less common with better occupational health, coal miner's pneumoconiosis is still seen. This gentleman has **pulmonary fibrosis** secondary to the inhalation of coal dust at work.

2 B The pallor and likely non-steroidal anti-inflammatory drug (NSAID) use make the diagnosis of **anaemia** most likely, secondary to occult gastrointestinal (GI) bleeding.

3 G The history of sudden-onset shortness of breath is most compatible with spontaneous **pneumothorax**, especially as the patient is likely to be a tall, young male.

4 C This unfortunate woman probably has antiphospholipid syndrome, leading to recurrent miscarriages and predisposing to arterial and venous thrombosis. The most likely diagnosis is therefore fatal **pulmonary embolism.**

5 J Inhaled **foreign bodies** often present in children, who inadvertently place small objects in their mouths. The history shows that it has most likely lodged within the right main bronchus, which is the most common location for foreign bodies, owing to its slightly sharper inclination.

5 CAUSES OF CLUBBING

1 A The history of weight loss, haemoptysis and smoking all point towards **bronchial carcinoma** as the cause of the clubbing.

2 F A prolonged fever with retinal haemorrhages (Roth spots) and microscopic haematuria in an intravenous drug user make the diagnosis of **subacute bacterial endocarditis** most likely – an echocardiogram is needed to confirm the diagnosis.

3 I **Congenital.** This accountant has symptoms consistent with influenza. The clubbing is probably long-standing and unrelated to his current problem.

4 J A malignancy is suggested by the profound weight loss. Given the fact that he does not smoke, **mesothelioma** secondary to occupational exposure to asbestos is the probable diagnosis.

5 G **Bronchiectasis** is irreversible dilatation of the airways and is a feature of cystic fibrosis, in which clubbing is universal.

6 COMPLICATIONS OF ANTITUBERCULOUS THERAPY

1 H It is not unusual for **rifampicin** to stain body secretions (including sweat, urine and tears) pink.

2 I Reduction in visual acuity and colour blindness are well-recognized side-effects of **ethambutol**: all patients should have their vision checked before commencing therapy.

3 E **Streptomycin** is only used as a second-line drug for tuberculosis: its major side-effect is damage to the vestibular nerve.

4 B Peripheral neuropathy is well-recognized with **isoniazid**, but usually prevented by the administration of pyridoxine at the same time.

5 F Hepatotoxicity can occur with many antituberculous drugs, but severe hepatotoxicity is most likely to be due to **pyrazinamide.**

7 COMPLICATIONS OF SMOKING

1 A This gentleman is having a myocardial infarction. Smoking considerably increases the risk of **ischaemic heart disease**: this is the major cause of mortality for smokers.

2 C **Bladder cancer.** Cancer of the urinary tract is associated with smoking and often presents as painless macroscopic haematuria: further investigation is mandatory.

3 G This heavy smoker has secondary **polycythaemia**. The high levels of carboxyhaemoglobin from smoking have stimulated the body to create more haemoglobin, giving the plethoric appearance.

4 B The history of impotence combined with buttock claudication suggests Leriche's syndrome, **peripheral vascular disease** of the iliac arteries leading to diminished blood supply to the genitalia and buttocks.

5 F **Bronchial carcinoma.** Smokers are at high risk of bronchial carcinoma – this gentleman has presented with some features of a Horner's syndrome (miosis and ptosis), indicating a probable Pancoast tumour invading the sympathetic chain at the right apex.

8 EXAMINATION FINDINGS IN RESPIRATORY DISEASE

1 D **Consolidated** lung transmits high-pitched sounds more clearly, leading to increased vocal resonance. Bronchial breathing is usually found over consolidated or collapsed lung.

2 E Hyper-resonant percussion with absent breath sounds indicates **pneumothorax**; these signs are due to the absence of underlying lung tissue.

3 C **Fibrosis**, a restrictive lung disease, leads to decreased chest wall movement with fine crackles as airways open. The thickened lung parenchyma conducts transmitted sounds better than normal tissue.

4 G A wheeze and prolonged expiratory phase are findings consistent with **obstructive lung disease**: the patient is unable to exhale quickly due to loss of elastic recoil and airway narrowing. While there may be a wheeze in asthma, chest wall movement is usually good.

5 B The characteristic finding of **pleural effusion** is the stony dull percussion note. Water does not transmit sound well, so vocal resonance is typically absent.

9 INVESTIGATION OF RESPIRATORY DISEASE 2

1 G **Arterial blood gas analysis** allows the level of hypoxia to be quantified, as well as measuring the concentration of carbon dioxide. An elevated P_{CO_2} with a low P_{O_2} indicates type II failure; a normal P_{CO_2} with a low P_{O_2} indicates type I failure.

2 J **Pleural aspiration** of an effusion is mandatory in cases such as this when the aetiology is unclear: this will allow determination of whether the effusion is a transudate or exudate, and may hint at an underlying pathological process (e.g. if malignant cells are seen within the effusion).

3 A Pulmonary embolism is the most likely diagnosis given the long-haul flight and sudden onset shortness of breath. Chest radiography rarely shows an abnormality in pulmonary embolism. A **CT pulmonary angiogram** is likely to show a pulmonary artery filling defect.

4 D The combination of renal failure and haemoptysis in a young person suggests the diagnosis of Goodpasture's syndrome, an autoimmune disease where antibodies are directed against type IV collagen in the glomerular basement membrane and alveolus. The diagnostic test is the **anti-GBM antibody**.

5 F **Sputum analysis.** This immigrant probably has tuberculosis, as suggested by constitutional symptoms and upper lobe shadowing. The diagnosis can be confirmed by showing the presence of acid-fast bacilli (AFB) in the sputum.

10 HAEMOPTYSIS

1 H **Wegener's granulomatosis** is a systemic vasculitis that often presents with haemoptysis and epistaxis due to nasal ulceration. The lesion on the chest X-ray is a granuloma: these are classically seen to migrate with time.

2 D This woman has **mitral stenosis** causing left ventricular failure. The mitral facies and mid-diastolic murmur at the apex are characteristic of this condition.

3 A **Pulmonary embolism** is the most likely diagnosis here. The wedge-shaped lesion on the chest X-ray is an infarct: this is a relatively uncommon sign of pulmonary embolism, occurring in only about 10 per cent of cases.

4 I This gentleman has Kartagener's syndrome, a congenital disease of cilia, leading to **bronchiectasis**, subfertility and situs inversus. The GP could not find the patient's heart as all the organs, including the heart, are transposed to the other side of the body.

5 C The fever and cough with signs of consolidation indicate **pneumonia** is most likely. Streptococcal pneumonia is associated with the production of rusty-coloured sputum.

11 PLEURAL EFFUSION

1 I **Acute pancreatitis** is most likely here: the multiple spider naevi and suspicion of alcohol abuse make alcohol the presumptive aetiology. Abdominal pain in pancreatitis is not always severe, and the condition may present more insidiously.

2 J This gentleman is thrombophilic due to his malignancy. The sudden-onset shortness of breath with right axis deviation on ECG makes **pulmonary embolism** most probable.

3 G The combination of gradual-onset shortness of breath, an elevated JVP and bibasal crackles make pulmonary oedema secondary to **cardiac failure** the best diagnosis.

4 C This woman demonstrates the three hallmarks of **nephrotic syndrome**: oedema, proteinuria and hypoalbuminaemia. Her pleural effusions are transudates secondary to the low protein in her blood. Hyperlipidaemia is usually also found in addition.

5 F **Tuberculosis** often presents insidiously with constitutional symptoms such as weight loss and night sweats. *M. tuberculosis* has a predilection for the upper lobes, and the chest X-ray confirms this.

12 COMPLICATIONS OF DRUGS USED IN RESPIRATORY MEDICINE

1 H Inhaled steroids such as **beclometasone** can promote the growth of fungi in the oropharynx. This patient has oral candidiasis, which usually responds well to anti-fungal therapy such as nystatin.

2 J Long-term steroid use causes osteoporosis, which manifests itself as a propensity to fracture bones. This woman has vertebral fractures as a result of the **prednisolone** tablets used to control her respiratory disease.

3 A β_2-agonists such as **salbutamol** cause a fine tremor, and are causing this patient's difficulties.

4 B **Ipratropium bromide** is an anticholinergic and blocks parasympathetic bodily functions such as salivation, resulting in a dry mouth.

5 E **Theophylline** is a bronchodilator that is used for respiratory disease that is resistant to other treatments. It has a narrow therapeutic index and can cause life-threatening arrhythmias in even small overdoses.

13 RESPIRATORY FAILURE

1 A The combination of fatigue, ptosis, and a superior mediastinal mass – probably a thymoma – in a young female make **myasthenia gravis** the most likely diagnosis.

2 J The slow progressive decline in this patient, combined with fasciculation and global muscle wasting, suggests **motor neurone disease.**

3 E **Drug reaction.** Opioid toxicity is characterized by pinpoint pupils and respiratory depression – in this case the patient is only taking 7 breaths/min. Intravenous naloxone would be indicated for treatment.

4 B **Guillain–Barré syndrome** is characterized by a progressive demyelinating neuropathy, sometimes preceded by a gastrointestinal infection, classically *Campylobacter*. In severe cases, assisted ventilation may be required.

5 I **Extrinsic allergic alveolitis** is a hypersensitivity reaction to environmental antigens. This farmer has unfortunately developed lung disease as a result of spores typically found in mouldy hay.

14 PULMONARY OEDEMA

1 A The cause of this woman's respiratory difficulties is left ventricular failure secondary to **mitral stenosis.** This cardiac lesion typically causes a mid-diastolic murmur, louder on expiration, which is heard best at the apex.

2 F This unfortunate diver has developed **adult respiratory distress syndrome (ARDS)** after nearly drowning. The chest X-ray typically shows infiltrates in both lungs; the prognosis is usually poor.

3 I **Iatrogenic** fluid overload after blood transfusion is sometimes seen: in those at risk, furosemide can be given with the blood to diurese the patient.

4 H Elevated ST segments on the ECG and central chest pain are highly suggestive of **myocardial infarction**, which is more common in certain ethnic subgroups. The patient here has developed cardiogenic shock, resulting in pulmonary oedema.

5 D The history of smoking makes it likely that this gentleman is an arteriopath. The recently started antihypertensive medication is likely to be an angiotensin-converting enzyme (ACE) inhibitor, which on the background of bilateral **renal artery stenosis** has precipitated flash pulmonary oedema.

15 COMPLICATIONS OF LUNG CANCER

1 D **Superior vena cava obstruction** is caused when a tumour causes extrinsic compression of the superior vena cava. This results in venous congestion in the head and thorax, giving rise to dilated veins and facial plethora. Treatment is with stenting or radiotherapy.

2 C **Hypercalcaemia** is a well-recognized side-effect of bronchial carcinoma, usually due to ectopic parathyroid hormone-related peptide (PTHrP) secretion from the malignant cells. This patient has both physical and psychological signs of hypercalcaemia.

3 E An apical (Pancoast's) tumour can cause **Horner's syndrome** (ptosis, miosis, hemifacial anhidrosis, apparent enophthalmos) and hand weakness by invasion of the sympathetic trunk and brachial plexus.

4 B The characteristic X-ray appearance indicates **hypertrophic pulmonary osteo-arthropathy** (HPOA), a non-metastatic manifestation of bronchial carcinoma. Patients usually present with pain or stiffness of the wrists or ankles.

5 G This is a myasthenic picture, with drooping eyelids. The **Eaton–Lambert syndrome** is caused by antibodies to voltage-gated calcium channels in patients with small-cell lung cancer. Characteristically the weakness improves with repeated activity, in contrast to myasthenia gravis where power decreases.

X-RAY ANSWERS

1 Film A is a posteroanterior (PA) projection, whereas film B is anteroposterior (AP). In an AP film, the clavicles tend to be horizontal and the scapulae overlie the lung fields. A PA projection allows the heart size to be evaluated.

2 There is a left basal pleural effusion, with the classic hallmark of a concave upper border. The aetiology of this effusion is most likely to be malignant.

3 There is a mass in the left upper lobe. With a history of chronic cough and haemoptysis in an elderly patient, a peripheral bronchial carcinoma is the most likely explanation.

4 The abnormality demonstrated on the chest X-ray is significant bilateral hilar lymphadenopathy. The combination of erythema nodosum, the rash found by the GP, and hilar lymph node enlargement is pathognomonic of sarcoidosis.

5 a) There is a right sided pneumothorax, where air has entered the pleural cavity. The lung edge can be seen, beyond which there are no lung markings.
  b) Initial treatment for a symptomatic spontaneous pneumothorax in a patient without underlying lung disease is oxygen and needle aspiration. Only if aspiration is unsuccessful is a chest drain needed.

6 a) There is dense consolidation of the right upper lobe, with bulging of the horizontal fissure. Given the clinical history, pneumonia is the most probable diagnosis.
  b) *Klebsiella* pneumonia classically causes bulging of the fissures on chest X-ray. In addition, when contracted as a community-acquired infection, it usually affects the debilitated such as the homeless and alcoholics.

7 a) The combination of ptosis and miosis (a small pupil) suggests the possibility of Horner's syndrome. Anhidrosis is rarely elicited in clinical practice.

   b) There is a large tumour at the left apex. This has presumably invaded the sympathetic nervous system leading to the Horner's syndrome. Lung cancers that behave in this way are referred to as Pancoast's tumours.

8 a) There are multiple round shadows, which are most likely to be metastases.

   b) Pulmonary metastases are most commonly seen in association with malignancy of the breast, thyroid, kidney, lung, colon and prostate.

9 a) The CT scan of the thorax shows a normal left lung and extensively thickened right pleura. The most likely cause of this is mesothelioma.

   b) Exposure to asbestos is aetiologically linked to the development of mesothelioma. Industries such as shipbuilding and construction had workers exposed to large quantities of asbestos fibres before it was recognized that it was a potent carcinogen.

10 a) The chest X-ray demonstrates a tension pneumothorax. The left lung has completely collapsed and the mediastinum has shifted away from the affected side, causing cardiovascular embarrassment. This is a clinical diagnosis – requesting a chest X-ray in these circumstances is inappropriate.

    b) Immediate treatment is required to prevent cardiac arrest and death. Decompression of the left hemithorax can be easily and rapidly achieved by the insertion of a cannula in the second intercostal space, mid-clavicular line.

11 The chest X-ray shows features of emphysema: the lungs are hyperexpanded with a flattened diaphragm and a small cardiac silhouette. Note the paucity of lung markings within both mid- and upper zones, due to the presence of bullae.

12 This patient has undergone bilateral breast augmentation previously, giving rise to the two well-defined circular opacities on the chest X-ray. Further imaging is not required!

13 a) This patient has had a thoracoplasty: the resection of several ribs to collapse the chest wall.

    b) This was commonly undertaken in the pre-antibiotic era as a treatment for pulmonary tuberculosis. The fact that many patients who had this surgery are still alive is a testament to the fact that it was a successful treatment.

14 The X-ray shows consolidation with cavitating lesions in the right upper lobe. These appearances are typical of active tuberculosis. The tender lesions on the patient's legs are probably erythema nodosum, which is associated with this condition.

Neurology

MULTIPLE CHOICE QUESTIONS

1 The following statements are true of subarachnoid haemorrhage:
   a) Arteriovenous malformation is the commonest cause
   b) Onset of symptoms is usually over a few hours
   c) Cerebrospinal fluid (CSF) examination may be a useful diagnostic tool
   d) Polycystic kidneys are associated with cerebral berry aneurysms
   e) Nimodipine decreases mortality

2 The following statements are true of multiple sclerosis:
   a) High-dose β-interferon is curative
   b) It occurs predominantly in old age
   c) Brain computed tomography (CT) is the most useful diagnostic investigation
   d) It is associated with smoking
   e) Short courses of steroids are useful for relapses

3 Causes of vertigo include:
   a) Vestibular neuronitis
   b) Salbutamol
   c) Poliomyelitis
   d) Ménière's disease
   e) Brainstem infarction

4 Causes of bulbar palsy include:
   a) Syringobulbia
   b) Cerebellar infarction
   c) Poliomyelitis
   d) Cauda equina syndrome
   e) Motor neurone disease

5 Causes of coma include:
   a) Uraemia
   b) Hypokalaemia
   c) Hyponatraemia
   d) Hyperlipidaemia
   e) Hypercalcaemia

6   Risk factors for stroke include:
   a) Atrial fibrillation
   b) Statins
   c) Thrombolysis post-myocardial infarction
   d) Hypertension
   e) Renal failure

7   Manifestations of a seventh cranial nerve palsy include:
   a) Loss of taste
   b) Loss of hearing
   c) Impaired blinking
   d) Impaired swallowing
   e) Impaired lacrimation

8   Regarding subdural and extradural haemorrhage:
   a) Subdural haemorrhage typically presents within 24 h of a major head injury in the elderly
   b) Conservative management is usually most suitable for an extradural haemorrhage
   c) There is usually a clear history of trauma in extradural haemorrhage
   d) Extradural haemorrhage is usually due to bleeding from the internal carotid artery
   e) Subdural haemorrhage is an important cause of confusion in the elderly

9   Examples of generalized seizures are:
   a) Absences
   b) Jacksonian seizures
   c) Temporal lobe seizures
   d) Tonic–clonic seizures
   e) Myoclonic seizures

10 Causes of vertigo include:
   a) Phenytoin
   b) Bulbar palsy
   c) Multiple sclerosis
   d) Amoxicillin
   e) Acoustic neuroma

11 The following statements are true of anticonvulsants:
   a) They are safe in pregnancy
   b) Rapid withdrawal is safe in young patients
   c) Ataxia is a side-effect
   d) Gabapentin is the treatment of choice in partial and generalized seizures
   e) In epilepsy, permission to drive a motor vehicle in the UK is dependent on compliance with anticonvulsant therapy

12 The following statements are true of Parkinson's disease:
   a) Most cases are iatrogenic
   b) It is a disease of westernized developed countries
   c) It is inherited in an autosomal recessive fashion
   d) It is usually caused by reduced acetylcholine levels in the substantia nigra (in the basal ganglia)
   e) It is incurable

13 The following statements are true of meningitis:
   a) Viral meningitis is more detrimental than bacterial meningitis
   b) The commonest offending bacterium in the UK is *Haemophilus influenzae*
   c) A basal skull fracture is a risk factor for pneumococcal meningitis
   d) Antibiotic administration should be delayed until after CSF examination in likely meningococcal meningitis
   e) Rifampicin is useful for prophylaxis in contacts of a patient with meningococcal meningitis

14 The following statements are true regarding treatment of Parkinson's disease:
   a) Drug treatment should start when symptoms of Parkinson's disease first appear
   b) Carbidopa should not be administered with levodopa
   c) Involuntary movements are a side-effect of levodopa
   d) The duration of action of levodopa declines over time
   e) On–off syndrome is a recognized problem associated with levodopa

15 Lumbar puncture examination typically reveals the following in acute bacterial meningitis:
   a) Low opening pressure
   b) Clear CSF appearance
   c) Lymphocytes as the predominant cell type
   d) Reduced glucose level
   e) Reduced protein level

16 Clinical features of Parkinson's disease include:
   a) Spasticity
   b) Progressive distal sensory loss
   c) Intention tremor
   d) Bradykinesia
   e) Expressionless face

17 The following statements are true of Bell's palsy:
   a) It commonly presents with a bilateral facial palsy
   b) In the majority of cases the palsy is permanent
   c) Antibiotics hasten recovery
   d) Corneal ulceration may be a sequela
   e) Prednisolone is of value in treating the condition

18 Features of Horner's syndrome include ipsilateral:
   a) Pupil dilatation
   b) Facial sensory loss
   c) Complete ptosis
   d) Impaired eye abduction
   e) Excessive facial sweating

19 Causes of polyneuropathy include:
   a) Charcot–Marie–Tooth syndrome
   b) Myasthenia gravis
   c) Guillain–Barré syndrome
   d) Diabetes mellitus
   e) Vitamin B_6 deficiency

20 A complete third cranial nerve palsy produces the following features:
   a) Constricted pupil
   b) Loss of sensation below the mouth and along the jaw
   c) Partial ptosis
   d) Complete blindness
   e) The eye is fixed in adduction

21 Cerebellar lesions may cause:
   a) Resting tremor
   b) Pressure of speech
   c) Nystagmus
   d) Hypotonia
   e) Ipsilateral sensory loss

22 The following statements are true of headaches:
   a) There is often associated focal neurology
   b) A chronic, band-like, bilateral headache is most likely to be due to cluster headache
   c) Headache secondary to raised intracranial pressure is typically worse in the early morning
   d) Sudden-onset severe headache with associated neck stiffness is most often due to subdural haemorrhage
   e) Facial tenderness, post-nasal drip and coryza is a typical presentation for cranial arteritis

23 Proximal myopathy occurs in:
   a) Thyrotoxicosis
   b) Polymyalgia rheumatica
   c) Alcohol excess
   d) Pseudogout
   e) Cushing's syndrome

24 A high thoracic complete spinal cord transection causes:
   a) Diaphragmatic paralysis
   b) Spastic tetraparesis
   c) Bladder disturbance
   d) Brown-Séquard syndrome
   e) Glove-and-stocking sensory loss

25 The following statements are true of myasthenia gravis:
   a) The disease is characterized by a deficiency of acetylcholine
   b) Weakness improves on repeated muscle use
   c) Anticholinesterases are useful in the treatment of the condition
   d) There is an association with cardiac tumours
   e) The eye muscles are spared

26 Causes of dysarthria include:
   a) Pseudobulbar palsy
   b) Infarct of Broca's area
   c) Parkinson's disease
   d) Acute confusional state
   e) Ill-fitting dentures

27 Regarding speech function, the following statements are true:
a) In the majority of people, language is controlled by the right cerebral hemisphere
b) Dysphasia is a disorder of speech articulation
c) Damage to Wernicke's area results in impaired fluency of speech
d) Speech is not affected by cerebellar lesions
e) Broca's area is located in the parietal lobe

28 The following are causes of blackouts:
a) Transient ischaemic attack (TIA)
b) Hyperthyroidism
c) Hyperventilation
d) Hypoglycaemia
e) Guillain–Barré syndrome

29 The following are features of the listed type of neurological gait:
a) Broad-based walking; spastic gait
b) Positive Romberg's test; cerebellar ataxia
c) Waddling; common peroneal palsy
d) High-stepping; sensory ataxia
e) Foot slapping the ground; parkinsonian

30 Features of a parkinsonian gait include:
a) Festinant walking
b) Hemiballismus
c) Shuffling
d) Retropulsion
e) High stepping

31 The following statements are true of cluster headaches:
a) They typically occur once a week for a period of several months
b) The pain is usually bilateral
c) Blindness may ensue if steroids are not administered soon after the onset of an acute attack
d) Sumatriptan is a useful treatment
e) There is an association with subarachnoid haemorrhage

32 The following are manifestations of a trigeminal nerve lesion:
a) Absent gag reflex
b) Inability to frown
c) Brisk jaw jerk reflex
d) Masseter wasting
e) Absent corneal reflex

33 Features of cauda equina syndrome include:
a) Urine retention
b) Buttock anaesthesia
c) Extensor plantar responses
d) Reduced anal tone
e) Leg weakness

34 Causes of delirium include:
  a) Morphine
  b) Faecal impaction
  c) Hypoxia
  d) Scurvy
  e) Urinary infection

35 The following statements are true of Guillain–Barré syndrome:
  a) It is an inheritable condition
  b) Respiratory failure is a recognized complication
  c) Immunoglobulin administration is a useful treatment
  d) Numbness starts proximally and moves distally
  e) It is usually a complication of malignancy

36 The following are recognized causes of dementia:
  a) Hypothyroidism
  b) Lewy bodies
  c) Hirschsprung's disease
  d) Syphilis
  e) Mononeuritis multiplex

37 The following can cause dementia:
  a) Pick's disease
  b) HIV
  c) von Willebrand's disease
  d) Huntington's disease
  e) Normal pressure hydrocephalus

38 Causes of chorea include:
  a) Crohn's disease
  b) Rheumatic fever
  c) Horner's syndrome
  d) Systemic lupus erythematosus
  e) Wilson's disease

39 Features of Parkinson's disease include:
  a) Constipation
  b) Simian posture
  c) Large handwriting
  d) Frequent blinking
  e) Slurred speech

40 The following are recognized complications of bacterial meningitis:
  a) Brain abscess
  b) Sensorineural deafness
  c) Creutzfeldt–Jakob disease
  d) Venous sinus thrombosis
  e) Mental retardation

41 Multiple sclerosis affects the following parts of the nervous system:
   a) Optic nerve
   b) Cerebellum
   c) Peripheral nerves
   d) Brainstem
   e) Cervical spinal cord

42 Causes of delirium include:
   a) Vitamin B_6 deficiency
   b) Alcohol withdrawal
   c) Unfamiliar surroundings
   d) Pott's disease
   e) Acute urinary retention

43 The following are indications for a CT scan after head injury:
   a) Headache
   b) Seizures
   c) Scalp laceration
   d) Glasgow coma scale of 10
   e) Depressed skull fracture

44 Causes of seizures include:
   a) Head injury
   b) Hypoglycaemia
   c) Hyperkalaemia
   d) Brain tumour
   e) Cerebrovascular disease

45 The following statements are true of strokes:
   a) 40 per cent are haemorrhagic
   b) Neuroimaging must be available before administering thrombolysis
   c) Management in a specialist stroke unit reduces mortality
   d) Carotid endarterectomy is generally indicated in internal carotid stenoses occluding >40 per cent of the lumen
   e) Clopidogrel is the initial treatment of choice in ischaemic stroke

46 The Glasgow Coma Scale (GCS) is formulated from the following components:
   a) Pupil size
   b) Verbal responses
   c) Core temperature
   d) Motor responses
   e) Respiratory rate

47 Causes of coma include:
   a) Hypoglycaemia
   b) Liver failure
   c) Eosinophilia
   d) Hypoalbuminaemia
   e) Hypothyroidism

48 The following are detectable on a brain CT scan:
  a) Brain abscess
  b) Cerebral infarction
  c) Cerebral toxoplasmosis
  d) Tuberculoma
  e) Extradural haemorrhage

49 Causes of pseudobulbar palsy include:
  a) Budd–Chiari syndrome
  b) Stroke
  c) Alzheimer's disease
  d) Multiple sclerosis
  e) Motor neurone disease

50 A lesion of the ninth and tenth cranial nerves may produce the following:
  a) Spastic tongue
  b) Dysphagia
  c) Hoarse voice
  d) Deviated uvula
  e) Weakness of trapezius

51 Clinical features of multiple sclerosis include:
  a) Ataxia
  b) Urinary incontinence
  c) Diplopia
  d) Spastic paraparesis
  e) Impotence

52 Causes of spastic paraplegia include:
  a) Vertebral metastasis
  b) Multiple sclerosis
  c) Poliomyelitis
  d) Guillain–Barré syndrome
  e) Syringomyelia

53 State whether these deep tendon reflexes are paired with their correct segmental innervations:
  a) Knee; L1, L2
  b) Triceps; C7
  c) Biceps; C8
  d) Ankle; L3, L4
  e) Supinator; C6

54 Features of a vestibular nerve defect may include:
  a) Deafness
  b) Nystagmus
  c) Loss of balance
  d) Vomiting
  e) Vertigo

55 Examination of cranial nerve II should involve:
    a) Testing for conjugate gaze
    b) Ishihara plates
    c) Fundoscopy
    d) Assessing pupillary reflexes
    e) Snellen chart

56 The following are causes of cerebellar impairment:
    a) Diabetes mellitus
    b) Friedreich's ataxia
    c) Excessive alcohol consumption
    d) Statins
    e) Multiple sclerosis

57 The following statements are true of the spinothalamic sensory tracts:
    a) They are responsible for vibration sense
    b) They transmit temperature sensation
    c) Decussation occurs in the brainstem
    d) They transmit joint position sense
    e) They are responsible for pain transmission

58 Features of cerebellar lesions include:
    a) Flaccid paralysis
    b) Broad-based gait
    c) Hyperreflexia
    d) Dysdiadochokinesis
    e) Staccato speech

59 Manifestations of extrapyramidal lesions include:
    a) Spasticity
    b) Bradykinesia
    c) Hemiplegia
    d) Rigidity
    e) Chorea

60 Features of an upper motor neurone lesion are:
    a) Flaccid weakness
    b) Clonus
    c) Positive Babinski sign
    d) Muscle wasting
    e) Hyporeflexia

61 Causes of a lower motor neurone lesion of the facial nerve include:
    a) Ramsay-Hunt syndrome
    b) Mumps
    c) Multiple sclerosis
    d) Acoustic neuroma
    e) Otitis media

62 Causes of dysarthria include:
  a) Alzheimer's dementia
  b) Myasthenia gravis
  c) Infarct of Wernicke's area
  d) Cerebellar tumour
  e) XII nerve palsy

63 Causes of syncope include:
  a) Micturition
  b) Sudden standing
  c) Charcot–Marie–Tooth syndrome
  d) Vertebrobasilar arterial insufficiency
  e) Stokes–Adams attack

64 The following statements are true of motor neurone disease:
  a) Ocular movements are affected early
  b) Fasciculation is a feature
  c) Sensory loss affects distal body parts first
  d) Short courses of steroids slow the progression of the disease
  e) Spastic paraparesis is a consequence

65 Precipitants of syncope include:
  a) Fear
  b) Coughing
  c) Head-turning
  d) Sleep
  e) Aortic stenosis

66 The following are causes of an isolated third cranial nerve palsy:
  a) Kallmann's syndrome
  b) Raised intracranial pressure
  c) Diabetes mellitus
  d) Posterior communicating artery aneurysm
  e) Bell's palsy

67 The following statements are true of giant cell arteritis:
  a) There is an association with polymyositis
  b) It is predominantly a disease of the elderly
  c) Non-steroidal anti-inflammatory drugs (NSAIDs) are the treatment of choice
  d) Anaemia is a frequent finding
  e) Diagnosis is by internal carotid artery biopsy

68 The following are causes of Horner's syndrome:
  a) Syringomyelia
  b) Cervical rib
  c) Bell's palsy
  d) Apical lung tumour
  e) Brainstem infarction

69 Clinical features of giant cell arteritis include:
   a) Hearing loss
   b) Scalp tenderness
   c) Amaurosis fugax
   d) Temporary hemiparesis
   e) Jaw claudication

70 Regarding head injuries:
   a) Extradural haemorrhages are not amenable to surgery
   b) A patient with open eyes, withdrawing to pain and uttering unintelligible sounds has a GCS of 11
   c) A nasogastric tube is contraindicated in basal skull fracture
   d) Recurrent post-traumatic seizures should not be treated with anti-epileptic medication
   e) Post-traumatic hypotension is usually due to intracranial haemorrhage

Answers: see pages 72–82

EXTENDED MATCHING QUESTIONS

1 THE GLASGOW COMA SCALE

Calculate the correct Glasgow Coma Scale (GCS) score for each of the patients below

A	4	F	9
B	5	G	10
C	6	H	11
D	7	I	12
E	8	J	13

1 A 41-year-old woman is brought in to hospital unconscious. The doctor on-call tries to perform a sternal rub to get her to open her eyes, but is unsuccessful. She does however try to push his hand away from her chest, at the same time making strange noises that no one can quite understand.

2 A driver of a car is brought in after an accident. The ambulance crew have been able to intubate him without any sedatives or muscle relaxants. The registrar cannot make him open his eyes or make any sound. While still in resus he begins to flex his arms and legs.

3 A 17-year-old girl is brought to the emergency department after taking some illicit drugs in a nightclub. She is extremely drowsy and does not know where she is. After repeatedly shouting loudly in her left ear, the doctor gets her to open her eyes and squeeze his hand.

4 An 89-year-old man is brought to hospital from his nursing home with a suspected stroke. He can only manage to say words such as 'dog' and 'holiday', which seem to have no context. His eyes are open spontaneously. When the doctor tries to take some blood from his left arm, he withdraws his whole body suddenly.

5 A 37-year-old man is brought into hospital by ambulance after having a fit in the street. The triage nurse recognizes him as being a frequent attendee with pseudoseizures. He does not make any sound, and the doctor cannot make him open his eyes. However, he localizes well to pain.

2 INTRACRANIAL HAEMORRHAGE

Each of the patients below has suffered an intracranial haemorrhage. Choose the best diagnosis from the options given for each of the clinical scenarios below

A Subdural haemorrhage
B Cerebellar haemorrhage
C Subarachnoid haemorrhage
D Extradural haemorrhage
E Intraventricular haemorrhage
F Intracerebral haemorrhage: anterior cerebral artery
G Intracerebral haemorrhage: middle cerebral artery
H Intracerebral haemorrhage: posterior cerebral artery
I Pontine haemorrhage
J Thalamic haemorrhage

1 A baby is born early, at 30 weeks gestation, and taken to the special care baby unit. One of the paediatricians gravely informs the parents that an ultrasound scan has shown a bleed into the brain. They are a little relieved when he says that this is a frequent occurrence in premature babies.

2 A 72-year-old man is found collapsed on the street. Before he lapses into a coma, he initially tells the ambulance crew that he cannot move his arms or legs. On arrival in hospital his pupils are small and unreactive. An urgent CT scan shows haemorrhage extending into the fourth ventricle.

3 An alcoholic man, well known to the emergency department, is brought in by one of his friends, who says that he is confused despite not having drunk any alcohol that day.

4 A 66-year-old woman presents to her general practitioner (GP) with unsteadiness, nausea and vomiting. He examines her thoroughly and elicits left-sided nystagmus, an intention tremor and a broad-based gait. He tells her that he suspects that she has had a stroke and sends her immediately to hospital.

5 A 42-year-old woman goes to see her doctor with a headache. A CT scan is normal but her lumbar puncture is positive for xanthochromia.

3 HEADACHE

Each of the patients below complains of a headache. Choose the best diagnosis from the options given for each of the clinical scenarios below

A   Cluster headache
B   Migraine
C   Iatrogenic
D   Trigeminal neuralgia
E   Tension headache

F   Brain tumour
G   Temporal arteritis
H   Subarachnoid haemorrhage
I   Sinusitis
J   Meningitis

1   A 22-year-old woman goes to see her GP complaining of a unilateral headache with nausea and vomiting. She is photophobic and says that she can see flashing and shimmering lights when she closes her eyes. Her pulse is 70 beats/min, temperature 36.7°C with neurological examination entirely unremarkable.

2   A 73-year-old man goes to see his GP with a right-sided headache. He says the pain gets worse when he eats.

3   A 53-year-old woman complains of short attacks of what she says feels like an electric shock over her left cheek. She says that the pain is intolerable and can be triggered by brushing her teeth.

4   A 33-year-old man goes to see his doctor with a severe headache. It affects the left side of his head and is associated with a red eye, ptosis and a running left nostril. He says that he suffers from the same symptoms every March.

5   A 29-year-old man is brought to see his GP by his wife. She is worried as he is having headaches every morning when he wakes up. They seem to get better through the course of the day by themselves. While examining the patient, the GP asks him to touch his toes, which seems to make the headache worse.

4 NEUROANATOMY

Select the area of the brain most likely to be responsible for the defects described below

A   Broca's area
B   Pituitary
C   Pons
D   Aqueduct of Sylvius
E   Cerebellum

F   Temporal lobe
G   Wernicke's area
H   Pineal gland
I   Olfactory bulb
J   Substantia nigra

1   A 76-year-old man is admitted with non-communicating hydrocephalus.

2   An 84-year-old woman is admitted after having had a stroke. She can understand the instructions of the doctor but is unable to speak.

3   A 61-year-old woman with Parkinson's disease wants to know where the defective neurones in her brain are.

4   A 29-year-old man, who lost his sense of smell after a car accident, wants to know which part of his brain isn't working.

5   A 59-year-old woman goes to see her GP asking for some sleeping tablets to help her with jet-lag. He patiently explains to her that part of the brain has a clock to help the body know whether it is day or night.

5 CRANIAL NERVE LESIONS

Each of the patients below has a cranial nerve lesion. Choose the defective nerve from the options given

A II
B III
C IV
D V
E VI

F VII
G VIII
H IX
I X
J XI

1 An obese 23-year-old woman goes to see her GP with headache and visual loss that is worse after bending over. The cranial nerve examination reveals that she cannot look to the right with her right eye.

2 An 83-year-old woman presents to the emergency department with a stroke. The doctor touches the back of her throat with a tongue depressor; the patient says that she can feel nothing.

3 A 69-year-old man complains that his sense of taste has gone. Careful examination reveals no taste sensation in the anterior two-thirds of his tongue. The posterior one-third functions normally.

4 An 83-year old man complains of diarrhoea. His GP says that this is the result of one of his nerves being cut when he had an operation for an ulcer 40 years ago.

5 A 71-year-old man tells his GP that he has been unable to lift his right shoulder after having had a stroke 6 months ago.

6 DRUGS USED IN NEUROLOGICAL DISEASE

Select the most appropriate drug for each of the indications below

A Riluzole
B Temazepam
C Fluoxetine
D Carbamazepine
E Lorazepam

F Amitriptyline
G Prochlorperazine
H Methylphenidate
I Donepezil
J Ethosuximide

1 A 31-year-old epileptic woman has been having a witnessed seizure for the past 30 min. The ambulance crew have helpfully sited an intravenous cannula.

2 A 22-year-old man with amyotrophic lateral sclerosis.

3 A 7-year-old boy with attention-deficit hyperactivity disorder.

4 A 9-year-old girl who suddenly seems to stop concentrating in class for 3 or 4 seconds before she returns to normal.

5 A 43-year-old woman who attends the emergency department with dizziness, tinnitus and vomiting. The doctor diagnoses benign paroxysmal positional vertigo and offers her some medication which he says will help.

7 DRUGS USED IN MOVEMENT DISORDERS

Select the most appropriate drug for each of the indications below

A   Cabergoline
B   Entacapone
C   Levodopa
D   Amantadine
E   Tetrabenazine

F   Propranolol
G   Benserazide
H   Apomorphine
I   Selegiline
J   Piracetam

1 A 37-year-old man with Huntington's disease presents to his neurologist with hemi-ballismus. He has not taken any medication to control his symptoms to date.

2 An 81-year-old man reads the patient information leaflet with his L-dopa tablets. It says that there are two drugs in the medication: he wants to know the name of the other one.

3 A 29-year-old doctor pops into neurology clinic to see the consultant. He explains that he has had a tremor all his life but has managed perfectly well until now. However his consultant, a plastic surgeon, is becoming increasingly frustrated with his suturing abilities.

4 A 71-year-old woman with newly diagnosed Parkinson's disease is started on L-dopa therapy. She tolerates this poorly and discontinues the medication. Her GP says that he will give her a different sort of tablet which he calls a dopamine agonist.

5 A 75-year-old man has end-stage Parkinson's disease. His wife is extremely frustrated as he just sits in a chair all day long. He is on a cocktail of oral medications, which only slightly improve his symptoms. The neurologist says that he thinks it may be time to move on to a powerful injection.

Answers: see pages 82–84

X-RAY QUESTIONS

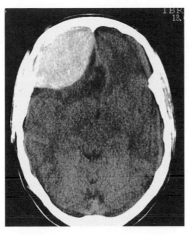

1

1   A 24-year-old man is brought to the emergency department by his friends after becoming involved in an altercation in the local pub. He complains of severe headache and drowsiness. The doctor requests a CT scan of his brain. Explain the patient's symptoms from the appearances of the CT scan.

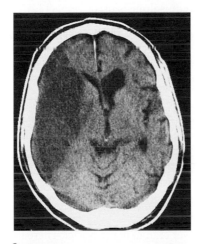

3

2   A 74-year-old man is brought into hospital by ambulance from his nursing home, having been found slumped over in bed. He cannot move one side of his body. An urgent CT scan is requested.
a) What is the diagnosis?
b) Which artery has been affected?
c) On which side would you expect neurological signs?

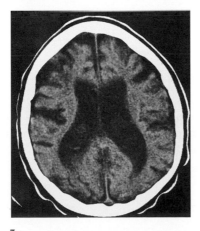

2

3   An 87-year-old man is taken to his GP by his wife, who complains that she has noticed that his short term memory is extremely poor. The GP requests a CT scan of his brain. What does the CT scan show?

Answers: see page 85

ANSWERS

MCQ ANSWERS

1 a) False. Berry aneurysm is the most frequent cause, accounting for approximately 70 per cent.
   b) False. The onset of severe headache is sudden.
   c) True. Haemorrhagic CSF turns xanthochromic after a few hours.
   d) True.
   e) True. A calcium channel antagonist, it reduces the vasospasm that follows a haemorrhage.

2 a) False. The drug can reduce the relapse rate by one-third, but does not cure the disease.
   b) False. The mean age of onset is 30 years.
   c) False. Magnetic resonance imaging (MRI) is the imaging investigation of choice.
   d) False.
   e) True. Intravenous (i.v.) methylprednisolone is used.

3 a) True. This is an acute attack of vertigo, believed to be triggered by a viral infection of the vestibular system.
   b) False.
   c) False. This is a viral disease affecting anterior horn cells.
   d) True. This is a disorder involving dilatation of the endolymphatic spaces of the labyrinth. Vertigo, deafness and tinnitus occur.
   e) True. A number of cranial nerves may be affected.

4 a) True. There is cavity formation in the brainstem.
   b) False. Bulbar palsy is due to a lesion in cranial nerves IX to XII, not the cerebellum.
   c) True. It affects the motor fibres within the brainstem.
   d) False.
   e) True. This produces defects of lower cranial nerve nuclei. There may be mixed lower and upper motor neurone features.

5 a) True.
   b) False. This causes arrhythmias.
   c) True.
   d) False.
   e) True.

6 a) True. It predisposes to cardiac thromboemboli.
   b) False. These lower serum cholesterol, thereby reducing cardiovascular risk.
   c) True. It is associated with a 1 per cent risk of stroke.
   d) True. This is an important treatable risk factor.
   e) False.

7 a) True. The chorda tympani branch supplies taste to the anterior two-thirds of the tongue.

    b) False. A paralysed stapedius muscle leads to a lack of sound damping, causing hyper-acusis.

    c) True. The orbicularis oculi muscle is innervated by the facial nerve (VII).

    d) False. Swallowing is controlled by nerves IX and X.

    e) True. The nervus intermedius branch of the facial nerve supplies parasympathetic fibres to the lacrimal gland.

8 a) False. Subdural bleeds can develop over weeks and months, often after trivial head injury.

    b) False. Haematoma evacuation through burr-holes is required.

    c) True. Trauma involves fracture of the temporal or parietal bone.

    d) False. Bleeding is from the middle meningeal artery and its branches.

    e) True. The bridging veins are more prone to tearing in the elderly. Alcoholics and epileptics are other high-risk groups.

9 a) True. They are also known as petit mal. The child stops, pauses for a short while, and then carries on what he was doing before.

    b) False. These are focal motor seizures.

    c) False. This is an example of partial seizures.

    d) True. They are also known as grand mal. There is loss of consciousness, followed by generalized rigidity, and then convulsions.

    e) True. There is sudden jerking, usually of the arms.

10 a) True. Phenytoin toxicity causes vertigo, nystagmus and ataxia.

     b) False. This is a motor defect of the ninth to the twelfth cranial nerves.

     c) True.

     d) False. Vertigo is not a recognized side-effect.

     e) True. This is an eighth nerve sheath neurofibroma at the cerebellopontine angle.

11 a) False. They are generally teratogenic.

     b) False. They may trigger rebound seizures.

     c) True.

     d) False. Valproate and carbamazepine are first-line agents.

     e) False. It is dependent on the patient's seizure-free period.

12 a) False. While some drugs, e.g. some neuroleptics, produce a parkinsonian syndrome, most cases are idiopathic.

     b) False. It is a worldwide condition.

     c) False. It is not an inheritable condition.

     d) False. A deficiency of dopamine in this region is responsible.

     e) True. Drug therapy may achieve symptomatic control, but does not delay the progression of the disease.

13 a) False. Viral meningitis is usually benign and self-limiting, while bacterial meningitis can be fatal within hours.
    b) False. This form of meningitis has largely been eradicated in the UK due to the childhood vaccination programme.
    c) True. As are sinusitis, otitis media, mastoiditis, cranial surgery – all presenting means of bacterial entry into the CNS.
    d) False. Antibiotics must be administered immediately.
    e) True.

14 a) False. Initiation of treatment is delayed until symptoms interfere with daily life.
    b) False. Carbidopa reduces the peripheral side-effects associated with levodopa.
    c) True.
    d) True. This is known as end-of-dose deterioration.
    e) True. This is alternation of 'freezing' with exaggerated involuntary movements.

15 a) False. Opening pressure is raised.
    b) False. The fluid usually appears turbid.
    c) False. Neutrophils are the most abundant.
    d) True. The level is typically reduced to less than half the plasma glucose level.
    e) False. Protein level is increased.

16 a) False. Rigidity is a cardinal feature, present throughout the entire range of motion (lead-pipe).
    b) False. The sensory pathways are unaffected.
    c) False. The tremor occurs at rest, classically 4–6 Hz, described as pill-rolling.
    d) True. This describes slow movements.
    e) True. This is a result of akinesia.

17 a) False. The facial palsy is unilateral.
    b) False. 10–15 per cent of cases remain permanent.
    c) False. A bacterial cause is not implicated in the aetiology.
    d) True. This may result from long-standing inability to close the eye.
    e) True. This may be helpful if given early in the course of the palsy.

18 a) False. There is pupil constriction. The syndrome is caused by a lesion of the sympathetic pathway.
    b) False. Sensation is unaffected.
    c) False. There is a partial ptosis.
    d) False. The abducens nerve is not affected.
    e) False. Sweating is impaired.

19 a) True. This is an example of a hereditary sensorimotor neuropathy, primarily affecting the peroneal muscles.
    b) False. This is a disease of the neuromuscular junction.
    c) True. This is an acute post-infective polyneuropathy.
    d) True.
    e) True. This is usually a consequence of isoniazid therapy. Vitamin B_1 and B_{12} deficiencies also cause polyneuropathy.

20 a) False. The pupil is fixed and dilated due to interruption of the parasympathetic fibres.
   b) False. The oculomotor nerve does not carry sensation.
   c) False. There is complete ptosis due to paralysis of the levator palpebrae superioris.
   d) False. Acuity is controlled by the optic nerve.
   e) False. The eye faces down and out.

21 a) False. This is a sign of Parkinson's disease. Cerebellar lesions cause an intention tremor with past-pointing.
   b) False. This is a term used in psychiatric disorders, where the patient's thoughts are racing faster than they can be verbalized.
   c) True. There is a horizontal nystagmus towards the side of the lesion.
   d) True.
   e) False. Sensory pathways are not involved.

22 a) False. The majority of headaches are benign. Headache in association with a demonstrable neurological deficit may indicate a serious underlying disease.
   b) False. This is the classic description of a tension headache.
   c) True.
   d) False. Subarachnoid haemorrhages present in this way.
   e) False. This is more suggestive of sinusitis.

23 a) True.
   b) False. Pain occurs in the limb girdles but weakness is not a feature.
   c) True.
   d) False. This is an arthropathy caused by calcium pyrophosphate deposits in the joints, commonly the knee.
   e) True.

24 a) False. The diaphragm is innervated by C3, 4 and 5 (phrenic nerve).
   b) False. There will be a spastic paraparesis. Full use of the upper limbs is possible.
   c) True. There is urinary incontinence.
   d) False. This occurs in hemisection of the cord, with ipsilateral weakness and contra-lateral loss of pain and temperature sensation.
   e) False. There is complete sensory loss below the level of a spinal cord transection.

25 a) False. Antibodies cause a decrease in functioning acetylcholine receptors at the neuromuscular junction.
   b) False. Fatigability is a characteristic of the disease.
   c) True. For example, pyridostigmine.
   d) False. Thymoma is associated with myasthenia. Thymectomy enhances the prognosis.
   e) False. The extraocular muscles are most likely to be affected.

26 a) True. This is caused by bilateral lesions above the pons, affecting muscles of speech and swallowing.
   b) False. This is a cause of dysphasia.
   c) True. There is a monotonous speech quality.
   d) False. The mechanism of speech articulation is unaffected.
   e) True.

27 a) False. The language centres are located in the dominant hemisphere, which is the left in most people.
   b) False. It is an impairment of language due to cerebral hemisphere damage.
   c) False. Wernicke's area is responsible for speech comprehension. Damage gives rise to nonsensical but fluent speech (receptive dysphasia).
   d) False. Cerebellar lesions cause scanning or staccato speech.
   e) False. This is the area concerned with speech formation; it is located in the frontal lobe.

28 a) True. Although loss of consciousness is unusual in TIA.
   b) False.
   c) True. Hypocapnia reduces cerebral blood flow.
   d) True. Especially in diabetics.
   e) False. This is a post-infective ascending polyneuropathy.

29 a) False. It is a feature of ataxic gait.
   b) False. The patient stands up with feet together and then closes his eyes. This is a test for impaired proprioception.
   c) False. Waddling is associated with proximal muscle (i.e. hip girdle) weakness.
   d) True. The patient feels as if he is walking 'on cotton wool'.
   e) False. It is a feature of foot drop.

30 a) True. This describes taking hurried steps.
   b) False. This is the wild, flinging, unilateral limb movements caused by a lesion in the contralateral subthalamic nucleus.
   c) True.
   d) True. Small backward steps on stopping.
   e) False. This is a feature of sensory ataxia.

31 a) False. Classically they occur at the same time every day for several months, interspersed by pain-free spells of months to years.
   b) False. The pain is always unilateral, and affects the same side each time.
   c) False. This may be true in giant cell arteritis.
   d) True. This is the drug of choice.
   e) False.

32 a) False. This is controlled by cranial nerves IX and X.
   b) False. Muscles of facial expression are innervated by the facial nerve.
   c) True. This is produced by a bilateral upper motor neurone lesion, e.g. a pseudo-bulbar palsy of the trigeminal nerve above the level of the pons.
   d) True. The trigeminal nerve innervates the muscles of mastication.
   e) True. There is impairment of the ophthalmic division (V_i).

33 a) True. Bladder disturbance is a feature.
   b) True. The distribution is described as 'saddle anaesthesia'.
   c) False. This is a sign of spinal cord damage, i.e. upper motor neurone lesion.
   d) True. This is a feature of anal sphincter disturbance.
   e) True. This is a flaccid weakness, i.e. lower motor neurone-type.

34 a) True. Analgesic needs must be finely balanced with the potential to cause confusion.
    b) True. This is not infrequent in post-operative patients.
    c) True.
    d) False. Vitamin C deficiency does not affect cognition.
    e) True. Urinary sepsis is a common cause of delirium in hospitals.

35 a) False. It is acquired.
    b) True. This occurs as a result of paralysis of respiratory muscles.
    c) True. Plasma exchange is also of benefit.
    d) False. It begins distally, and subsequently ascends.
    e) False. It is a post-infective condition.

36 a) True.
    b) True. Lewy body dementia is associated with fluctuating cognitive impairment, visual hallucinations, and parkinsonism.
    c) False. This is a paediatric cause of constipation.
    d) True. Dementia, or general paralysis of the insane, is one presentation of neurosyphilis.
    e) False. This is mononeuropathy of at least two peripheral nerves, for example in diabetes mellitus.

37 a) True. This is fronto-temporal dementia.
    b) True. The AIDS–dementia complex is a diffuse encephalopathy.
    c) False. This is a bleeding disorder involving von Willebrand's factor.
    d) True. This is an autosomal dominant inherited form of dementia.
    e) True. Features include urinary incontinence and gait disturbance.

38 a) False.
    b) True. Sydenham's chorea.
    c) False.
    d) True.
    e) True. Copper deposition in the basal ganglia may give rise to extrapyramidal movement disorders.

39 a) True. Resulting from slowed peristalsis.
    b) True. This describes the stooped, immobile stance.
    c) False. The handwriting becomes smaller – micrographia.
    d) False. Blinking is reduced.
    e) True.

40 a) True.
    b) True.
    c) False. This is a rare form of degenerative encephalopathy, transmissible by prions.
    d) True.
    e) True. As a consequence of cerebral parenchymal involvement.

41 a) True.
    b) True.
    c) False.
    d) True.
    e) True.

42 a) False. Pyridoxine deficiency is rare; it causes a polyneuropathy.
    b) True. This is known as delirium tremens. Visual hallucinations are a feature.
    c) True. A rapid change in environment can precipitate acute confusion in prone, elderly individuals.
    d) False. This is tuberculosis of the spine.
    e) True. This is a problem that is often encountered in post-operative patients.

43 a) False.
    b) True. Seizures or focal neurological deficit are an indication.
    c) False.
    d) True. National Institute for Clinical Excellence (NICE) guidelines recommend CT scanning if the Glasgow Coma Scale (GCS) is less than 13 at any time, or 13–14 at 2 h post-injury.
    e) True. An open, depressed, or basal skull fracture is an indication.

44 a) True.
    b) True.
    c) False.
    d) True.
    e) True.

45 a) False. Approximately 80–85 per cent are ischaemic, the remainder being haemorrhagic.
    b) True. This is to exclude haemorrhagic stroke.
    c) True.
    d) False. >70–80 per cent is a good indication for endarterectomy.
    e) False. Aspirin is started initially.

46 a) False. Eye opening is a component, graded out of 4.
    b) True. It is graded out of 5.
    c) False.
    d) True. It is graded out of 6.
    e) False.

47 a) True
    b) True. Hepatic encephalopathy grade IV is a comatose state.
    c) False.
    d) False.
    e) True.

48 a) True.
    b) True.
    c) True.
    d) True.
    e) True.

49 a) False. This is hepatic vein thrombosis.
    b) True. The palsy is produced by bilateral corticobulbar (upper motor neurone) lesions of the lower cranial nerves.
    c) False. This is a common form of dementia.
    d) True.
    e) True. This is one of the most important causes. There may be features of both upper and lower motor neurone defects.

50 a) False. The motor function of the tongue is controlled by the hypoglossal nerve (XII).
    b) True. There is palatal and pharyngeal paralysis.
    c) True. There is dysphonia due to vocal cord paresis.
    d) True. A vagal nerve lesion will cause the uvula to deviate away from the side of the lesion, on elevation of the soft palate.
    e) False. This muscle is innervated by the accessory nerve (XI).

51 a) True.
    b) True.
    c) True.
    d) True.
    e) True.

52 a) True. This is a cause of spinal cord compression.
    b) True.
    c) False. This affects the anterior horn cells, thereby causing flaccid paralysis.
    d) False. This is a form of polyneuropathy, causing distal weakness (flaccid type).
    e) True. Fluid-filled cavities in the spinal cord cause gradual destruction of the neural pathways, including the corticospinal tracts.

53 a) False. L3, L4.
    b) True.
    c) False. C5.
    d) False. S1, S2.
    e) True.

54 a) False. Hearing is controlled by the cochlear nerve.
    b) True.
    c) True. Balance relies on the vestibular system, cerebellum, vision and proprioception.
    d) True. Vomiting frequently accompanies vertigo.
    e) True. There is an illusion of movement of the patient or surroundings.

55 a) False. The optic nerve does not control eye movements.
    b) True. This is a test for colour vision.
    c) True. For viewing of the optic disc (head of the optic nerve).
    d) True. The afferent pathway of the pupillary light and accommodation reflexes is carried by the optic nerve.
    e) True. For assessment of visual acuity.

56 a) False. Somatic and autonomic neuropathies may be a feature. The cerebellum is not affected.
    b) True. This is an autosomal recessive spinocerebellar degenerative disorder.
    c) True.
    d) False. It is not a recognized side-effect.
    e) True. This is an important cause.

57 a) False. The dorsal columns carry vibration sense.
    b) True.
    c) False. Decussation occurs at a spinal level close to the fibres' entry into the cord.
    d) False. The dorsal columns transmit proprioception sense.
    e) True.

58 a) False. Weakness is not a feature.
    b) True. It is a sign of ataxia.
    c) False. Reflexes may be depressed.
    d) True. This is poor coordination of rapidly alternating movements.
    e) True. Cerebellar dysarthria is variously described as staccato, scanning, or slurred.

59 a) False. This is resistance to passive movement, with sudden give (clasp-knife) – an upper motor neurone lesion sign.
    b) True. There is reduction in the speed of movements.
    c) False. This is a pyramidal upper motor neurone pattern of weakness.
    d) True. There is resistance to passive movements throughout the range of motion (lead-pipe feel).
    e) True. There are rapid, jerky, involuntary movements – e.g. Huntington's, Sydenham's chorea.

60 a) False. This is a lower motor neurone lesion sign.
    b) True. This is a sign of hypertonia.
    c) True. This is an upgoing plantar response.
    d) False. This is a lower motor neurone lesion sign.
    e) False. Hyperreflexia is found.

61 a) True. This is herpes zoster of the geniculate ganglion. A facial palsy and herpetic vesicles in the external acoustic meatus occur.
    b) True. The facial nerve pierces the parotid gland, which is affected by the mumps virus.
    c) False. This is an upper motor neurone disorder.
    d) True. A tumour occurring at the cerebellopontine angle may compress the seventh nerve, among others.
    e) True. This affects the facial nerve during its course through the petrous temporal bone.

62 a) False. The mechanism of speech articulation is unaffected.
    b) True. Speech fatigues over time, becoming quieter.
    c) False. This causes receptive dysphasia.
    d) True. There may be scanning speech.
    e) True. The hypoglossal nerve controls tongue movements, involved in speech articulation.

63 a) True. It usually occurs in men, after emptying the bladder at night.
    b) True. Syncope occurs in those with impaired vasomotor reflexes.
    c) False. This is a hereditary sensorimotor neuropathy causing peroneal muscle atrophy.
    d) True. Impaired posterior cerebral circulation can cause transient brainstem ischaemia.
    e) True. This is syncope due to a cardiac arrhythmia, e.g. paroxysmal bradycardia.

64 a) False. Ocular control is never affected.
    b) True.
    c) False. The sensory pathways are unaffected.
    d) False.
    e) True. This is a feature of amyotrophic lateral sclerosis, one form of presentation of motor neurone disease.

65 a) True. Fear, pain and prolonged standing are all causes of vasovagal syncope.
    b) True. A prolonged bout of coughing can precipitate syncope, e.g. in patients with chronic obstructive pulmonary disease.
    c) True. This is suggestive of carotid sinus sensitivity.
    d) False.
    e) True. The impaired cardiac output gives rise to syncope on exertion.

66 a) False. This is a genetic disorder with deficiency of gonadotrophin-releasing hormone and anosmia.
    b) True. It causes tentorial coning, with compression of the third nerve.
    c) True. The pupil is spared.
    d) True. Compression of the nerve occurs.
    e) False. This is a seventh nerve palsy.

67 a) False. It is associated with polymyalgia rheumatica.
    b) True.
    c) False. High-dose prednisolone must be administered immediately.
    d) True.
    e) False. Superficial temporal artery biopsy is the standard diagnostic test.

68 a) True. The syrinx interrupts the sympathetic pathway during its course through the cervical spinal cord.
    b) True. There is compression of the sympathetic trunk at the thoracic outlet.
    c) False. This is an idiopathic facial nerve palsy.
    d) True. This is known as a Pancoast tumour.
    e) True. Horner's syndrome is a feature of the lateral medullary syndrome.

69 a) False.
    b) True. This is often noticed when combing the hair.
    c) True. There is sudden loss of vision in one eye.
    d) False.
    e) True. This is jaw pain that becomes worse on eating.

70 a) False. Evacuation is possible using a bone flap or burr-hole.
    b) False. The score is 10 (eyes 4, motor 4, speech 2).
    c) True. Intracranial placement is a risk.
    d) False.
    e) False. Because the skull is a fixed compartment, intracranial blood loss cannot be sufficient to account for hypotension. In addition, cerebral ischaemia triggers the Cushing reflex, causing hypertension and bradycardia.

EMQ ANSWERS

1 THE GLASGOW COMA SCALE

1 E   This patient scores **8** (eyes 1, verbal 2, motor 5).

2 B   This patient scores **5** (eyes 1, verbal 1, motor 3).

3 J   This patient scores **13** (eyes 3, verbal 4, motor 6).

4 H   This patient scores **11** (eyes 4, verbal 3, motor 4).

5 D   This patient scores **7** (eyes 1, verbal 1, motor 5).

The scale is as follows:

Eye opening	
Spontaneous	4
To speech	3
To pain	2
None	1
Best verbal response	
Orientated	5
Confused	4
Inappropriate words	3
Incomprehensible sounds	2
None	1
Best motor response	
Obeys commands	6
Localizes to pain	5
Withdraws from pain	4
Abnormal flexion	3
Extension	2
None	1
Total	/15

2 INTRACRANIAL HAEMORRHAGE

1 **E** **Intraventricular haemorrhage** – where fragile vessels in the brain at the lateral wall of the lateral ventricle rupture – is a complication of prematurity. It is a serious condition and indicates a greater probability of later developmental problems.

2 **I** **Pontine haemorrhage** results in coma, quadriplegia and small pupils which are un-reactive to light. The bleeding usually extends into the fourth ventricle; the prognosis is extremely poor.

3 **A** In alcoholics there has to be a high index of suspicion for chronic **subdural haemor-rhage**. These patients often have a coagulopathy and are predisposed to falling down, without necessarily recollecting the event. A CT scan is usually diagnostic.

4 **B** This patient has multiple signs of cerebellar disease: nystagmus, intention tremor, ataxia and vomiting. A **cerebellar haemorrhage** is likely.

5 **C** After a **subarachnoid haemorrhage**, blood degrades in the cerebrospinal fluid leading to bilirubin formation. The presence of xanthochromia, or yellow CSF, can be used to diagnose the condition.

3 HEADACHE

1 **B** This young woman has a typical history for **migraine** with teichopsia, nausea and vomiting associated with a unilateral headache. The lack of fever makes meningitis unlikely.

2 **G** Jaw claudication is a specific sign of **temporal arteritis**: urgent treatment with steroids is indicated.

3 **D** An electric shock-like pain over one of the branches of the trigeminal nerve is a feature of **trigeminal neuralgia**. Attacks can be triggered by light touch, shaving, face washing, or even brushing the teeth. The pain lasts up to 2 min, after which time it spon-taneously stops.

4 **A** Sufferers of **cluster headache** experience unilateral episodic, short attacks with no aura (unlike migraine). There is often associated ipsilateral lacrimation with nasal con-gestion.

5 **F** This patient has signs of raised intracranial pressure: morning headaches resolving through the day, worse on stooping. The only option which is compatible with a long history and raised intracranial pressure is **brain tumour**.

4 NEUROANATOMY

1 **D** The **aqueduct of Sylvius**, the communicating canal between the third and fourth ventricles, is particularly narrow and therefore susceptible to blockage, resulting in hydrocephalus.

2 **A** This patient has an expressive dysphasia: she is able to understand but unable to speak. The lesion is in **Broca's area**, in the dominant (usually the left) frontal lobe.

3 **J** The **substantia nigra** is an area of the midbrain with predominantly dopaminergic neurones. It is involved in the control of voluntary movement. Degeneration of this area leads to the characteristic features of Parkinson's disease.

4 **I** The **olfactory bulb** is located in the limbic system and is involved in the recognition of smell.

5 **H** A physiological function of the **pineal gland** is to secrete melatonin, a hormone which controls the body's diurnal rhythm. This hormone is available as a drug in other countries for jet-lag, but is not licensed in the UK.

5 CRANIAL NERVE LESIONS

1 E   The history here is suggestive of benign intracranial hypertension. The inability to gaze laterally occurs with an abducens (**VI**) nerve palsy, a false localizing sign of raised intracranial pressure.

2 H   There are two components to the gag reflex. The afferent (sensory) part involves the glossopharyngeal (**IX**) nerve, whereas the motor component is mediated via the vagus nerve.

3 F   The facial nerve (**VII**) is responsible for taste in the anterior two-thirds of the tongue; the rest of the tongue is innervated by the glossopharyngeal nerve.

4 I   Before the advent of medication such as H_2-blockers (e.g. ranitidine) and proton pump inhibitors (e.g. omeprazole), highly selective vagotomy (**X**) was a well-recognized treatment to reduce acid secretion.

5 J   The accessory nerve (**XI**) innervates the trapezius and sternocleidomastoid. The trapezius is responsible for elevating the shoulders.

6 DRUGS USED IN NEUROLOGICAL DISEASE

1 E   This patient is in status epilepticus, a medical emergency. First-line treatment, if intravenous access is available, is with **lorazepam**. An alternative is rectal diazepam.

2 A   **Riluzole** is an approved treatment for amyotrophic lateral sclerosis. It can prolong the time that patients have before they are dependent on mechanical ventilation.

3 H   **Methylphenidate** (also known as Ritalin, Novartis) is a stimulant that paradoxically works in attention-deficit hyperactivity disorder. It should only be used as part of an overall strategy to treat the condition.

4 J   The history here is suggestive of absence seizures, with a temporary loss of awareness of the surroundings. **Ethosuximide** can be used to treat simple absence seizures.

5 G   **Prochlorperazine**, a phenothiazine, is a dopamine antagonist and works in the central nervous system to suppress nausea and vomiting.

7 DRUGS USED IN MOVEMENT DISORDERS

1 E   **Tetrabenazine** is thought to deplete nerve endings of dopamine and can improve symptoms in some patients with Huntington's disease.

2 G   Levodopa is always given with a dopamine decarboxylase inhibitor such as **benserazide**, which does not cross the blood–brain barrier. This stops the peripheral metabolism of the levodopa and permits the utilization of smaller doses, which have fewer side-effects.

3 F   The history sounds like benign essential tremor given its long history and lack of progression. **Propranolol** (and alcohol) can give symptomatic relief.

4 A   **Cabergoline** is an oral dopamine receptor agonist and is sometimes used as a first-line therapy for idiopathic Parkinson's disease.

5 H   **Apomorphine** is a powerful dopamine agonist that is only used in advanced Parkinson's disease owing to its need to be administered parenterally, and its potential to cause severe vomiting.

X-RAY ANSWERS

1   There is an area of increased density in the right frontal area, with a convex inner border. This represents an area of new bleeding within the cranial vault. The convex inner border signifies an extradural haematoma, probably originating from a torn middle meningeal artery. Subdural haematomas have concave inner borders.

2   a) The CT scan confirms the clinical suspicion of stroke, with a large low density area on the right side indicating cerebral infarction.
    b) The territory of the infarction corresponds to the area supplied by the right middle cerebral artery.
    c) Neurones from the right cerebral cortex control the motor activity of the left side of the body – a left hemiparesis or hemiplegia would be expected here.

3   There is widespread atrophy of the brain, with enlargement of the sulci and ventricular dilatation. The symptoms that this patient's wife describes may be indicative of dementia; the CT scan would support this diagnosis.

CHAPTER 4

Rheumatology and orthopaedics

MULTIPLE CHOICE QUESTIONS

1 The following bone tumours are malignant:
   a) Osteosarcoma
   b) Osteoid osteoma
   c) Chondroma
   d) Ewing's sarcoma
   e) Osteochondroma

2 Indications for a hip replacement include:
   a) Rheumatoid arthritis
   b) Meralgia paraesthetica
   c) Osteoarthritis
   d) Avascular necrosis of the femoral head
   e) Neck of femur fracture

3 Local steroid injection is helpful for the following conditions:
   a) Tennis elbow
   b) Septic arthritis
   c) Frozen shoulder
   d) Acromioclavicular joint osteoarthritis
   e) Knee osteoarthritis

4 The following statements are true of posterior hip dislocation:
   a) It is less common than anterior dislocation
   b) Usually the leg lies in external rotation
   c) Reduction often occurs spontaneously
   d) Avascular necrosis of the femoral head is a complication
   e) The sciatic nerve may be damaged

5   Features of systemic lupus erythematosus include:
  a) Pleural effusion
  b) Appendicitis
  c) Fever
  d) Pityriasis rosea
  e) Glomerulonephritis

6   Early fracture complications include:
  a) Avascular necrosis
  b) Non-union
  c) Compartment syndrome
  d) Chronic osteomyelitis
  e) Haemarthrosis

7   Complications of a supracondylar fracture of the elbow include:
  a) Cubitus varus
  b) Axillary nerve lesion
  c) Brachial artery damage
  d) Axillary artery damage
  e) Median nerve lesion

8   Examples of traction apophysitis include:
  a) Sever's disease
  b) Achondroplasia
  c) Still's disease
  d) Osgood–Schlatter's disease
  e) Golfer's elbow

9   The following are tests used to examine the knee:
  a) McMurray's test
  b) Trendelenburg test
  c) Thomas' test
  d) Lachman test
  e) Schober test

10   Pathological fractures can be caused by:
  a) Paget's disease
  b) Osteoarthritis
  c) Acromegaly
  d) Bone metastasis
  e) Osteoporosis

11   Late fracture complications include:
  a) Myositis ossificans
  b) Compartment syndrome
  c) Malunion
  d) Avascular necrosis
  e) Osteoarthritis

12   Regarding shoulder dislocation:
   a)   Posterior dislocation is more common than anterior dislocation
   b)   The dislocated shoulder should be reduced after a period of 3 days
   c)   Patients with recurrent dislocation are able to reduce the shoulder themselves
   d)   Axillary nerve damage is a complication of anterior dislocation
   e)   Surgery is useful for recurrent traumatic dislocation

13   The following statements are true of systemic lupus erythematosus:
   a)   Blood count may reveal a lymphopenia
   b)   The oral contraceptive pill is useful in controlling symptoms
   c)   Complement levels are typically raised during flare-ups
   d)   It is more common in females
   e)   Corticosteroids have a useful role

14   Causes of hip pain include:
   a)   Trochanteric bursitis
   b)   Adhesive capsulitis
   c)   de Quervain's tenosynovitis
   d)   Polymyalgia rheumatica
   e)   Meralgia paraesthetica

15   The following statements are true of rheumatoid arthritis:
   a)   The joint most commonly affected is the hip
   b)   Rheumatoid factor is present in at least 95 per cent of cases
   c)   It is more common in females
   d)   Human leucocyte antigen (HLA)-B27 correlates with a poor prognosis
   e)   It is more common in occupations involving repetitive joint stress

16   Extra-articular manifestations of rheumatoid arthritis include:
   a)   Splenomegaly
   b)   Retinopathy
   c)   Urethral stricture
   d)   Lung fibrosis
   e)   Peripheral neuropathy

17   Extra-articular features of rheumatoid arthritis include:
   a)   Renal amyloidosis
   b)   Pancreatitis
   c)   Episcleritis
   d)   Psoriasis
   e)   Pericarditis

18   The following statements are true of gout:
   a)   It affects men and women equally
   b)   An acute attack should be treated with allopurinol
   c)   The diagnosis can be excluded by a normal serum urate level
   d)   Microscopy reveals positively birefringent crystals
   e)   Bendroflumethiazide can precipitate an attack

19 The following investigations are useful in polymyositis:
   a) Muscle biopsy
   b) Serum alkaline phosphatase
   c) Electromyography
   d) Visual evoked potentials
   e) Serum creatine kinase

20 Risk factors for osteoporosis include:
   a) Cushing's syndrome
   b) The oral contraceptive pill
   c) Hyperthyroidism
   d) Smoking
   e) High alcohol intake

21 The following tests are useful in the investigation of Paget's disease of the bone:
   a) Serum lactate dehydrogenase (LDH)
   b) Serum electrophoresis
   c) Calcitonin level
   d) Serum alkaline phosphatase
   e) Urine hydroxyproline

22 Causes of osteomalacia include:
   a) Chronic renal failure
   b) Salmonella infection
   c) Malabsorption
   d) Haemolytic anaemia
   e) Being bedbound

23 Clinical features of a median nerve injury include:
   a) Absence of wrist extension
   b) Hypothenar muscle wasting
   c) Loss of thumb abduction
   d) Sensory loss over the palmar surface of the little finger
   e) Thenar muscle wasting

24 Causes of carpal tunnel syndrome include:
   a) Acromegaly
   b) Meralgia paraesthetica
   c) Motor neurone disease
   d) Hypothyroidism
   e) Pregnancy

25 Causes of scoliosis include:
   a) Cerebellar ataxia
   b) Acromegaly
   c) Poliomyelitis
   d) Spondylolisthesis
   e) Syringomyelia

26 The following statements are true of ankylosing spondylitis:
   a) It only occurs in men
   b) Buttock pain is relieved by rest
   c) There is an association with HLA-B27
   d) Iritis is a complication
   e) The disease often regresses in old age

27 Manifestations of rheumatoid arthritis in the hands and wrists include:
   a) Tophi
   b) Swan-neck deformity
   c) Heberden's nodes
   d) Ulnar deviation of the fingers
   e) Bouchard's nodes

28 Causes of bone avascular necrosis include:
   a) Steroids
   b) Gaucher's disease
   c) Trauma
   d) Sickle cell disease
   e) Hypertension

29 The following factors delay union of a fractured bone:
   a) Malignancy
   b) Distraction of the fragments
   c) Young patient age
   d) Local infection
   e) Poor blood supply

30 Features of systemic lupus erythematosus include:
   a) Pericarditis
   b) Psychosis
   c) Gallstones
   d) Mouth ulceration
   e) Raynaud's phenomenon

31 The following are fractures of the wrist:
   a) Monteggia fracture
   b) Barton's fracture
   c) Smith's fracture
   d) Colles' fracture
   e) Pott's fracture

32 Complications of hip replacement surgery include:
   a) Immunosuppression
   b) Loosening of the prosthesis
   c) Malignant bone tumour
   d) Prosthetic infection
   e) Peri-prosthetic fracture

33 Complications of pelvic fracture include:
   a) Deep vein thrombosis (DVT)
   b) Lumbosacral plexus nerve damage
   c) Bladder rupture
   d) Vaginal perforation
   e) Urethral rupture

34 Causes of lumbar back pain include:
   a) Myeloma
   b) Ankylosing spondylitis
   c) Osgood–Schlatter's disease
   d) Osteoporosis
   e) Spondylolisthesis

35 Causes of knee pain include:
   a) Torsion of the hydatid cyst of Morgagni
   b) Pseudogout
   c) Osteochondritis dissecans
   d) Baker's cyst
   e) Pott's disease

36 Radiological features of osteoarthritis include:
   a) Increased joint space
   b) Bone cysts
   c) Looser's zones
   d) Subchondral sclerosis
   e) Pepperpot skull

37 The following are risk factors for osteoarthritis:
   a) Smoking
   b) Sport
   c) Obesity
   d) Osteoporosis
   e) Joint trauma

38 Complications of acute haematogenous osteomyelitis include:
   a) Osteoid osteoma
   b) Growth interruption
   c) Paget's disease
   d) Septic arthritis
   e) Chronic osteomyelitis

39 Regarding congenital dislocation of the hip:
   a) It is more common in males than females
   b) It may be bilateral
   c) Most hips that are dislocatable at birth will become stable within 3 weeks
   d) It is assessed by Thomas' test
   e) It may be diagnosed by ultrasound scan

40 Examples of brachial plexus injuries include:
   a) Pseudobulbar palsy
   b) Klumpke's palsy
   c) Bell's palsy
   d) Erb's palsy
   e) Supranuclear palsy

41 Signs of a basal skull fracture include:
   a) Cheyne–Stokes respiration
   b) Periorbital haematoma
   c) Absent doll's head reflex
   d) Cerebrospinal fluid rhinorrhoea
   e) Mastoid bruising

42 Regarding scaphoid fractures:
   a) Ulnar nerve injury is a complication
   b) Plain X-ray often shows the fracture more clearly after a few weeks than initially
   c) Wrist osteoarthritis is a complication
   d) Plaster cast is unnecessary
   e) Avascular necrosis is a complication

43 The following statements are true of osteomalacia:
   a) It predisposes to malignant bone tumours
   b) Radiographs of affected areas may reveal Looser's zones
   c) Treatment should include increasing sunlight exposure
   d) Alkaline phosphatase levels are reduced
   e) Proximal myopathy is a feature

44 Causes of pes cavus include:
   a) Lower limb venous insufficiency
   b) Charcot–Marie–Tooth disease
   c) Congenital defect
   d) Hallux valgus
   e) Poliomyelitis

45 Complications of Paget's bone disease include:
   a) Deafness
   b) Osteosarcoma
   c) Dementia
   d) Iritis
   e) Heart failure

46 Causes of a Charcot joint include:
   a) Osteoarthritis
   b) Syphilis
   c) Hyperthyroidism
   d) Diabetes mellitus
   e) Leprosy

47 Causes of spinal kyphosis include:
   a) Tuberculosis
   b) Osteoporosis
   c) Guillain–Barré syndrome
   d) Fixed flexion deformity of the hip
   e) Ankylosing spondylitis

48 The following are forms of seronegative spondyloarthritis:
   a) Rheumatoid arthritis
   b) Psoriatic arthritis
   c) Gout
   d) Reiter's syndrome
   e) Ankylosing spondylitis

49 The following conditions are associated with Dupuytren's contracture:
   a) Rheumatoid arthritis
   b) Chronic liver disease
   c) Chronic obstructive pulmonary disease
   d) Diabetes mellitus
   e) Cushing's disease

Answers: see pages 106–112

EXTENDED MATCHING QUESTIONS

1 ANTIBODIES IN RHEUMATOLOGICAL DISEASE

Choose the antibody test most likely to be both positive and diagnostic in each of the patients below

A   Anti-Jo 1
B   Anti-nuclear antibody (ANA)
C   Rheumatoid factor
D   Anti-histone
E   Anti-topoisomerase 1

F   pANCA (anti-neutrophil cytoplasmic antibody, myeloperoxidase [MPO])
G   cANCA (proteinase-3 [PR 3])
H   Anti-cardiolipin
I   Anti-dsDNA
J   Anticentromere

1   A 34-year-old woman goes to her general practitioner (GP) complaining of arthralgia and fatigue. He is about to dismiss her as having non-specific pains when he notices an unusual rash on her cheeks and bridge of her nose.

2   A 30-year-old woman is referred to hospital for investigation of her recurrent miscarriages: she has had three spontaneous abortions in the past 5 years. Her past medical history includes migraine and a deep venous thrombosis 2 years ago.

3   A 27-year-old woman attends her GP surgery. She is on long-term disability allowance as she says she cannot work due to general weakness, fatigue, and now shortness of breath. When the GP examines her, he finds she has proximal muscle weakness and wasting. He also notes that she takes a minute to rise from her chair in his office.

4   A 56-year-old woman presents to the emergency department in acute renal failure, having had no history of kidney trouble in the past. Despite being a lifelong non-smoker she has also noticed that she has begun to cough up blood. A chest X-ray shows multiple cavitating lesions.

5   A 41-year-old man attends rheumatology outpatients as he has been having difficulty with his hands. He has suffered from severe Raynaud's phenomenon for many years, and has recently noticed that the skin over his fingers feels tight. The consultant notes the presence of telangiectasia on the hands, and orders some blood tests.

2 MONOARTHRITIS

Each of the patients below presents with a swollen, tender joint. Choose the most likely diagnosis from the options given

A   Psoriatic arthritis
B   Pseudogout
C   Enteropathic arthritis
D   Gonococcal arthritis
E   Tuberculous arthritis

F   Reactive arthritis
G   Gout
H   Behçet's syndrome
I   Rheumatoid arthritis
J   Ankylosing spondylitis

1   A 73-year-old woman presents to the emergency department with a painful knee. There is a large effusion, so the doctor on-call removes 30 mL of fluid for analysis. Microscopy reveals weakly positively birefringent crystals.

2   A 31-year-old is travelling in Asia with two friends. He unfortunately contracts dysentery which resolves spontaneously after a few days. Two weeks later, he calls a doctor complaining of ulceration of his penis and a swollen right ankle. He vehemently denies any recent sexual contacts, and his friends readily confirm this.

3   A 23-year-old hairdresser presents to the emergency department with a fever and a painful, swollen left knee. An aspiration reveals plentiful white cells and Gram-negative diplococci.

4   A 57-year-old man presents to the emergency department with a painful ankle. There is an effusion evident, so the junior on-call doctor removes a small volume of fluid for analysis. Microscopy reveals strongly negatively birefringent crystals.

5   A 46-year-old woman goes to the emergency department with a swollen wrist. The doctor takes a careful history and finds that she also suffers from recurrent mouth ulcers, which come and go. She was seen in gastroenterology clinic last week for this, and had some routine blood tests. When the doctor goes to bleed her again, he notices a pustule over the site of the previous venepuncture.

3 VASCULITIS

Each of the patients below has vasculitis. Choose the most likely diagnosis for each of the clinical scenarios below

A   Wegener's granulomatosis
B   Polyarteritis nodosa
C   Churg–Strauss syndrome
D   Microscopic polyangiitis
E   Henoch–Schönlein purpura

F   Takayasu's arteritis
G   Goodpasture's syndrome
H   Kawasaki disease
I   Giant cell arteritis
J   Polymyalgia rheumatica

1 A 34-year-old man presents to his GP with rhinitis. He sees the doctor regularly for asthma. On further questioning, he reports that he has noticed an unusual rash over his trunk, which the GP suspects is vasculitic. Blood tests reveal an elevated eosinophil count and positive MPO antineutrophil cytoplasmic antibody (ANCA).

2 A 21-year-old woman goes to the emergency department with some chest pain. The registrar is troubled that he cannot feel either radial pulse, even though the triage sheet shows the patient to be hypertensive.

3 A woman takes her 3-year-old child to the emergency department as she has noticed peeling skin on the soles of his feet. The child has had a fever for a week now, with no specific cause. The doctor finds cervical lymphadenopathy and a red tongue, and immediately arranges for the child to be admitted.

4 A 23-year-old man presents to the emergency department with haemoptysis and acute renal failure. He is a smoker, but has never coughed up any blood before. A chest X-ray shows blotchy shadowing in both lungfields; two days later his initial blood tests reveal a positive anti-glomerular basement membrane (GBM) antibody.

5 A 76-year-old man goes to see his GP as he says it hurts him when he eats and combs his hair. The GP finds a prominent left temporal artery and immediately refers him to hospital.

4 COMPLICATIONS OF RHEUMATOID ARTHRITIS

Each of the patients below presents with a complication of their rheumatoid arthritis. Select the most likely diagnosis from the options given

A   Amyloidosis
B   Pericarditis
C   Atlanto axial subluxation
D   Sjögren's syndrome
E   Scleromalacia

F   Felty's syndrome
G   Septic arthritis
H   Carpal tunnel syndrome
I   Pulmonary fibrosis
J   Mononeuritis multiplex

1   A 63-year-old woman presents to her GP with loss of sensation over the upper outer part of her left arm. When asked to abduct the arm, the doctor grades her power as 4/5.

2   A 45-year-old man goes to see his doctor complaining of a gritty feeling in his eyes. He is carrying a bottle of mineral water with him, which he keeps sipping during the consultation, saying his mouth is very dry.

3   A 61-year-old woman, who has had her rheumatoid arthritis for 30 years, goes to see her doctor because she is feeling tired, and she has swollen legs. Blood tests reveal a normocytic anaemia, low albumin and high cholesterol. Urinalysis shows protein +++.

4   A 73-year-old woman presents with easy bruising. The GP examines her and can feel a large spleen, extending halfway to the umbilicus. He performs some blood tests, which show a normocytic anaemia, and quite marked neutropenia.

5   A 58-year-old man complains of tingling in his thumb, index and middle fingers, which he notices especially when he drives his car. On examination, his grip is weakened and he has wasting of the thenar eminence.

5 PHARMACOLOGICAL TREATMENT OF RHEUMATOLOGICAL DISEASE

Choose the most appropriate medication for each of the scenarios below

A   Calcium supplementation
B   Hydroxychloroquine
C   Etanercept
D   Cyclophosphamide
E   Prednisolone

F   Celecoxib
G   Alendronate
H   Allopurinol
I   Hypromellose
J   Methotrexate

1   A patient with Sjögren's syndrome, who complains of persistently dry eyes.

2   A patient with severe rheumatoid arthritis, who has tried every oral medication her rheumatologist can prescribe. He wants to try a new therapy which he says works against tumour necrosis factor (TNF) α.

3   A patient who has had three severe attacks of gout in the past year.

4   A patient newly diagnosed with systemic lupus erythematosus (SLE), with mild skin disease.

5   A patient with multiple crush fractures of her vertebral column.

6 COMPLICATIONS OF DRUGS USED TO TREAT RHEUMATOLOGICAL DISEASE

Each of the patients below presents with complications of medications prescribed by their doctor to treat their rheumatological disease. Select the medication most likely to cause each of the side-effects in the clinical scenarios below

A	Calcium supplementation	F	Celecoxib
B	Hydroxychloroquine	G	Alendronate
C	Etanercept	H	Allopurinol
D	Cyclophosphamide	I	Hypromellose
E	Prednisolone	J	Methotrexate

1 A 27-year-old returns to clinic a few days after her treatment complaining of macroscopic haematuria. The registrar says that this is a rare complication of the medication.

2 A 35-year-old develops active pulmonary tuberculosis while being treated for her arthritis. Her consultant tells her that the medication may well have been responsible for this.

3 A 76-year-old woman with temporal arteritis is seen in clinic after 9 months of treatment. She complains of easy bruising and weight gain. In his letter to the GP, the rheumatologist notes the presence of an interscapular fat pad.

4 A 56-year-old man is seen in rheumatology clinic as a follow-up. He complains of symptoms of oesophageal reflux and is referred for an oesophagogastroduodenoscopy (OGD). This shows severe oesophagitis with some oesophageal ulceration.

5 A 48-year-old woman is sent back to rheumatology clinic by her GP after some abnormal blood tests. She has a megaloblastic anaemia, with leucopenia and thrombocytopenia.

7 DRUGS USED TO TREAT RHEUMATOID ARTHRITIS

Each of the drugs below is used in the treatment of rheumatoid arthritis. Choose the best match for each of the statements below

A	Methotrexate	F	Leflunomide
B	Prednisolone	G	Sulfasalazine
C	Hydroxychloroquine	H	Etanercept
D	Sodium aurothiomalate	I	Penicillamine
E	Azathioprine	J	Ibuprofen

1 Commonly referred to as 'gold' injections.

2 A 5-aminosalicylic acid derivative, also used to treat inflammatory bowel disease.

3 Also used as an antimalarial.

4 Used in the treatment of Wilson's disease.

5 Inhibits the production of folate by inhibition of the enzyme dihydrofolate reductase.

8 RAYNAUD'S PHENOMENON

Each of the patients below presents to their GP with symptoms characteristic of Raynaud's phenomenon. Select the most likely cause from the options given

A   Scleroderma
B   Sjögren's syndrome
C   Dermatomyositis
D   Idiopathic
E   Occupational

F   SLE
G   Cryoglobulinaemia
H   Iatrogenic
I   Myeloma
J   Rheumatoid arthritis

1   A 22-year-old intravenous drug user with hepatitis B presents with a purpuric rash, arthralgia and glomerulonephritis. He is wearing thick gloves, which he says stops him suffering from such bad pain in his hands.

2   A 39-year-old housewife makes an appointment with her GP, complaining of sore eyes, and an inability to swallow food without drinking water at the same time. He notes from his computer that she has been seen three times in the last year complaining of Raynaud's phenomenon.

3   A 31-year-old lawyer seeks medical attention, complaining of painful fingertips when she goes outside in the cold. She says her fingers first go white and then turn red.

4   A 26-year-old construction worker presents to his GP with painful hands, which are worse in the cold.

5   A 67-year-old retired engineer goes to see his doctor complaining of weakness and hand pain. Over the past few months, he has found it increasingly difficult to climb the stairs. On examination, he has roughened papules over the dorsal surfaces of his fingers.

9 EPONYMS

Each of the eponyms below is used to describe a fracture, syndrome or sign in orthopaedics. Choose the correct eponym to match the descriptions given

A   Colles
B   Barlow
C   Trendelenburg
D   Lachman
E   Ortolani

F   Osgood–Schlatter
G   Battle
H   Smith
I   Baker
J   Garden

1   Bruising over the mastoid process 24–48 h after a basal skull fracture.

2   Fracture of the distal radius with volar displacement of the distal fragment.

3   Classification scheme for intracapsular fractures of the neck of femur.

4   A swelling in the popliteal fossa, associated with osteoarthritis of the knee.

5   An attempt to forcibly dislocate the hip of a child.

10 COMPLICATIONS OF FRACTURES

Each of the patients below has suffered a complication of a fracture. For each of the cases below, choose the best answer from the options given

A   Delayed union
B   Compartment syndrome
C   Wound infection
D   Non-union
E   Osteomyelitis

F   Fat embolism
G   Deep vein thrombosis
H   Osteoarthritis
I   Reflex sympathetic dystrophy
J   Malunion

1   A 34-year-old banker breaks his tibia and fibula after coming off his motorbike at 40 mph. He is placed in a cast overnight while awaiting surgery. The doctor is called to see him in the early hours of the morning as his pain is becoming intolerable. When she gently dorsiflexes his foot, the patient's screams wake the other patients in the bay.

2   A 79-year-old woman fractures her neck of femur and is brought to hospital with a shortened, externally rotated leg. She undergoes surgery the next day, but during the operation suddenly has a cardiac arrest and dies.

3   A 39-year-old woman fractures her tibia after falling from her horse. Open reduction and internal fixation are performed and she goes home 3 days later in a cast. When the cast is removed 6 weeks later, the leg is red and hot.

4   A 52-year-old man presents to hospital with a Colles' fracture of his left wrist. He is treated successfully in a cast, but returns 6 months later complaining of an intense burning pain over the wrist when he is lightly touched.

5   A 43-year-old man falls over and breaks his ulna. An operation is performed to attach a metal plate to the bone, and the surgeon notes that there has been good reduction. One month later, the patient returns with pain and swelling of the arm. A plain X-ray is reported as showing a sequestrum.

Answers: see pages 112–116

X-RAY QUESTIONS

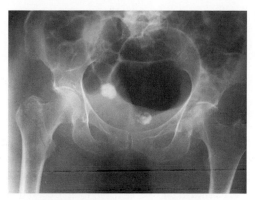

1

1 A 79-year-old woman is brought to hospital after having tripped on a paving stone and fallen over. She has been unable to walk since the accident.
a) What injury has this woman sustained?
b) What is the best treatment for this condition?

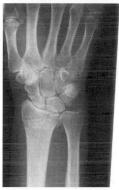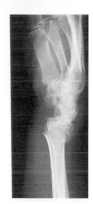

2

2 A 68-year-old man is walking his dog and slips on an icy path. He walks to the emergency department complaining of a swollen and painful wrist. What injury has been sustained?

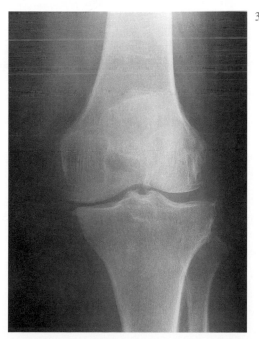

3

3 A 72-year-old man seeks medical attention for a painful knee. He says that he has had difficulty walking for the past 6 months. His doctor requests an X-ray.
a) What is the likely cause of this patient's knee pain?
b) What treatment options are available?

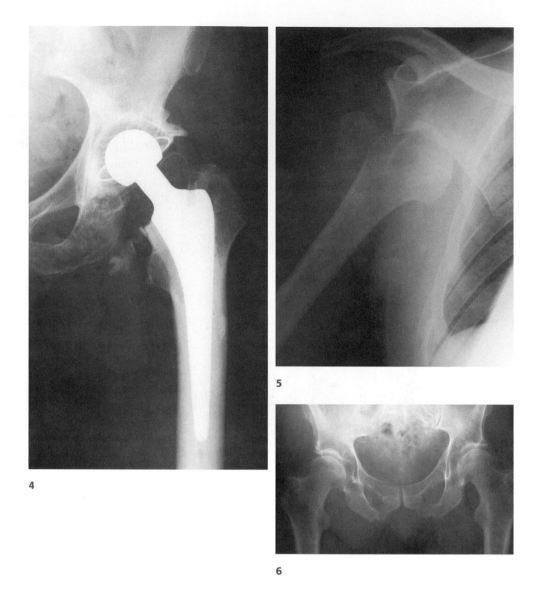

4

5

6

To answer the questions below, please refer to the corresponding numbered X-ray images above.

4   A 64-year-old woman complains of pain in her left hip. Her doctor requests an X-ray.
   a) What procedure has been performed?
   b) What is the most common indication for this operation?

5   A 27-year-old rugby player comes to hospital with a painful shoulder. An X-ray is taken.
   a) What injury has this man sustained?
   b) How should he be treated? Which nerve may be damaged?

6   A 92-year-old demented woman is brought to hospital by her concerned relatives, as she is unable to weight bear after a fall. She indicates vaguely where her pain is; the emergency department doctor requests an X-ray.
   a) Why can this patient not walk?
   b) How are these injuries usually treated?

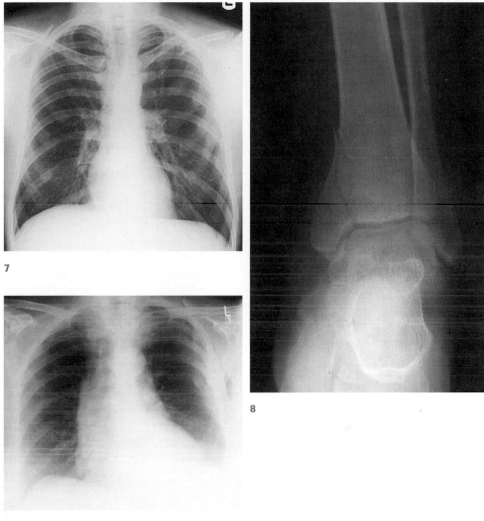

To answer the questions below, please refer to the corresponding numbered X-ray images above.

7   A 37-year-old man is brought to the emergency department by ambulance after having been involved in a road traffic accident. A trauma X-ray series is taken, including a chest X-ray.
   a) What injury has this patient sustained?
   b) How is this usually treated?

8   A 22-year-old man sustains an eversion injury to his ankle while playing basketball. On examination, the ankle is swollen and tender. What injury has this man sustained?

9   A 51-year-old man goes to see his doctor complaining of chest pain, which is worse on inspiration. He admits having being involved in an altercation. Why is this patient experiencing chest pain?

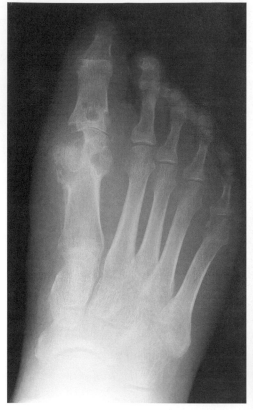

10

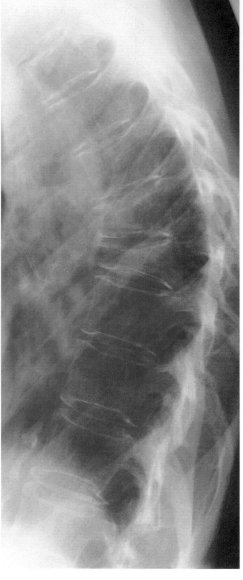

11

To answer the questions below, please refer to the corresponding numbered X-ray images above.

10 A 57-year-old man goes to see his GP complaining of pain in his right foot. The GP requests an X-ray.
   a) What is the likely diagnosis?
   b) What medical treatments can be offered to this patient?

11 An 89-year-old woman complains of back pain to her GP. He organizes an X-ray of her spine. Why is this patient suffering from back pain?

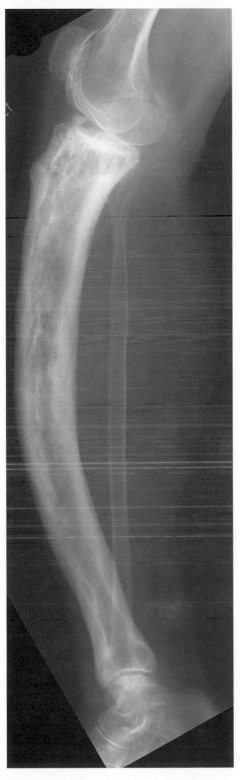

12 An 81-year-old man complains of difficulty and pain on walking. An X-ray is taken of his tibia. What is the most likely cause of these appearances?

12

Answers: see pages 116–117

ANSWERS

MCQ ANSWERS

1. a) True. A tumour of adolescents, it affects the metaphysis of long bones, often at the knee.
   b) False. This is a painful round tumour affecting young males.
   c) False. This affects the tubular bones of the hands and feet.
   d) True. This presents in adolescents and affects the diaphysis of long bones.
   e) False. This is the commonest benign bone tumour.

2. a) True.
   b) False. This is compression of the lateral cutaneous nerve of the thigh.
   c) True.
   d) True.
   e) True.

3. a) True. This is lateral epicondylitis of the elbow.
   b) False. Steroids impair the immune response and predispose to avascular necrosis.
   c) True. This is adhesive capsulitis.
   d) True.
   e) True.

4. a) False. Anterior dislocation is uncommon.
   b) False. It is typically internally rotated.
   c) False. Reduction under general anaesthetic is necessary.
   d) True.
   e) True.

5. a) True.
   b) False.
   c) True.
   d) False. This is a rash occurring on the trunk in young adults and adolescents.
   e) True.

6. a) False. This is a late complication.
   b) False. This is a late complication.
   c) True.
   d) False. This is a long-term complication.
   e) True. A fracture involving a joint can lead to bleeding into the joint – haemarthrosis.

7. a) True. Malunion can result in a permanent cubitus varus deformity.
   b) False.
   c) True.
   d) False.
   e) True. Loss of function is usually temporary.

8   a) True. This affects the calcaneus.
    b) False. This is a genetic disorder involving reduced cartilaginous bone growth, causing short stature.
    c) False. This is juvenile chronic arthritis.
    d) True. This is traction apophysitis of the tibial tuberosity.
    e) False. This is medial epicondylitis of the elbow.

9   a) True. This is a test for meniscal tears of the knee.
    b) False. This tests the stability of the hip.
    c) False. This assesses the presence of a fixed flexion deformity of the hip.
    d) True. This tests the stability of the cruciate ligaments.
    e) False. This assesses lumbar spine flexion.

10 a) True.
    b) False.
    c) False.
    d) True.
    e) True. Reduced bone density predisposes to fractures.

11 a) True. An area of damaged muscle can ossify, producing a bony lump.
    b) False. This is an early complication.
    c) True. This occurs when the fragments rejoin in an undesirable position.
    d) True. This occurs most commonly at the head of the femur, the talus, and the proximal scaphoid bone.
    e) True. A fracture involving an articular surface is vulnerable to osteoarthritis.

12 a) False. Posterior dislocation is rare; it may occur after an epileptic seizure or electric shock.
    b) False. It should be replaced immediately.
    c) True. Over time, reduction is possible with increasing ease.
    d) True.
    e) True. The shoulder capsule is repaired.

13 a) True. There may be a haemolytic anaemia, leucopenia, lymphopenia, thrombocytopenia.
    b) False. It is a trigger for flare-ups.
    c) False. They are reduced.
    d) True.
    e) True.

14 a) True. There is inflammation in the bursa lateral to the greater trochanter.
    b) False. This is also known as a frozen shoulder.
    c) False. This is inflammation of the sheath containing the extensor pollicis brevis and abductor pollicis longus tendons – occurring near the wrist.
    d) True. This causes pain and stiffness in the limb girdles.
    e) True. This is caused by entrapment of the lateral cutaneous nerve beneath the inguinal ligament.

15 a) False. The hips are usually spared early on.
    b) False. The figure is approximately 70 per cent.
    c) True.
    d) False. HLA-DR4 is associated with a poor prognosis.
    e) False. The condition has an autoimmune pathogenesis.

16 a) True. When combined with lymphadenopathy and neutropenia, this is known as Felty's syndrome.
    b) False.
    c) False.
    d) True.
    e) True.

17 a) True. This causes nephrotic syndrome and renal failure.
    b) False.
    c) True. Scleritis may also occur.
    d) False.
    e) True. Pericarditis, myocarditis and endocarditis are all cardiac manifestations of rheumatoid arthritis.

18 a) False. It is commoner in males.
    b) False. Non-steroidal anti-inflammatory drugs (NSAIDs) or colchicine are used. Allopurinol must not be started within 3–4 weeks of an acute attack.
    c) False. Up to 10 per cent of individuals presenting with an acute attack have a normal urate level.
    d) False. Sodium urate crystals are negatively birefringent and needle-shaped.
    e) True. Thiazide diuretics impair excretion of uric acid.

19 a) True. It reveals inflammatory infiltrate and muscle necrosis.
    b) False.
    c) True.
    d) False.
    e) True. It is usually raised, reflecting muscle damage.

20 a) True. Increased levels of corticosteroids, whether endogenous or exogenous, pre-dispose to osteoporosis.
    b) False.
    c) True.
    d) True.
    e) True.

21 a) False.
    b) False. This is useful in myeloma.
    c) False.
    d) True. This is raised in Paget's disease, reflecting increased bone turnover.
    e) True. This is an indicator of osteoclastic activity.

22 a) True. There is reduced hydroxylation of vitamin D.
   b) False.
   c) True. This leads to vitamin D deficiency.
   d) False.
   e) True. There is inadequate exposure to sunlight, causing insufficient skin synthesis of vitamin D.

23 a) False. Wrist extension is controlled by the radial nerve.
   b) False. This is a feature of an ulnar nerve lesion.
   c) True. The abductor pollicis brevis is affected.
   d) False. There is loss of sensation over the palmar surface of the lateral three and a half fingers.
   e) True.

24 a) True. Enlargement of the soft tissues surrounding the carpal tunnel compresses the median nerve.
   b) False. This is a mononeuropathy of the lateral cutaneous nerve of the thigh as it passes below the inguinal ligament.
   c) False.
   d) True
   e) True. Soft tissue swelling in pregnancy causes median nerve compression.

25 a) False.
   b) False.
   c) True. This is due to unequal pull on the spine because of muscular paralysis.
   d) True.
   e) True.

26 a) False. The disease presents earlier in men.
   b) False. The lower back and buttock pain and stiffness are worse in the morning, and relieved by exercise.
   c) True. This is a feature of all the seronegative spondyloarthritides.
   d) True.
   e) False. It is a progressive disease.

27 a) False. These are urate deposits found in gout.
   b) True. This is hyperextension of the proximal interphalangeal joint and flexion of the distal interphalangeal joint.
   c) False. This is nodal osteoarthritis of the distal interphalangeal joint.
   d) True. This occurs as a result of subluxation of the metacarpo-phalangeal joints.
   e) False. This is nodal osteoarthritis of the proximal interphalangeal joint.

28 a) True.
   b) True. This is a familial disorder affecting the Ashkenazi Jews; the femoral head is prone to avascular necrosis.
   c) True. For example, an intracapsular fracture of the neck of femur, or fractures of the scaphoid or talus bone.
   d) True. Microthrombi cause infarction of the bone.
   e) False.

29 a) True. Generalized malignancy impairs the patient's ability to heal. Malignant bone has less healing potential than healthy bone.
   b) True.
   c) False. Children's bones heal faster than adults'.
   d) True.
   e) True.

30 a) True.
   b) True.
   c) False.
   d) True.
   e) True.

31 a) False. This is fracture of the proximal half of the ulna with dislocation of the radial head.
   b) True. This is a distal radius fracture with the fracture line extending into the joint and anterior displacement of the fragment.
   c) True. This is a distal radius fracture with volar angulation.
   d) True. This is a distal radius fracture with dorsal displacement and angulation.
   e) False. This is a fracture of the ankle.

32 a) False.
   b) True.
   c) False.
   d) True.
   e) True.

33 a) True. Pelvic fractures confer a high risk of DVT.
   b) True.
   c) True. The rupture may be intraperitoneal or extraperitoneal.
   d) True. This is uncommon.
   e) True. This may be suggested by bleeding at the urethral meatus.

34 a) True. This is a malignancy of plasma cells in the bone marrow.
   b) True. This is a seronegative spondylitis affecting the sacroiliac joints and the spine.
   c) False. This is traction apophysitis of the patellar tendon.
   d) True. A vertebral crush fracture can cause immense pain.
   e) True. There is displacement of a vertebral body over the underlying vertebra, usually L5/S1 or L4/L5.

35 a) False. This is torsion of the embryological remnant of the Müllerian duct attached to the superior pole of the testis.
   b) True. This is a calcium pyrophosphate crystal arthritis, commonly affecting the knee in the elderly, causing a painful effusion and synovitis.
   c) True. A fragment of cartilage and bone separates from the knee joint, causing pain and locking. It usually affects young males.
   d) True. This is a popliteal cyst that occurs secondary to a knee effusion.
   e) False. This is spinal tuberculosis.

36 a) False. The joint space is reduced.
    b) True.
    c) False. These are pseudofractures occurring in osteomalacia.
    d) True. This is a reaction to increased stress exerted on the articular bone.
    e) False. This occurs in multiple myeloma.

37 a) False.
    b) True. Repetitive stress on joints predisposes to osteoarthritis.
    c) True. Increased weight-bearing by joints increases articular stress.
    d) False.
    e) True. A fracture through a joint increases the risk of osteoarthritis.

38 a) False. This is a benign bone tumour.
    b) True. If the growth plate is involved.
    c) False.
    d) True. Infection may track into the adjacent joint.
    e) True. Inadequate treatment may lead to persistent infection.

39 a) False.
    b) True.
    c) True.
    d) False. This is a test for fixed flexion deformity of the hip. The Barlow and Ortolani tests are useful for congenital dislocation.
    e) True.

40 a) False. This is an upper motor neurone lesion of the bulbar muscles, affecting swallowing and talking.
    b) True. Acquired as a birth injury, it affects the inferior trunk of the brachial plexus.
    c) False. This is a lower motor neurone facial nerve palsy.
    d) True. This is a birth injury affecting the superior trunk of the brachial plexus.
    e) False. This consists of dementia and absent vertical gaze.

41 a) False. This is deep breathing combined with apnoea, seen in coma.
    b) True. This occurs in anterior and middle fossae fractures.
    c) False. Loss of this reflex occurs in brainstem death.
    d) True. This is found in anterior fossa fractures.
    e) True. Found in posterior fossa fractures.

42 a) False.
    b) True.
    c) True. This may occur after avascular necrosis or non-union.
    d) False. The fracture needs to be immobilized in a long-arm cast extending to the proximal thumb phalanx.
    e) True. The proximal fragment is prone to this common complication.

43 a) False.
    b) True. These are pseudofractures running perpendicular to the bone surface.
    c) True. To increase skin synthesis of vitamin D. Oral intake should also be increased.
    d) False. They are increased.
    e) True. This gives rise to a waddling gait.

44 a) False.
    b) True. This is a hereditary sensorimotor neuropathy causing peroneal muscular atrophy.
    c) True.
    d) False. This is lateral deviation of the big toe.
    e) True. This causes peripheral neuropathy.

45 a) True. Due to compression of the VIIIth cranial nerve.
    b) True. Occurs in 1 per cent of cases.
    c) False.
    d) False.
    e) True. Increased blood supply to the bone leads to high-output heart failure.

46 a) False.
    b) True. Tabes dorsalis gives rise to neuropathic joints.
    c) False.
    d) True. Diabetic neuropathy is the commonest cause in the UK.
    e) True.

47 a) True. Spinal tuberculosis may give rise to kyphosis.
    b) True. Osteoporotic spinal fractures are a common cause of kyphosis in the elderly.
    c) False.
    d) False. This may be compensated for by a hyperlordosis of the back.
    e) True. Due to fusion of the vertebrae.

48 a) False. Rheumatoid factor is present in 70 per cent of cases.
    b) True.
    c) False. This is a crystal arthritis.
    d) True. This is a combination of urethritis, arthritis and conjunctivitis.
    e) True. This is predominantly a disorder of the back, affecting young adults.

49 a) False.
    b) True.
    c) False.
    d) True.
    e) False.

EMQ ANSWERS

1 ANTIBODIES IN RHEUMATOLOGICAL DISEASE

1 B A rash over the cheeks and bridge of the nose is typically found in systemic lupus erythematosus. Ninety-five per cent of patients with this condition have a positive **ANA.**

2 H Features of the antiphospholipid syndrome include recurrent miscarriages and arterial and venous thrombosis. **Anti-cardiolipin** antibodies point to the diagnosis.

3 A The insidious history of progressive weakness, proximal myopathy and respiratory problems suggests the diagnosis of polymyositis. **Anti-Jo 1** antibodies are typically found in patients with polymyositis with respiratory involvement.

4 G Cavitating lesions on the chest X-ray combined with acute renal failure make the most likely diagnosis Wegener's granulomatosis. The vast majority of patients with Wegener's are **cANCA (proteinase-3)** positive.

5 J This gentleman has severe Raynaud's phenomenon, sclerodactyly and telangiectasia, suggesting limited cutaneous scleroderma. **Anti-centromere** antibodies are usually found in this condition.

2 MONOARTHRITIS

1 B The presence of positively birefringent crystals in a joint aspirate is pathognomonic of **pseudogout**. The most common presentation is with a large joint monoarthritis.

2 F This patient has ulceration of the glans and a monoarthritis. Given the preceding gastrointestinal infection, and the lack of any recent sexual contacts, **reactive arthritis** is the best diagnosis.

3 D **Gonococcal arthritis**. This is a typical presentation of septic arthritis. The most common cause of this in young males is infection with *N. gonorrhoeae*, the Gram-negative diplococci seen under the microscope.

4 G The other common crystal-associated arthropathy is **gout**, characterized by the presence of negatively birefringent crystals on microscopy.

5 H Recurrent oral ulceration associated with arthritis and a positive pathergy test (the presence of a pustule at a site of sterile skin puncture) suggests **Behçet's syndrome**. Genital ulceration is also frequently seen.

3 VASCULITIS

1 C Asthma, eosinophilia and vasculitis are the hallmarks of **Churg–Strauss syndrome**. MPO ANCA is usually, but not always, found.

2 F Obliteration of the peripheral pulses is one of the key features of **Takayasu's arteritis**, a large vessel vasculitis which usually affects young women. The condition is sometimes referred to colloquially as pulseless disease.

3 H Desquamation of the palms, prolonged fever, cervical lymphadenopathy and a strawberry tongue are all signs of **Kawasaki disease**, a self-limiting idiopathic vasculitis. The most worrying complication of this disease is the development of coronary artery aneurysms.

4 G **Goodpasture's syndrome**, an autoimmune disease characterized by antibodies to the glomerular basement membrane, classically causes a combination of pulmonary haemorrhage and acute glomerulonephritis due to similarities in the collagen in both lung and kidney.

5 I **Giant cell arteritis**, or temporal arteritis, is a medical emergency affecting the elderly. Features such as a tender temporal artery or jaw claudication warrant immediate treatment with oral steroids (to prevent the feared complication of blindness) and an urgent temporal artery biopsy.

4 COMPLICATIONS OF RHEUMATOID ARTHRITIS

1 C This patient has both sensory and motor involvement of cervical nerve roots. **Atlanto-axial subluxation** can cause compression of the cervical cord resulting in a range of presentations from minor loss of nerve function to paralysis.

2 D Dry eyes and a dry mouth are the initial presenting symptoms of **Sjögren's syndrome**, which may be associated with rheumatoid arthritis. Treatment is usually supportive.

3 A This woman has the triad of oedema, hypoalbuminaemia and proteinuria – the hallmarks of nephrotic syndrome. Renal **amyloidosis**, which can occur in any chronic inflammatory condition, is the likely cause.

4 F **Felty's syndrome**, the combination of splenomegaly and neutropenia on a background of rheumatoid arthritis often indicates severe disease.

5 H Tingling in the radial three and half fingers is characteristic of **carpal tunnel syndrome**. Swelling and synovitis quite commonly cause compression of the median nerve; surgical decompression may be required.

5 PHARMACOLOGICAL TREATMENT OF RHEUMATOLOGICAL DISEASE

1 I **Hypromellose** eye drops are used as a form of synthetic tear to lubricate the eyes in patients with chronic dry eyes secondary to Sjögren's syndrome.

2 C The monoclonal antibody **etanercept** binds to TNF α in the systemic circulation before it can bind to its receptor. It is a highly effective treatment and is used in disease refractory to conventional disease-modifying antirheumatic drugs (DMARDs).

3 H **Allopurinol** inhibits the enzyme xanthine oxidase, thereby preventing the accumulation of uric acid. It can decrease the frequency of attacks of gout in susceptible patients but must not be started during an acute attack as it may worsen symptoms initially.

4 B Antimalarials such as **hydroxychloroquine** are a good initial treatment for patients with mild SLE. Their mechanism of action is still unclear.

5 G The use of a bisphosphonate such as **alendronate** would be sensible in a patient with osteoporotic crush fractures in an effort to increase bone mineral density. Due to oesophageal toxicity, these drugs are contraindicated in patients who cannot remain upright for half an hour after taking their medication.

6 COMPLICATIONS OF DRUGS USED TO TREAT RHEUMATOLOGICAL DISEASE

1 D Haemorrhagic cystitis is an infrequent but important complication of **cyclophosphamide**. In high-risk patients the drug mesna is co-prescribed, which binds to the toxic metabolite and prevents inflammation of the urinary epithelium.

2 C It is critical that patients about to undergo therapy with anti-TNF agents, such as **etanercept** and infliximab, undergo screening for tuberculosis, as these drugs can exacerbate pre-existing disease.

3 E The features described are the typical signs and symptoms of Cushing's syndrome, the most common cause of which is an iatrogenic exogenous steroid administration. **Prednisolone** is widely used in rheumatology to suppress inflammatory activity; care should be exercised to keep the steroid dose as low as possible.

4 G **Alendronate**, a bisphosphonate used to increase bone mineral density is associated with oesophagitis and oesophageal ulceration.

5 J **Methotrexate** works by inhibiting the enzyme dihydrofolate reductase, which is involved in the synthesis of folate (thereby causing a macrocytic anaemia). Regular monitoring is required as it can cause bone marrow suppression, as in this case.

7 DRUGS USED TO TREAT RHEUMATOID ARTHRITIS

1 D **Sodium aurothiomalate** is the parenteral form of gold, sometimes used to treat rheumatoid arthritis. Side-effects such as pruritus, blood disorders and renal dysfunction often result in therapy being stopped.

2 G **Sulfasalazine** is the combination of a 5-ASA (aminosalicylic acid) molecule attached to the biologically inactive sulfonamide sulfapyridine, which acts as a carrier molecule to the gut.

3 C **Hydroxychloroquine** is also used both in the treatment of systemic lupus erythematosus and as an antimalarial. Many species of Plasmodium are now however resistant to chloroquine.

4 I **Penicillamine** is used as a chelating agent to remove excess copper from the body in Wilson's disease. It can cause renal and haematological side-effects.

5 A **Methotrexate** is often the first-line DMARD used in rheumatoid arthritis. It is highly effective in suppressing inflammation through its inhibition of the enzyme dihydrofolate reductase.

8 RAYNAUD'S PHENOMENON

1 G Hepatitis B infection is associated with **cryoglobulinaemia**, which can present with a palpable rash, joint pain and Raynaud's phenomenon.

2 B These symptoms of a dry mouth and dry eyes suggest **Sjögren's syndrome**. About 50 per cent of patients with this condition also suffer from Raynaud's phenomenon.

3 D Raynaud's phenomenon is extremely common in the general population, and the vast majority of cases are **idiopathic**. There are no features here to suggest any other underlying disease.

4 E **Occupational.** Transmitted vibration from tools at work can cause secondary Raynaud's phenomenon. In severe cases, neurological signs such as paraesthesiae and loss of proprioception may be found.

5 C The hand lesions being described here are Gottron's papules, which are pathognomonic of **dermatomyositis**. Raynaud's phenomenon is found in both this condition and polymyositis.

9 EPONYMS

1 G **Battle's sign.** Other features of a basal skull fracture include cerebrospinal fluid (CSF) rhinorrhoea, bilateral periorbital haematomas (raccoon's eyes) and haemotympanum (blood in the middle ear).

2 H **Smith's fracture** is sometimes referred to as a reverse Colles' fracture: the distal fragment is displaced towards the palm of the hand (in a Colles' fracture the distal fragment is displaced dorsally). The mechanism of injury is usually a fall onto a flexed hand.

3 J The **Garden classification** is used to describe the severity of a fractured neck of femur. It ranges from stage I, an impacted fracture, to stage IV, where the proximal fragment is completely displaced and no longer attached to the distal femur.

4 I A **Baker's cyst** is a synovial fluid sac extending posteriorly from the knee joint. If it ruptures it can cause calf pain and tenderness and clinically resemble a deep vein thrombosis (DVT).

5 B **Barlow's test** attempts to dislocate a susceptible femoral head from the acetabulum of a child with developmental dysplasia of the hip (DDH); Ortolani's test involves trying to relocate an already dislocated hip.

10 COMPLICATIONS OF FRACTURES

1 B **Compartment syndrome** is a feared complication of fractures occurring in closed fascial compartments, usually in the arm or the leg. Raised pressure leads to venous stasis and prevents further blood from entering, leading to muscle necrosis. Important signs are pain out of proportion to the injury, and pain on passive stretching. The loss of the pulse and paraesthesiae are late signs.

2 F **Fat embolism** may occur suddenly and cause cardiovascular collapse after fractures. The diagnosis is often made at autopsy.

3 G A swollen red limb in an orthopaedic patient is likely to be caused by **deep vein thrombosis**: it is too late after the operation for a wound infection to be likely. DVT is common after lower limb fractures.

4 I The sensation being described is allodynia, when seemingly innocuous stimuli produce pain. **Reflex sympathetic dystrophy** may produce a chronic pain syndrome due to nerve damage after a fracture. Successful treatment can be difficult.

5 E A sequestrum, an area of dead bone, is pathognomonic of **osteomyelitis**. If organisms are introduced into a fracture site at operation, they may infect the bone, resulting in bone death. A prolonged course of antibiotics is needed, with possible removal of the metal prosthesis.

X-RAY ANSWERS

1 a) There is a right undisplaced intertrochanteric fracture of the femoral neck.

   b) This is an extracapsular fracture, so there should not be difficulties with vascular compromise of the proximal fragment. Replacement of the femoral head with a hemiarthroplasty is therefore not required; a dynamic hip screw would hold the fracture together securely.

2 This is an example of a Colles' fracture: a fracture of the distal radius with posterior displacement of the distal fragment. The lateral projection best shows the characteristic 'dinner fork deformity'.

3 a) Osteoarthritis of the knee is common in the elderly population. Changes seen here on X-ray include loss of joint space, osteophyte formation and subchondral sclerosis.

   b) Initial treatment of osteoarthritis usually involves physiotherapy and simple analgesics. For refractory cases, joint replacement is often required.

4 a) This patient has had a left total hip replacement. The X-ray shows a prosthesis replacing the head and neck of the femur, and a cup replacing the acetabulum.

   b) Total hip replacements are most commonly carried out for osteoarthritis and are highly effective treatments, increasing mobility and decreasing pain substantially.

5 a) The X-ray shows a right shoulder dislocation, associated with a fracture of the greater tuberosity. The head of the humerus is lying abnormally, inferior to the coracoid process.

   b) Reduction of the joint will treat this patient's pain and loss of mobility. Care must be taken to document axillary nerve function (supplying the lateral upper arm) before and after reduction, as this may be damaged in the process.

6 a) The right pubic rami are fractured. This injury is typically seen in the elderly population after a fall.

   b) Treatment is usually conservative; operative intervention is rarely needed.

7 a) There is a left-sided displaced fracture of the clavicle.

   b) Clavicular fractures are often treated conservatively in a sling; however when there is significant displacement, internal fixation may be required.

8 There is a fracture of the medial malleolus of the right ankle. Typically, the medial malleolus is affected in eversion injuries, whereas inversion injuries usually cause damage to the lateral malleolus.

9 There are rib fractures of the left second and fourth to the seventh ribs posteriorly. These are common after trauma; the diagnosis is usually clinical. Analgesia is often the only treatment required.

10 a) There are bony erosions and soft tissue swelling around the first metatarsophalangeal joint. This is the classic site affected by gout, when it is known as podagra.

   b) Acutely, NSAIDs are used to relieve pain and inflammation; in the longer term, allopurinol can be given to prevent attacks.

11 There is a collapsed mid-thoracic vertebra – probably secondary to osteoporosis. Treatment is usually supportive with analgesia and physiotherapy, although intervention may be required if conservative measures fail to control pain.

12 There is grossly abnormal bone modelling within the tibia, with cortical thickening. Bowing results when load-bearing stress is placed on weakened bone. These changes are characteristic of Paget's disease.

CHAPTER 5

The gastrointestinal system

MULTIPLE CHOICE QUESTIONS

1   The following statements are true of nutritional support in hospitals:
   a) Intravenous nutrition should normally be instituted if a patient has not eaten for 3 days
   b) A gastroenterologist usually assesses patients' nutritional requirements
   c) Parenteral nutrition is safer than nasogastric feeding
   d) Total parenteral nutrition is normally given via a central venous catheter for long-term feeding
   e) A feeding nasogastric tube should be changed weekly

2   The following may give rise to constipation:
   a) Anal fissure
   b) Coeliac disease
   c) Myxoedema
   d) Anaemia
   e) Diabetes mellitus

3   Regarding gastric adenocarcinoma:
   a) Most are located in the cardia of the stomach
   b) It may present with a right-sided supraclavicular lymph node (Virchow's node)
   c) Acanthosis nigricans is an extra-gastrointestinal feature of the disease
   d) It may present with ascites
   e) Radiotherapy offers the best hope of a cure

4   With regard to coeliac disease:
   a) 90 per cent of cases present in teenage years
   b) There is an association with smoking
   c) Splenic atrophy may be a feature
   d) There is an association with autoimmune disease
   e) There is an association with dermatitis artefacta

5   The following may complicate Crohn's disease:
   a) Uveitis
   b) Rheumatoid arthritis
   c) Venous thrombosis
   d) Primary sclerosing cholangitis
   e) Acanthosis nigricans

6   The following are causes of constipation:
   a) Hyperthyroidism
   b) Magnesium-containing antacids
   c) Hirschsprung's disease
   d) Iron tablets
   e) Patient-controlled analgesia

7   The following are causes of constipation:
   a) Depression
   b) Non-steroidal anti-inflammatory drugs
   c) Parkinson's disease
   d) Colorectal carcinoma
   e) Syndrome of inappropriate antidiuretic hormone secretion (SIADH)

8   Causes of hypoalbuminaemia include:
   a) Dehydration
   b) Hyperparathyroidism
   c) Liver cirrhosis
   d) Malnutrition
   e) Nephrotic syndrome

9   The following statements are true of colorectal cancer:
   a) Metastasis occurs most commonly to the stomach
   b) The 5 year survival rate for a Dukes Stage B cancer is 30–40 per cent
   c) A prophylactic colectomy is offered to those with a positive family history of colo
       rectal cancer
   d) A universal screening programme exists for the over-65 population in the UK
   e) Tenesmus is suggestive of a rectal carcinoma

10   Regarding abnormalities of stool colour:
   a) Melaena can be caused by a bleeding sigmoid colon cancer
   b) Pale stools may be caused by haemolytic jaundice
   c) As much as 10 mL of blood is required to produce the appearance of melaena
   d) Bismuth therapy causes black stools
   e) Pale stools may be a sign of malabsorption

11   The following are complications of total parenteral nutrition:
   a) Pneumothorax
   b) Varicose veins
   c) Hyperglycaemia
   d) Fluid overload
   e) Sepsis

12 Regarding gastro-oesophageal varices:
   a) Bleeding usually stops spontaneously
   b) The first priority in the management of persistently bleeding varices is endoscopy
   c) Variceal banding should only be attempted in the operating theatre
   d) Terlipressin can be used to control bleeding in emergencies
   e) A Sengstaken–Blakemore tube is used to inject bleeding varices

13 The following are causes of malnutrition:
   a) Dementia
   b) Diabetes insipidus
   c) Hypothyroidism
   d) Malignancy
   e) Small bowel resection

14 Regarding acute upper gastrointestinal bleeding:
   a) Varices are the commonest cause
   b) Urgent endoscopy is always required
   c) A Mallory–Weiss tear usually requires urgent surgical repair
   d) Injection of oesophageal varices in the acute stage is contraindicated
   e) Aorto-enteric fistula is a cause

15 Recognized risk factors for gastric adenocarcinoma include:
   a) Crohn's disease
   b) Long-term omeprazole use
   c) *H. pylori*
   d) Long-term aspirin use
   e) Pernicious anaemia

16 The following are recognized risk factors for colorectal adenocarcinoma:
   a) Diverticular disease
   b) Irritable bowel syndrome
   c) Family history
   d) Pseudomembranous colitis
   e) Ulcerative colitis

17 The following statements are true of vomiting:
   a) Bile-stained vomitus is a sign of gastric outflow obstruction
   b) Faeculent vomit is normally a result of bowel perforation
   c) Uraemia is a cause
   d) Hyperkalaemia is a cause
   e) Hypocalcaemia is a cause

18 Regarding coeliac disease:
   a) It is caused by an anaphylactic response to gluten
   b) Anti-mitochondrial antibodies are a typical feature
   c) Jejunal biopsy classically shows villous hypertrophy
   d) Steroids form the mainstay of treatment
   e) There is an association with gastrointestinal malignancies

19 The following are recognized complications of gastro-oesophageal reflux disease:
   a) Oesophageal varices
   b) Oesophageal squamous cell carcinoma
   c) Barrett's oesophagus
   d) Hiatus hernia
   e) Oesophageal adenocarcinoma

20 The following statements are true about the plain abdominal X-ray:
   a) Diagnosis of toxic megacolon is possible
   b) Colonic haustra are seen to cross the entire lumen
   c) Small bowel valvulae conniventes are seen to cross the entire lumen
   d) Under normal circumstances the large bowel does not contain gas
   e) Faecal matter is generally not visible

21 The following statements are true of infective diarrhoea:
   a) Food poisoning is a notifiable disease in the UK
   b) *Salmonella* has a longer incubation period than *Campylobacter*
   c) The antibiotic of choice in bacterial dysentery is metronidazole
   d) Cholera classically produces explosive bloody diarrhoea
   e) *Bacillus cereus* has a predilection for undercooked meat

22 With regard to colorectal cancer:
   a) The disease is the commonest cause of death from cancer in the UK
   b) Familial adenomatous polyposis (FAP) and hereditary non-polyposis colorectal cancer (HNPCC) account for 30 per cent of cases
   c) The caecum and ascending colon are the sites most commonly affected
   d) Caecal cancer typically presents with altered bowel habit
   e) Barium enema is preferable to colonoscopy in the investigation of the disease

23 The following statements are true of achalasia:
   a) The condition is caused by vitamin B deficiency
   b) Dysphagia occurs for both liquids and solids
   c) Endoscopy reveals a 'bird's beak appearance'
   d) Balloon dilatation of the lower oesophageal sphincter is usually ineffective
   e) There is an increased risk of oesophageal cancer

24 Dysphagia may occur because of:
   a) Cervical spondylosis
   b) Diabetes mellitus
   c) Old age
   d) Depression
   e) Multiple sclerosis

25 Symptom relief in gastro-oesophageal reflux disease may be achieved by:
   a) Bed rest
   b) Smoking cessation
   c) Increasing oral fluid intake
   d) Eating before bedtime
   e) Reducing alcohol consumption

26 The following statements are true of colorectal cancer:
   a) Most rectal cancers cannot be felt on digital rectal examination
   b) Rectosigmoid cancers commonly present with a change in bowel habit
   c) Tenesmus refers to faeculent vomiting seen with some colorectal cancers
   d) Anaemia may be the only presenting feature of a caecal cancer
   e) Diverticular disease is a precursor to colonic malignancy

27 *Helicobacter pylori* infection can be diagnosed by:
   a) Blood culture
   b) Stool immunoassay
   c) Throat swab
   d) Serology
   e) Gastric biopsy investigation

28 Regarding Dukes' staging of colorectal tumours:
   a) A colonic cancer that has metastasized to the liver is a Stage C
   b) Stage A has a 5-year survival of at least 90 per cent
   c) Stage B comprises regional lymph node involvement
   d) Five-year survival for Stage D is 50 per cent
   e) Plain abdominal X-ray is useful in staging the disease

29 The following are associated with obesity:
   a) Addison's disease
   b) Prader–Willi syndrome
   c) Corticosteroid therapy
   d) Chronic renal failure
   e) Cushing's syndrome

30 Regarding peptic ulcer disease, the following statements are true:
   a) There is no association between socio-economic status and *H. pylori* infection
   b) The risk of acquiring *H. pylori* infection declines after childhood
   c) Gastric ulcers are more common than duodenal ulcers
   d) The pain of gastric ulcers is classically relieved by eating
   e) The Zollinger–Ellison syndrome has no known cause

31 Which of the following are risk factors for peptic ulcers?
   a) Naproxen
   b) Alcohol
   c) Prednisolone
   d) Paracetamol
   e) Smoking

32 Regarding diverticular disease:
   a) The caecum is most commonly affected
   b) Diet is implicated in the aetiology
   c) Right iliac fossa pain is the commonest symptom
   d) Antispasmodic drugs are contraindicated
   e) Young people are most affected

33 The following statements are true of mouth disorders:
    a) Oral hairy leucoplakia is caused by cytomegalovirus
    b) Phenytoin causes gingival hyperplasia
    c) Asthmatics who take inhaled steroids are at increased risk of oral candidiasis
    d) Iron tablets can cause glossitis
    e) Spicy food is a recognized cause of squamous cell carcinoma of the mouth

34 Causes of oral ulceration include:
    a) Behçet's disease
    b) Systemic lupus erythematosus
    c) Coeliac disease
    d) Neutropenia
    e) Inflammatory bowel disease

35 The following are extragastrointestinal manifestations of inflammatory bowel disease:
    a) Erythema multiforme
    b) Erythema nodosum
    c) Clubbing
    d) Dupuytren's contracture
    e) Pyoderma gangrenosum

36 Regarding inflammatory bowel disease:
    a) Skip lesions are present in the colon in ulcerative colitis
    b) The bowel inflammation in Crohn's disease is deeper than in ulcerative colitis
    c) Granulomas are not a feature of Crohn's disease
    d) Gastrointestinal tuberculosis (TB) is an important differential diagnosis in suspected Crohn's disease
    e) Smoking is a risk factor for Crohn's disease and ulcerative colitis

37 The following are gastrointestinal complications of Crohn's disease:
    a) Perianal abscess
    b) Vesico-colic fistula
    c) Anal fissure
    d) Small bowel stricture
    e) Anorectal fistula

38 The following statements are true of inflammatory bowel disease:
    a) Barium enema is contraindicated in toxic megacolon
    b) A biopsy is commonly needed to differentiate between Crohn's disease and ulcerative colitis
    c) Colorectal cancer develops more commonly in Crohn's disease than in ulcerative colitis
    d) Toxic megacolon may be diagnosed on a plain abdominal film
    e) Colonoscopy is contraindicated in severe acute ulcerative colitis

39 The following are risk factors for oesophageal cancer:
    a) Oesophageal candidiasis
    b) Achalasia
    c) Oesophageal reflux
    d) Alcohol
    e) Coeliac disease

40 In the treatment of inflammatory bowel disease:
 a) Long-term steroid therapy is usually recommended for maintaining remission
 b) An elemental diet is useful in active Crohn's disease
 c) Infliximab may be indicated in fistulating disease
 d) Intravenous hydrocortisone is indicated in acute severe ulcerative colitis
 e) Aminosalicylates are not useful in the maintenance of remission in ulcerative colitis

41 The following statements are true of the complications of diverticulosis:
 a) Haemorrhage is usually associated with severe colicky pain
 b) Bed rest is usually sufficient to control haemorrhage
 c) Vagino-colic fistula may occur
 d) Metronidazole is useful for treating diverticulitis
 e) Perforation is not a risk

42 The following are known causes of diarrhoea:
 a) Hypothyroidism
 b) Carcinoid syndrome
 c) Pseudomembranous colitis
 d) Hypercalcaemia
 e) Chronic pancreatitis

43 Dysphagia may be caused by the following:
 a) Anxiety
 b) Iron-deficiency
 c) Pyloric stenosis
 d) Systemic sclerosis
 e) Hiatus hernia

44 The following are features of irritable bowel syndrome:
 a) Explosive diarrhoea
 b) Bloating
 c) Rectal bleeding
 d) Weight loss
 e) Abdominal pain relieved by defecation

Answers: see pages 141–147

EXTENDED MATCHING QUESTIONS

1 UPPER GASTROINTESTINAL BLEEDING

Match the clinical scenarios below with the most likely cause of upper gastrointestinal bleeding

A   Oesophageal varices
B   Gastric carcinoma
C   Oesophageal rupture
D   Aorto-enteric fistula
E   Iatrogenic

F   Zollinger–Ellison syndrome
G   Mallory–Weiss tear
H   Peptic ulceration
I   Gastritis
J   Osler–Weber–Rendu syndrome

1   An 81-year-old man is brought to the emergency department by ambulance, having been found in bed by his wife in a pool of black faeces. She starts crying and says that he has only ever been in hospital before for his aneurysm. He is pale, hypotensive and peripherally shut down. Despite large volume fluid replacement, he dies 2 h later.

2   A 19-year-old medical student is brought to the emergency department by his friends after having drunk 20 shots of vodka during rag week. He has been vomiting several times and has now noticed streaks of blood in his vomit. When the doctor on-call examines his chest, she finds that his skin is crunchy under her fingers.

3   A 48-year-old milkman has been seen by his general practitioner (GP) for the last year with severe indigestion. He is currently taking high-dose omeprazole but still suffers from dyspepsia. An upper gastrointestinal (GI) endoscopy shows multiple ulcers throughout the duodenum; blood tests reveal a high serum gastrin.

4   A 51-year-old publican is brought in after vomiting a litre of blood over the bar. He has multiple spider naevi, gynaecomastia and a liver flap. Peripheral venous access is impossible, so a central line is inserted to stabilize the patient before the gastroenterologist can reach the hospital.

5   A 66-year-old man is being investigated for iron-deficiency anaemia. Unfortunately, he cannot tolerate upper GI endoscopy due to his severe chronic obstructive pulmonary disease (COPD). He attends the emergency department one afternoon after vomiting up about 20 mL of fresh blood. The registrar requests a computed tomography (CT) scan of his abdomen, which shows a gastric mass with regional lymphadenopathy.

2 CAUSES OF DYSPHAGIA 1

The patients below all complain of difficulty swallowing. Match the most likely cause of this with the clinical scenarios

A Oesophageal carcinoma
B Bulbar palsy
C Oesophageal web
D Benign oesophageal stricture
E Scleroderma

F Myasthenia gravis
G Pharyngeal pouch
H Goitre
I Achalasia
J Enlarged left atrium

1 A 42-year-old housewife returns to her GP for an appointment. She is a frequent attendee with menorrhagia and is always complaining of tiredness and general fatigue. Her complaint this time is that she is having difficulty swallowing. On examination, she has spoon-shaped nails and pale conjunctivae.

2 A 75-year-old woman goes to see her GP saying that she is having difficulty swallowing. Clinical examination is unremarkable apart from a mid-diastolic murmur heard best at the apex.

3 A 32-year-old cleaner presents to her GP with dysphagia. She has been to see him several times in the past few months for persistent Raynaud's phenomenon. On this visit, the GP notices that she has a small mouth and shiny skin over her fingers.

4 A 26-year-old actress presents to the emergency department with dysphagia, fatigue and shortness of breath. The doctor notices both her eyelids are droopy, and performs some blood tests and a chest X-ray. The chest X-ray shows a mass above the heart.

5 A 71-year-old retired bank manager presents to his GP with a 3-month history of dysphagia, regurgitation and cough. He has been admitted to hospital twice in the past year with aspiration pneumonia. On examination, there is a palpable neck swelling which seems to gurgle.

3 CAUSES OF DYSPHAGIA 2

Each of the patients below has presented with difficulty swallowing. Choose the most likely diagnosis from the options given

A Foreign body
B Oesophageal atresia
C Oesophageal carcinoma
D Plummer–Vinson syndrome
E Pharyngeal pouch

F Achalasia
G Oesophageal stricture
H Retrosternal goitre
I Hiatus hernia
J Scleroderma

1 Staff in a nursing home are concerned as a usually healthy 83-year-old resident with dementia develops sudden-onset difficulty in swallowing.

2 A 30-year-old woman presents to her GP complaining of worsening dysphagia, worse for liquids than solids. She has also noticed intermittent retrosternal chest pain.

3 An 80-year-old man complains of recent unintentional weight loss and sudden difficulty swallowing solids and liquids over the last few weeks.

4 A 60-year-old gives a long history of acid reflux and burning retrosternal pain, worse on lying down. She says that she can feel food 'sticking' after meals.

5 A 75-year-old woman presents with halitosis and a swelling in the neck. She regurgitates food on lying down.

4 CONDITIONS AFFECTING THE STOMACH

Select the most likely diagnosis for each of the scenarios below

A Erosive gastritis
B Sliding hiatus hernia
C Ménétrier's disease
D Gastric varices
E Pyloric stenosis

F Adenocarcinoma of the stomach
G Peptic ulceration
H Autoimmune gastritis
I Rolling hiatus hernia
J Dumping syndrome

1 An obese 53-year-old lorry driver presents to his GP with heartburn, only slightly improved by over-the-counter antacids. The GP sends him for a barium swallow, which is reported as showing part of the stomach, including the oesophagogastric junction, in the thorax.

2 A 4-week-old boy will not stop vomiting, and so his mother takes him to their GP. She describes the vomiting as projectile, saying it will often travel up to a metre. The GP examines the boy carefully and finds a small nodule in the epigastrium.

3 A 42-year-old teacher goes to her GP with fatigue and paraesthesiae in her fingers and toes. He finds that she has glossitis and angular stomatitis and orders an oesophago-gastroduodenoscopy (OGD) looking for a cause. This shows achlorhydria; histology from gastric biopsies shows gastritis throughout the stomach.

4 A 63-year-old man sees his GP for epigastric discomfort. He rarely comes to his GP surgery and the only medical history that the GP can find on his computer is a partial gastrectomy for an ulcer 20 years ago. On examination, the GP finds a mass in the epigastrium.

5 A 35-year-old air hostess has chronic back pain, for which she takes regular diclofenac. She attends her local GP surgery with epigastric pain. Examination is unremarkable, apart from some slight tenderness in the epigastrium.

5 MALABSORPTION

All of the patients below have malabsorption. Pick the most likely diagnosis from the options given

A   Crohn's disease
B   Coeliac disease
C   Dermatitis herpetiformis
D   Bacterial overgrowth
E   Whipple's disease

F   Chronic pancreatitis
G   Short bowel syndrome
H   Iatrogenic
I   Tropical sprue
J   Giardiasis

1   A 49-year-old Irish barman presents to his GP with malaise and tiredness. For 3 months he has been suffering from occasional abdominal pain, mouth ulcers and diarrhoea, which he says is often pale and offensive. The GP asks him to undergo an OGD, which shows subtotal villous atrophy.

2   A 28-year-old osteopath complains of fatigue and intermittent diarrhoea for the past 2 years. Examination reveals some aphthous ulceration of the mouth, but is otherwise unremarkable. Bloods reveal a macrocytic anaemia with low levels of vitamin B_{12}.

3   A 56-year-old security guard goes to see his GP complaining of pale stools that his wife complains do not flush away. The GP knows that the marriage is in jeopardy due to his heavy drinking, and fears that this may be the last straw. He orders an abdominal film which shows a calcified mass in the epigastrium.

4   A 31-year-old with Crohn's disease sees her gastroenterologist with intractable diarrhoea and an inability to put on weight. She has had eight laparotomies in the past for flare-ups of her disease refractory to medical therapy.

5   A 54-year-old shopkeeper sees his GP to complain about pale, frothy stools. He has type 2 diabetes mellitus and is on gliclazide and orlistat to maintain his glycaemic control. On examination, he is clinically obese, with no signs of gastrointestinal disease.

6 COMPLICATIONS OF INFLAMMATORY BOWEL DISEASE

The patients below all have complications of inflammatory bowel disease. Choose the most likely diagnosis for each of the clinical scenarios

A   Cirrhosis
B   Anterior uveitis
C   Pyoderma gangrenosum
D   Cholangiocarcinoma
E   Colorectal carcinoma

F   Sacroiliitis
G   Primary sclerosing cholangitis
H   Deep venous thrombosis
I   Episcleritis
J   Erythema nodosum

1   A 23-year-old writer with an 8-year history of inflammatory bowel disease presents to her GP as she has turned yellow. The GP performs some blood tests which show alkaline phosphatase (ALP) 230 IU/L, alanine transaminase (ALT) 34 IU/L, bilirubin 59 µmol/L, and pANCA (anti myeloperoxidase)-positive. An ultrasound of the liver shows that the biliary tree is not dilated.

2   A 56-year-old company director with a 20-year history of Crohn's disease suffers a flare-up of his disease and has diarrhoea and abdominal pain. He also complains of photophobia, blurred vision, eye pain and headache.

3   A 31-year-old photographer returns home after a photo shoot and notices a small red papule on his left shin. He is fit and well but suffers from ulcerative colitis, which was diagnosed 3 years ago. He is worried when the small lesion on his leg turns into a large painful ulcer over the course of the next two weeks.

4   A 48-year-old carpenter has had ulcerative colitis for the past 21 years. He suffers from flare-ups every 6 months when he passes blood and mucus: these usually settle with oral medication. He attends clinic for a persistent flare-up, where he is found to have lost 7 kg of weight in the past 3 months.

5   A 31-year-old dentist goes to his GP because he has developed some tender red areas on his shins. He is known to have Crohn's disease, which is usually well controlled.

7 CONSTIPATION

Select the most likely cause of constipation for each of the clinical scenarios below

A   Small bowel obstruction
B   Depression
C   Iatrogenic
D   Multiple sclerosis
E   Colorectal carcinoma

F   Hirschsprung's disease
G   Irritable bowel syndrome
H   Hypercalcaemia
I   Hypothyroidism
J   Large bowel obstruction

1   A 71-year-old woman presents to her GP with constipation. She has high cholesterol and high blood pressure and has recently started treatment with simvastatin and verapamil. He performs some routine blood tests, which are entirely normal.

2   A 41-year-old woman calls an ambulance because she is vomiting profusely and has abdominal pain. She tells the doctor that she has never been in hospital before apart from having an appendicectomy at the age of 21 years. Examination reveals a distended abdomen with hyperactive bowel sounds. An X-ray shows dilated bowel, with markings crossing the entire width.

3   A newborn baby is sent home with her mother 1 day after a normal birth. Three days later the mother returns to the emergency department saying that her daughter has not passed stool since birth and is vomiting. An X-ray shows a megacolon. The surgical registrar takes a biopsy, which the pathologist reports as devoid of ganglion cells.

4   A 32-year-old investment banker goes to her GP complaining of 6 months of intermittent abdominal pain relieved by defecation. She often feels bloated and has noticed mucus in her stool, but denies any blood. Her constipation is causing her great difficulties at work. Her GP performs some blood tests which are entirely normal.

5   A 46-year-old chef complains of constipation, fatigue and lethargy. On examination, her pulse is 54 beats/min, blood pressure 130/68 mmHg. Her skin is dry and coarse and she appears pale. Neurological examination reveals slow relaxing reflexes.

8 DIARRHOEA

Each of the following patients has diarrhoea. Select the most likely cause from the options given

A *Escherichia coli*
B Pancreatic tumour
C Malabsorption
D *Campylobacter jejuni*
E *Salmonella* spp

F Thyrotoxicosis
G Iatrogenic
H Overflow diarrhoea
I Colonic carcinoma
J Inflammatory bowel disease

1 A 9-year-old boy eats a hamburger at a barbecue and becomes unwell 24 h later with fever, diarrhoea and vomiting. His parents take him to hospital where he is given intravenous (i.v.) fluids and antibiotics. Three days later he develops haemolysis and renal failure and, despite being moved to the intensive therapy unit (ITU), unfortunately dies.

2 An 83-year-old nursing home resident tells his GP on his monthly visit that he is suffering from diarrhoea. The staff members complain that the patient has recently become incontinent of faeces. Examination reveals abdominal fullness, with a loaded rectum.

3 A 62-year-old woman complains of profuse watery diarrhoea. Her GP knows her well as she has recently been in the local neurosurgical unit for excision of a pituitary adenoma; 5 years ago she had her parathyroids excised for hyperparathyroidism. A 24 h stool collection shows a weight of 1.2 kg.

4 A 52-year-old office worker is diagnosed as being diabetic and is started on metformin. He returns to his GP a month later with diarrhoea which he finds quite debilitating. Physical examination is unremarkable.

5 A 68-year-old man is brought to the GP by his wife as he is suffering from a change in bowel habit. He has not noticed any blood in his stool. Examination, including rectal examination, reveals no abnormality. Blood tests show haemoglobin (Hb) 10.9 g/dL, mean corpuscular volume (MCV) 76 fL, white cell count (WCC) 6.2×10^9/L and platelets 297×10^9/L.

9 INFECTIVE DIARRHOEA

Select the most likely cause of infective diarrhoea for each of the clinical scenarios below

A *Campylobacter jejuni*
B *Staphylococcus aureus*
C *Bacillus cereus*
D *Shigella* spp
E *Salmonella enteritidis*

F *Escherichia coli*
G *Clostridium botulinum*
H *Clostridium difficile*
I *Vibrio cholerae*
J Norwalk-like virus

1 A 71-year-old woman suffers from repeated bouts of hospital-acquired pneumonia while waiting for social services input. She is treated with cefuroxime which resolves the pneumonia. Two days later she develops profuse watery diarrhoea and becomes incontinent of faeces.

2 A 23-year-old student returns from his travels in West Bengal. One day later he comes to hospital with profuse diarrhoea. He says his stools look like rice water. He is sent home by the emergency department doctor with advice to drink plenty of fluids. An ambulance brings the same patient in 12 h later with tachycardia and hypotension.

3 A ward sister rings the duty manager of the hospital saying that since a 68-year-old man was admitted to her ward with diarrhoea, eight of the other patients have begun to complain of the same symptoms. She recommends that her ward be closed.

4 A 36-year-old man orders a Chinese takeaway which he is unable to finish. The next day he eats the rice and noodles for lunch, warming them in the staff microwave. Two hours later, he becomes unwell with profuse vomiting, and presents to his GP.

5 A 49-year-old man eats some cooked cold salmon from a tin for dinner. One day later he becomes extremely concerned as he has diarrhoea and finds that he has blurred vision and diplopia. He calls an ambulance and is taken to hospital, where 12 h later he finds himself unable to move despite being fully conscious.

10 ABDOMINAL PAIN 1

Each of the following patients has abdominal pain. Select the most likely cause from the options given

A   Renal colic
B   Myocardial infarction
C   Irritable bowel syndrome
D   Pyelonephritis
E   Acute pancreatitis

F   Inflammatory bowel disease
G   Pneumonia
H   Gastritis
I   Sickle cell disease
J   Acute intermittent porphyria

1 A 6-year-old boy is brought to paediatric emergency department by his mother. He complains of severe left upper quadrant abdominal pain, which is refractory to treatment with Calpol (paracetamol) and Nurofen (ibuprofen), and requires opiates. Blood tests reveal Hb 7.5 g/dL, WCC 12.4×10^9/L, MCV 71 fL.

2 A 71-year-old man calls an ambulance because he has severe epigastric pain. On arrival at hospital he looks pale and sweaty, but has no abdominal tenderness. There is a sinus tachycardia; chest and abdominal X-rays are normal. Bloods show Hb 12.3 g/dL, WCC 7.3 $\times 10^9$/L, amylase 140 U/L, creatine kinase (CK) 870 U/L.

3 A 75-year-old man is admitted to hospital with a 2-day history of right upper quadrant pain, fever and cough. He denies any change in bowel habit. Examination of the abdomen is unremarkable.

4 A 21-year-old telephonist goes to her GP complaining of malaise and intermittent abdominal pain. She has felt fatigued for the past 6 months. She occasionally suffers from bouts of diarrhoea. Bloods tests show Hb 9.2 g/dL, WCC 8×10^9/L, MCV 104 fL, low vitamin B_{12}, normal folate and haematinics.

5 A 49-year-old policewoman presents to the emergency department with a 3-h history of pain in the left iliac fossa, which she says comes and goes. When seen by the doctor, she is writhing round on the bed, and says that the pain is equivalent to that she experienced when she gave birth to her two children. A urine dipstick shows ++ blood in the urine, but she denies dysuria.

11 ABDOMINAL PAIN 2

Each of the following patients has abdominal pain. Select the most likely cause from the options given

A   Ulcerative colitis
B   Acute pancreatitis
C   Crohn's disease
D   Ischaemic colitis
E   Diverticulitis

F   Mittleschmerz
G   Gastritis
H   Ruptured ectopic pregnancy
I   Intestinal obstruction
J   Acute appendicitis

1   A 20-year-old medical student is brought to the emergency department with severe right-sided lower abdominal pain. She is cold and clammy with blood pressure 90/40 mmHg and heart rate 120 beats/min. Her last menstrual period was 7 weeks ago.
2   A 45-year-old publican presents with sudden onset of severe epigastric pain radiating to the back, with nausea and vomiting. He has had several previous identical episodes.
3   A 75-year-old man presents to the emergency department with severe generalized abdominal pain. His blood pressure is 100/70 mmHg and pulse 95 beats/min and irregular. On examination, he is exquisitely tender throughout his abdomen with guarding.
4   An 18-year-old is seen in the emergency department with a 1-day history of right-sided lower abdominal pain and anorexia. Her temperature is 37.8°C. There is right-sided tenderness on rectal examination. Blood tests show an elevated C-reactive protein (CRP) and white cell count.
5   A 76-year-old woman had an open repair of an abdominal aortic aneurysm (AAA) 5 years ago. She now presents with a 48-h history of colicky abdominal pain, nausea and vomiting. She has not opened her bowels today.

12 INVESTIGATION OF ABDOMINAL PAIN

Choose the most appropriate next investigation for each of the patients below

A   Ultrasound of the abdomen
B   Chest X-ray
C   Urine dipstick
D   Abdominal X-ray
E   Endoscopic retrograde cholangiopancreatography (ERCP)

F   Echocardiogram
G   Blood glucose
H   Laparoscopy
I   Oesophagogastroduodenoscopy (OGD)
J   Intravenous urogram

1   A plump 40-year-old woman complains of right upper quadrant pain after eating fatty food.
2   An elderly man presents with a 4-h history of central abdominal pain radiating to the back. On examination, he is warm and well perfused with a blood pressure of 130/70 mmHg. He has an expansile, pulsatile mass in the epigastrium.
3   A 65-year-old man presents to the surgical assessment unit with a 2-day history of abdominal pain, vomiting and absolute constipation.
4   A 21-year-old student has a sudden onset of left loin pain radiating to the groin. She is rolling around the bed in agony. She has never had the pain before.
5   A 64-year-old man presents to the emergency department with epigastric pain. While he is in the department, he starts vomiting. A nurse comments that the vomit looks like coffee grounds.

13 DRUGS USED IN GASTROENTEROLOGY 1

Match the drugs below to the class to which they belong

A   Ranitidine
B   Loperamide
C   Sodium picosulfate
D   Lactulose
E   Metoclopramide

F   Magnesium hydroxide
G   Misoprostol
H   Omeprazole
I   Mesalazine
J   Mebeverine

1   Prostaglandin analogue
2   H$_2$-blocker
3   Stimulant laxative
4   5-aminosalicylic acid
5   Proton pump inhibitor

14 DRUGS USED IN GASTROENTEROLOGY 2

Each of the patients below is given a new prescription by their doctor. Select the most likely medication from the options given

A   Ranitidine
B   Loperamide
C   Sodium picosulfate
D   Lactulose
E   Metoclopramide

F   Magnesium hydroxide
G   Misoprostol
H   Lansoprazole
I   Mesalazine
J   Mebeverine

1   A 31-year-old man returns to his GP with symptoms of gastro-oesophageal reflux disease (GORD). He is currently on prescription medication; the GP says that she will try the most effective pill she has at her disposal for the suppression of gastric acid.
2   A 19-year-old woman is seen by her gastroenterologist with a new diagnosis of ulcerative colitis. He says that he is going to give her some medication that acts as an immuno-modulator.
3   A 52-year-old fast food chef has a particularly bad bout of food poisoning. His doctor gives him a prescription to help control his vomiting.
4   The 52-year-old chef returns a day later saying his vomiting has improved but that the diarrhoea is now causing him difficulty. He is due to leave for holiday the next day, so the GP gives him a prescription for a medicine that she says will treat this.
5   An 89-year-old woman is admitted to hospital for investigation of a change in bowel habit. The house officer on call is asked to come and prescribe an appropriate bowel-cleansing solution.

15 ORAL ULCERATION

Each of the patients below presents with oral ulceration. Choose the most likely cause of this from the options given

A   Trauma
B   Inflammatory bowel disease
C   Behçet's syndrome
D   Stevens–Johnson syndrome
E   Idiopathic

F   Reiter's syndrome
G   Coeliac disease
H   Systemic lupus erythematosus
I   Squamous cell carcinoma
J   Lichen planus

1   A 21-year-old receptionist goes to see her GP as she has a cold. She wants some antibiotics so she feels better more quickly, and leaves with a prescription for some amoxicillin. Three days later she returns, in considerable distress, as she has developed severe mouth ulcers and a rash all over her body.

2   A 32-year-old graphic designer makes an emergency appointment at his local surgery. He is horrified as he has developed two ulcers on his scrotum, along with a mouth ulcer. He insists that he has had no new sexual contacts for the past 6 months.

3   A 91-year-old woman is seen by her GP on his regular visit to her nursing home. He is a little impatient as he has to wait for her to put her dentures in (apparently they do not fit well), but she eventually tells him that her mouth ulcers are really quite troubling.

4   A 56-year-old plasterer goes to the emergency department on his way home. He is concerned because he has noticed a mouth ulcer which does not seem to be getting better. The doctor finds a 2 cm rough irregular lesion on the hard palate, and a black hairy tongue.

5   A 22-year-old man goes to see his doctor, complaining of recurrent oral ulceration. He has been to see the GP six times in the past year with the same problem. The GP examines him and finds two 5 mm ulcers inside the mouth, but can find no other abnormality.

16 RECTAL BLEEDING

All the patients below have presented with rectal bleeding. Choose the most likely cause of this from the options given

A   Angiodysplasia
B   Anal fissure
C   Dysentery
D   Colonic polyp
E   Meckel's diverticulum

F   Colonic carcinoma
G   Intussusception
H   Haemorrhoids
I   Diverticulosis
J   Ulcerative colitis

1   A 28-year-old woman goes to her GP, very concerned about some rectal bleeding. She has noticed some fresh blood in the pan and on the toilet paper after defecation. Physical examination is entirely unremarkable.

2   A 31-year-old woman goes to her doctor with a 3-month history of abdominal pain, diarrhoea, and rectal bleeding. She says that the diarrhoea is so debilitating it is affecting her work. She is passing stool approximately 15 times per day.

3   A 26-year-old man goes to see his GP complaining of rectal bleeding. He says that he is frightened to go to the toilet to defecate, as each time he does it feels as if he is passing razor blades. He refuses to let the GP perform a rectal examination as he says it would simply be too painful.

4   A 63-year-old man goes to see his GP with cramping lower abdominal pain and diarrhoea. He says that he has noticed some blood mixed in with the stool. The GP takes a careful history and notes with interest that he returned from Borneo one week ago.

5   A 4-year-old girl is taken to the emergency department by her father, complaining of severe abdominal pain and vomiting. He mentions that he has noticed blood in her stool. The paediatric registrar performs a digital rectal examination, which reveals a full rectum with what looks like redcurrant jelly. A subsequent abdominal X-ray reveals dilated loops of bowel.

17 INVESTIGATION OF RECTAL BLEEDING

Select the most useful investigation for each of the patients below, all of whom have presented with rectal bleeding

A   CT colography
B   Rigid sigmoidoscopy
C   Abdominal X-ray
D   CT of the abdomen/pelvis
E   Barium follow through

F   Visceral angiography
G   Upper GI endoscopy
H   Colonoscopy
I   Technetium nuclear medicine scan
J   Arterial blood gas analysis

1   A 27-year-old man goes to see his GP with rectal pain and bleeding. He says that he has had this before and has been diagnosed with a solitary rectal ulcer in the past.

2   A 93-year-old woman is referred to hospital because a GP has incidentally found her to have a microcytic anaemia. Examination is unremarkable apart from pale conjunctivae. The consultant is concerned as he feels an invasive procedure may be too risky, given her age.

3   A 7-year-old boy, with no prior medical history, presents with a 12-h history of intermittent nausea, vomiting, and bloody stools. An abdominal X-ray is unremarkable. The paediatrician suspects Meckel's diverticulum and informs the parents he is arranging a test to confirm the diagnosis.

4   A 43-year-old homeless man is brought to the emergency department after being found on the pavement in a puddle of blood. He smells strongly of alcohol, and has multiple spider naevi. While in the department, he has a further massive rectal bleed consisting of fresh blood with some clots.

5   An 82-year-old man is admitted to hospital with rectal bleeding. Endoscopy is unremarkable, and the surgeon suspects angiodysplasia. However, he is loath to operate without pinpointing the source of bleeding.

18 PERIANAL CONDITIONS

Choose the best diagnosis from the options given for each clinical scenarios below

A   Rectal cancer
B   Fistula-in-ano
C   Pilonidal sinus
D   Anal warts
E   Perianal abscess

F   Perianal haematoma
G   Anal fissure
H   Rectal prolapse
I   Haemorrhoids
J   Anal cancer

1   A 53-year-old lorry driver goes to the emergency department as he finds it excruciatingly painful to sit down. The doctor diagnoses an abscess at the top of the natal cleft.

2   A 61-year-old man goes to see his doctor. He complains that he often feels the urge to go to the toilet to pass stool, but finds that there is nothing there. A rectal examination reveals a mass at the tip of the GP's finger.

3   A 26-year-old man makes an emergency appointment at his local GP surgery, complaining of excruciating anal pain. When the GP examines him, he finds a small purple lump at the anal verge.

4   A 32-year-old woman sees a general surgeon after she is diagnosed with a perianal abscess. She is very relieved when he drains it under general anaesthetic. At her follow-up appointment 4 months later, however, she is quite irate, complaining of chronic perianal discharge.

5   A 28-year-old hairdresser goes to see his GP, with new symptoms of perianal discomfort. The GP examines him and finds several small fleshy growths around the anus.

Answers: see pages 147–153

X-RAY QUESTIONS

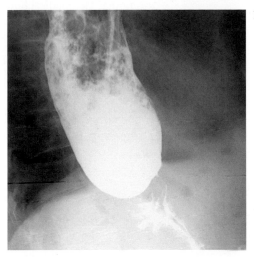

1

1   A 62-year-old man goes to see his doctor with a 2-year history of retrosternal chest pain and dysphagia. He has been admitted to hospital three times in the past year with suspected aspiration pneumonia. His GP refers him for a barium meal. Why is this patient having difficulty swallowing?

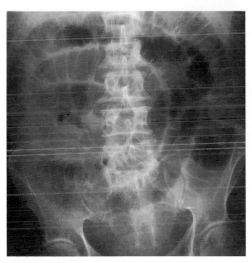

2

2   A 29-year-old woman goes to hospital complaining of abdominal distension and vomiting. She has only been in hospital once before, for a perforated appendix. A plain abdominal X-ray is requested.
a) What is the cause of this patient's symptoms?
b) Why has this patient developed this condition?

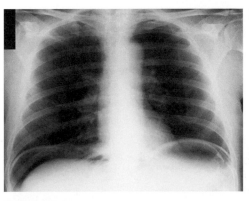

3

3   A 47-year-old man comes to hospital, complaining of severe abdominal pain. The doctor requests a chest X-ray after feeling his abdomen. What is the likely cause of this patient's abdominal pain?

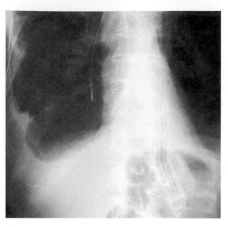

4

4 A 75-year-old man is admitted to hospital for treatment of his oesophageal carcinoma. The medical house officer on call is asked to check the position of his nasogastric feeding tube.
   a) Is the tube correctly positioned?
   b) How has the oesophageal carcinoma been treated?

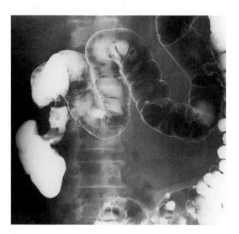

5

5 A 77-year-old woman was incidentally found by her GP to have a microcytic anaemia. She was not however keen on a colonoscopy; the GP was able to compromise on a barium enema.
   a) What is the likely cause of the anaemia?
   b) Where is the lesion?

6

6 An 86-year-old man calls an ambulance, complaining of abdominal distension. An abdominal X-ray is performed in the emergency department.
   a) Describe the abnormality seen on the X-ray.
   b) What is the treatment for this condition?

Answers: see page 154

ANSWERS

MCQ ANSWERS

1 a) False. Parenteral nutrition should be considered if the gastrointestinal tract is not functional for at least 7 days.
   b) False. A dietitian usually provides input regarding nutritional support for most relevant inpatients. Gastroenterologists may become involved in complicated cases.
   c) False. Enteral nutrition is generally preferable to parenteral nutrition due to the risks involved.
   d) True. A central line lasts longer and is safer than a peripheral line.
   e) False.

2 a) True. The intense pain of an anal fissure creates a profound fear of passing stools.
   b) False.
   c) True.
   d) False.
   e) True. Diabetic neuropathy can cause constipation.

3 a) False. The antrum is the commonest location.
   b) False. Virchow's node is left-sided.
   c) True. This is a blackening of the axillae.
   d) True. Metastasis to the liver can occur.
   e) False. Surgery is the best mode of treatment for operable gastric cancers.

4 a) False. It presents at any age, including infancy.
   b) False.
   c) True.
   d) True. There is an increased incidence of type 1 diabetes, thyroid disease etc.
   e) False. There is an association with dermatitis herpetiformis.

5 a) True.
   b) False.
   c) True.
   d) True.
   e) False.

6 a) False. Hypothyroidism is a cause.
   b) False. These cause diarrhoea. Aluminium-containing antacids are constipating.
   c) True. This is a congenital condition featuring an aganglionic segment of large bowel.
   d) True.
   e) True. Opiate analgesics are a common cause.

7 a) True.
   b) False.
   c) True.
   d) True. This causes large bowel obstruction.
   e) False.

8 a) False.
   b) False.
   c) True. There is reduced hepatic protein synthesis.
   d) True. There is reduced protein intake.
   e) True. There is increased renal excretion of albumin.

9 a) False. The liver is most commonly involved.
   b) False. The survival rate is approximately 75–85 per cent for this group.
   c) False. Individuals found to be affected with familial adenomatous polyposis should be offered this operation.
   d) False.
   e) True. This is the sensation of incomplete evacuation of the bowels after defecation.

10 a) False. Melaena results from upper gastrointestinal haemorrhage, from a site proximal to the transverse colon.
   b) False. Obstructive jaundice gives rise to pale stools.
   c) False. At least 50 mL of blood is needed.
   d) True. This drug is occasionally used for the treatment of peptic ulceration.
   e) True. Steatorrhoea involves the passage of pale, bulky, offensive stools.

11 a) True. This may occur during insertion of the central line.
   b) False.
   c) True. Insulin therapy is often needed.
   d) True. Fluid balance must be checked meticulously.
   e) True. This is the most important complication. Pathogens may enter the blood at the site of tube insertion.

12 a) False. Bleeding varices are an emergency and should be treated aggressively.
   b) False. The patient must always be adequately resuscitated before endoscopy.
   c) False. This procedure may be performed in an endoscopy unit.
   d) True. This is a vasoconstrictor (an antidiuretic hormone [ADH] analogue), useful for controlling variceal bleeds.
   e) False. The tube uses balloon tamponade to compress varices and control a bleed.

13 a) True. Due to inadequate intake of food.
   b) False.
   c) False.
   d) True. Causing anorexia.
   e) True. Causing malabsorption of nutrients.

14 a) False. The commonest cause is peptic ulceration.
   b) False. Urgent endoscopy is indicated if there is continued bleeding, liver disease, or shock.
   c) False. Most heal spontaneously.
   d) False. Varices are often injected at the first endoscopy.
   e) True. This may occur after aortic graft surgery.

15 a) False.
   b) False.
   c) True. Long-standing infection gives rise to chronic gastritis, which predisposes to gastric cancer.
   d) False.
   e) True. The atrophic gastritis in this condition confers a small increased risk of gastric cancer.

16 a) False.
   b) False. This is a functional disorder.
   c) True. The inherited colonic polyp syndromes predispose to colorectal cancer.
   d) False. This is caused by *Clostridium difficile*, and may occur after broad-spectrum antibiotic therapy.
   e) True. There is an increased risk of colorectal cancer in those with extensive ulcerative colitis for over 10 years.

17 a) False. Bile-stained vomitus requires an obstruction distal to the pylorus.
   b) False. A gastrocolic fistula gives rise to faeculent vomit. Distal intestinal obstruction is another cause.
   c) True.
   d) False.
   e) False. Hypercalcaemia is a cause.

18 a) False. Anaphylaxis is not a feature.
   b) False. Serology for anti-endomysial antibodies, tissue transglutaminase antibodies and anti-gliadin antibodies are useful investigations.
   c) False. Flattened mucosa with subtotal villous atrophy is the typical finding.
   d) False. Treatment is largely by avoidance of gluten-containing foods.
   e) True. Oesophageal and small bowel carcinoma, and gastrointestinal lymphoma are complications.

19 a) False. These are a complication of hepatic portal vein hypertension.
   b) False.
   c) True. This is a premalignant lesion, in which squamous epithelium is transformed into columnar epithelium in the lower oesophagus.
   d) False. This is a cause of gastro-oesophageal reflux disease (GORD).
   e) True. This may follow on from Barrett's oesophagus.

20 a) True. This is seen as gross dilatation of the colon.
   b) False.
   c) True.
   d) False. Colonic gas is almost always present.
   e) False. Faeces give a mottled appearance in the colon.

21 a) True.
   b) False. The incubation period of Salmonella is 12–48 h, while that for Campylobacter is 48–96 h.
   c) False. Ciprofloxacin is the drug of choice.
   d) False. Profuse watery diarrhoea, or 'rice water' stools, are typical.
   e) False. The organism has a preference for reheated rice.

22 a) False. It is the second commonest, behind lung cancer.
    b) False. These genetic syndromes account for less than 5 per cent of cases. Most cancers are sporadic.
    c) False. The rectum is the commonest site, followed by the sigmoid colon.
    d) False. Right-sided cancers may be asymptomatic. Patients may present with anaemia, weight loss, or an abdominal mass.
    e) False. Biopsies are possible with colonoscopy.

23 a) False. The aetiology is unknown in the majority of cases. The condition is an oesophageal motility disorder.
    b) True.
    c) False. This finding is noted on barium swallow investigation.
    d) False. This intervention succeeds in 80 per cent of cases.
    e) True. Squamous cell carcinoma of the oesophagus is a complication.

24 a) False. This is a degeneration of the cervical vertebrae and intervertebral discs.
    b) True. Oesophageal motility may be affected.
    c) True. This is known as presbyoesophagus.
    d) True. This can cause a functional dysphagia.
    e) True. Dysphagia may occur if the brainstem is affected.

25 a) False. Lying down worsens symptoms.
    b) True.
    c) False.
    d) False. This exacerbates symptoms at night.
    e) True.

26 a) False. Approximately 90 per cent can be palpated.
    b) True.
    c) False. It is the persistent sensation of a full rectum despite attempts at defecation, caused by a rectal tumour.
    d) True. Right-sided tumours often present with weight loss and anaemia; left-sided tumours usually present with obstructive symptoms.
    e) False.

27 a) False.
    b) True. Proton pump inhibitors (PPIs) need to be halted for 1 week before the test is performed.
    c) False.
    d) True. IgG antibodies are present.
    e) True. Biopsy analysis may involve culture, histology, or the rapid urease test.

28 a) False. Stage D involves distant metastases.
    b) True.
    c) False. Stage B describes a tumour that extends across the bowel wall. Stage C involves regional lymph nodes.
    d) False. The prognosis is poor – 5-year survival is less than 5 per cent.
    e) False. Computed tomography (CT) scanning is an excellent investigation for staging.

29 a) False. Weight loss occurs.
   b) True. This is a genetic disorder involving obesity, mental retardation and small genitalia.
   c) True. Weight gain is a very common side-effect.
   d) False.
   e) True. Excess corticosteroid causes weight gain.

30 a) False. The infection is linked with low socio-economic status.
   b) True. It seems that the infection is transmitted mainly during childhood.
   c) False. Duodenal ulcers are more common.
   d) False. This is true of duodenal ulcers.
   e) False. This is caused by a pancreatic adenoma that secretes gastrin, causing excessive acid production.

31 a) True. Non steroidal anti-inflammatory drugs (NSAIDs) are a common cause of peptic ulceration.
   b) True.
   c) True. Corticosteroids are a risk factor.
   d) False.
   e) True.

32 a) False. The sigmoid colon is most frequently involved.
   b) True. A low-fibre diet is thought to be the cause.
   c) False. The colicky pain tends to be left-sided.
   d) False. Antispasmodic drugs are useful for colicky pain in diverticular disease. Antimotility drugs are contraindicated.
   e) False. The disease is more common as age increases.

33 a) False. Epstein–Barr virus is the responsible pathogen. The disorder occurs in HIV infection.
   b) True.
   c) True. Mouth rinsing after inhalation is preventative.
   d) False. Glossitis is caused by anaemia due to B_{12}, folate or iron deficiency.
   e) False. Alcohol, tobacco, and the betel nut are implicated in the aetiology.

34 a) True. This is a multisystem disorder involving oral and genital ulceration, inflammatory eye lesions and neurological involvement.
   b) True.
   c) True.
   d) True.
   e) True. Oral ulceration is a well-recognized feature of Crohn's disease.

35 a) False.
   b) True. This describes tender lesions on the shins.
   c) True.
   d) False.
   e) True. This is an ulcerating skin condition.

36 a) False. Skip lesions are a feature of Crohn's disease.
   b) True.
   c) False. Granulomas are present in Crohn's disease but absent in ulcerative colitis.
   d) True. TB and Crohn's disease both have a predilection for the terminal ileum.
   e) False. Smoking is a risk factor for Crohn's disease but appears to be protective against ulcerative colitis.

37 a) True.
   b) True.
   c) True.
   d) True.
   e) True.

38 a) True. Because of the risk of perforation.
   b) True.
   c) False. This complication is more common in ulcerative colitis.
   d) True.
   e) True. There is a serious risk of perforation.

39 a) False.
   b) True. For squamous cell carcinoma.
   c) True. For adenocarcinoma.
   d) True. For squamous cell carcinoma.
   e) True. For squamous cell carcinoma.

40 a) False. Steroid therapy is usually tailed off in favour of steroid-sparing agents.
   b) True.
   c) True. An anti-tumour necrosis factor (TNF)-α antibody.
   d) True.
   e) False. They are the treatment of choice for maintenance of remission in ulcerative colitis.

41 a) False. Haemorrhage is typically painless.
   b) True.
   c) True. Fistulae may occur between the colon and small bowel, vagina, or bladder.
   d) True. A combination of cefuroxime and metronidazole is a typical regime.
   e) False.

42 a) False. Hyperthyroidism causes diarrhoea. Hypothyroidism is a cause of constipation.
   b) True.
   c) True.
   d) False. This is a cause of constipation. Hypocalcaemia may cause diarrhoea.
   e) True. Malabsorption syndromes can cause diarrhoea or steatorrhoea.

43 a) True. Globus hystericus.
   b) True. A post-cricoid web may occur. This is known as the Paterson–Brown-Kelly or Plummer–Vinson syndrome.
   c) False. This causes projectile vomiting.
   d) True. Oesophageal motility is impaired.
   e) False. Reflux is a feature.

44 a) False. Diarrhoea or constipation may occur. Explosive diarrhoea suggests an infective cause.
   b) True.
   c) False. This is a feature of organic disease, not a functional disorder.
   d) False.
   e) True. This is one of the diagnostic criteria.

EMQ ANSWERS

1 UPPER GASTROINTESTINAL BLEEDING

1 D This gentleman has had a massive and ultimately fatal gastrointestinal bleed. With the history of an aneurysm operation, an **aorto-enteric fistula**, a communication between the repaired aorta and the GI tract must be considered.

2 C Crunchy skin is a sign of surgical emphysema, air in the subcutaneous tissues. The differential diagnosis of haematemesis after forceful vomiting includes **oesophageal rupture** and Mallory–Weiss tear. The latter does not cause surgical emphysema.

3 F Multiple ulcers within the duodenum are unusual. A high serum gastrin can be attributed to a gastrinoma, causing the **Zollinger–Ellison syndrome**, which causes recurrent GI ulceration often refractory to proton pump inhibitor therapy.

4 A Signs of chronic liver disease combined with massive haematemesis suggest bleeding from **oesophageal varices**. These patients have an extremely high mortality.

5 B **Gastric carcinoma** is an uncommon cause of haematemesis, but is the only option given that would result in a mass with lymphadenopathy. Note that smoking is associated with stomach cancer.

2 CAUSES OF DYSPHAGIA 1

1 C Koilonychia (spoon-shaped nails) is a sign of iron-deficiency anaemia, which is probably secondary to menorrhagia in this patient. This patient has Paterson–Brown–Kelly (Plummer–Vinson) syndrome: an **oesophageal web** secondary to iron-deficiency anaemia.

2 J This patient has signs of mitral stenosis, which causes an **enlarged left atrium**. If the chamber becomes significantly dilated, it can compress the oesophagus resulting in dysphagia.

3 E This patient has four features of **scleroderma**: oesophageal involvement, microstomia (a small mouth), Raynaud's phenomenon and sclerodactyly. Others include telangiectasia and calcinosis.

4 F **Myasthenia gravis** often presents with ptosis and fatigue, which typically worsens with repeated activity. In this case, this is associated with a thymoma, as evidenced by the superior mediastinal mass on chest radiography.

5 G A **pharyngeal pouch** is an idiopathic weakness of the pharyngeal mucosa through Killian's dehiscence, a triangular area in the wall of the pharynx. As the pouch grows in size, it can cause pressure on the oesophagus resulting in difficulty swallowing.

3 CAUSES OF DYSPHAGIA 2

1 A This patient has probably swallowed a **foreign body**: in the elderly false teeth are common culprits, while young children mostly swallow coins.

2 F **Achalasia** is a disorder where there is degeneration of the oesophageal myenteric plexus. Peristaltic contractions of the oesophagus are lost and there is failure of relaxation of the lower oesophageal sphincter. Patients tend to be between 30 and 50 years old. Dysphagia is intermittent and tends to be worse for liquids. Occasionally, fluid regurgitation at night results in aspiration pneumonia.

3 C This story is worrying and **oesophageal carcinoma** is the most likely cause. There may also be a history of Barrett's oesophagus or achalasia.

4 G Patients with **oesophageal strictures** will have a history of GORD or hiatus hernia. The pain of the reflux is worse on lying flat. The stricture is secondary to an inflammatory process.

5 E Patients with a **pharyngeal pouch** tend to be elderly and may have noticed a swelling in the posterior triangle of the neck. Other symptoms include recurrent sore throat, aspiration pneumonia, lung abscesses and gurgling noises in the neck.

4 CONDITIONS AFFECTING THE STOMACH

1 B A **sliding hiatus hernia** occurs when the oesophagogastric junction moves into the thorax with part of the stomach. This contrasts with a rolling hiatus hernia, where the position of the oesophagogastric junction is preserved.

2 E The finding of an 'olive' in the epigastrium is characteristic of **pyloric stenosis**, which is associated with projectile vomiting in children 3–6 weeks of age.

3 H A pan-gastritis is typical of pernicious anaemia, an **autoimmune gastritis**; this patient also has symptoms of a peripheral neuropathy from the B_{12} deficiency associated with this condition.

4 F Partial gastrectomy is a risk factor for **adenocarcinoma of the stomach**, with a greater than 5-fold increased chance of developing this condition after 20 years.

5 A NSAIDs commonly cause **erosive gastritis**, manifested by epigastric pain. Cyclo-oxygenase-2 (COX-2) inhibitors such as rofecoxib were developed to reduce this complication, but many have been withdrawn because of an excess in cardiac mortality detected after they were launched.

5 MALABSORPTION

1 B **Coeliac disease** is extremely common in the Irish population, and often presents insidiously. In this case, the presentation is with malabsorption and steatorrhoea. The typical findings on duodenal biopsy are subtotal villous atrophy and crypt hypertrophy.

2 A **Crohn's disease** often presents with non-specific symptoms of lethargy and malaise. It has a predilection for the terminal ileum, the site of absorption of vitamin B_{12}, and may therefore cause signs of malabsorption.

3 F Calcification of the pancreas is a sign of **chronic pancreatitis**. This patient has malabsorption secondary to this condition, which is probably due to his excessive alcohol intake.

4 G Surgery is usually the last resort in Crohn's disease. This patient has had multiple laparotomies, and probably multiple bowel resections. She now presents with symptoms of **short bowel syndrome**: there is not enough small bowel left to allow enough nutrients to be absorbed.

5 H **Iatrogenic.** Orlistat is a pancreatic lipase inhibitor which prevents the breakdown of fats in the intestinal lumen. A common side-effect is therefore steatorrhoea.

6 COMPLICATIONS OF INFLAMMATORY BOWEL DISEASE

1 G **Primary sclerosing cholangitis** is an autoimmune disease associated with inflammatory bowel disease, particularly ulcerative colitis. The biliary tree is frequently not dilated despite a cholestatic picture from the liver function tests. pANCA is often positive.

2 B **Anterior uveitis**, inflammation of the anterior chamber of the eye, can occur with both Crohn's disease and ulcerative colitis. Diagnosis is made with a slit lamp. Episcleritis can also occur, but presents with scleral injection rather than visual disturbance.

3 C **Pyoderma gangrenosum** is an ulcerating lesion, usually affecting the lower limbs.

4 E Ulcerative colitis strongly predisposes to **colorectal carcinoma**: the lifetime risk is around 5 per cent. Surveillance colonoscopy is used to detect lesions whilst still at an early stage. Diagnosis by clinical symptoms alone can be difficult, as many (such as abdominal pain, iron-deficiency anaemia, and diarrhoea) overlap with ulcerative colitis.

5 J Inflammatory bowel disease is a cause of **erythema nodosum**, which presents as tender red nodules, particularly over the shins.

7 CONSTIPATION

1 C **Iatrogenic.** The most common side-effect of verapamil is constipation.

2 A Previous abdominal surgery predisposes to adhesions causing **small bowel obstruction**. The valvulae conniventes are the markings traversing the entire diameter of the small intestine, and are useful in differentiating small from large bowel obstruction.

3 F **Hirschsprung's disease** occurs when neural cells fail to migrate into the colon, leaving a segment of aganglionic bowel. The presentation is usually with a congenital mega-colon and symptoms of bowel obstruction.

4 G Abdominal pain relieved by defecation, the passage of mucus, and bloating are all part of the Rome criteria for the diagnosis of **irritable bowel syndrome**. Women are two to three times more likely to develop irritable bowel syndrome than men.

5 I This patient has many signs and symptoms of **hypothyroidism**, which is an important diagnosis to make as it is an eminently treatable cause of constipation.

8 DIARRHOEA

1 A Haemolysis and renal failure make up the haemolytic uraemic syndrome, which is strongly associated with *Escherichia coli* O157 infection. *E. coli* is commonly transmitted from undercooked beef products.

2 H **Overflow diarrhoea** is a common cause of diarrhoea and faecal incontinence in the elderly. Treatment is by faecal disimpaction.

3 B A stool weight of 1.2 kg is significantly elevated, indicating secretory diarrhoea. The most likely underlying diagnosis here is multiple endocrine neoplasia (MEN) type 1, with the triad of an anterior pituitary tumour, parathyroid adenoma and **pancreatic tumour**, probably a VIPoma.

4 G **Iatrogenic.** Metformin frequently causes gastrointestinal upset. This is usually transient and settles spontaneously.

5 I A microcytic anaemia in the elderly is presumed to be **colonic carcinoma** until proven otherwise. The change in bowel habit also supports this diagnosis.

9 INFECTIVE DIARRHOEA

1 H Diarrhoea starting shortly after broad-spectrum antibiotic therapy is often due to *Clostridium difficile*; the eradication of the usual bowel flora allows these spores to infect the GI tract. The rise in the use of ineffective alcohol gels, instead of hand washing with soap and water, has contributed to an increase in the rates of *Clostridium difficile* infection.

2 I Rice water stool (looking like the white water produced when rice is washed) is the characteristic description of the diarrhoea produced after infection with *Vibrio cholerae*. Cholera is endemic in West Bengal.

3 J Viral gastroenteritis is highly infectious, and causes particular problems in institutions where outbreaks may spread rapidly. **Norwalk-like virus** is often the culprit.

4 C *Bacillus cereus* typically infects contaminated rice, producing a toxin that can cause either vomiting or diarrhoea.

5 G The paralysis affecting this gentleman is caused by infection with *Clostridium botulinum*. Initially, this presents as gastrointestinal upset progressing to cranial nerve palsies, and sometimes paralysis. Treatment is with antitoxin and respiratory support if needed.

10 ABDOMINAL PAIN 1

1 I The positive findings in this history are severe left hypochondrial pain and a microcytic anaemia. **Sickle cell disease** can produce both of these findings in a sickle cell crisis affecting the spleen.

2 B **Myocardial infarction** can present as epigastric pain. The elevated creatine kinase in this patient is derived from damaged myocardium.

3 G Part of the right lower lobe is posterior to the liver. **Pneumonia** can therefore give rise to pain seemingly derived from the abdomen.

4 F The long history of constitutional symptoms and gastrointestinal upset combined with clinically significant vitamin B_{12} deficiency makes **inflammatory bowel disease** most probable. The likely diagnosis is Crohn's disease affecting the terminal ileum.

5 A Few conditions produce pain as severe as that of childbirth! **Renal colic** presents with undulating abdominal pain and haematuria. The diagnosis can be made by abdominal radiography, or by low dose CT of the kidney, ureters and bladder.

11 ABDOMINAL PAIN 2

1 H This young woman is shocked and unwell; she potentially has a **ruptured ectopic pregnancy**. This diagnosis should always be considered in patients of childbearing age with abdominal pain.

2 B **Acute pancreatitis** is the likely diagnosis in this patient. In the UK, the most common causes of acute pancreatitis are gallstones and alcohol excess.

3 D **Ischaemic colitis** is becoming increasingly common due to the ageing population. Causes include embolic events (e.g. atrial fibrillation) and low-flow states (e.g. shock). The pain is often preceded by a few episodes of mild, transient abdominal pain (much like that of diverticulitis) progressing to peritonitis. Investigations will reveal a leucocytosis, raised lactate and profound acidosis.

4 J Right-sided abdominal pain, low grade fever and a systemic inflammatory response all point towards the likely diagnosis of **acute appendicitis**. In difficult cases, ultrasound scanning can sometimes provide additional information.

5 I **Intestinal obstruction** is a common surgical emergency which carries a good prognosis if recognized promptly. At least 80 per cent of cases are due to small bowel obstruction, usually caused by adhesions, hernias or neoplasia. An abdominal X-ray will confirm the diagnosis in most cases, showing dilated gas-filled loops.

12 INVESTIGATION OF ABDOMINAL PAIN

1 A This history is very suggestive of gallstones; an **ultrasound of the abdomen** is the best way of confirming this diagnosis. Although the patient here is stereotypically fat, fertile, female and 40, gallstones are common in the entire adult population.

2 A This man probably has an abdominal aortic aneurysm but is cardiovascularly stable. Ideally he would have a CT of the abdomen, but in this case, an **ultrasound of the abdomen** would suffice. Had he been shocked, investigations would be inappropriate: he would need an emergency laparotomy and aneurysm repair.

3 D An **abdominal X-ray** would show dilated loops of bowel typical of bowel obstruction.

4 C The history sounds like ureteric colic. A **urine dipstick** will typically show blood, and helps to verify the diagnosis. It is important to confirm haematuria in cases of suspected ureteric colic, to avoid unnecessary radiation exposure from an intravenous urogram.

5 I **OGD** is the most useful investigation as it is both diagnostic and therapeutic. This patient is probably suffering from gastric erosions or peptic ulceration.

13 DRUGS USED IN GASTROENTEROLOGY 1

1 G **Misoprostol** is a prostaglandin analogue, which is used to protect the gastric mucosa from NSAID-associated ulceration in vulnerable populations.

2 A **Ranitidine** is an H_2-blocker, used to decrease gastric acid secretion.

3 C **Sodium picosulfate** is a stimulant laxative, usually used as bowel preparation in patients before colonoscopy or colonic surgery.

4 I **Mesalazine**, 5-aminosalicylic acid, is used in the management of inflammatory bowel disease. Derivatives include balsalazide and olsalazine.

5 H **Omeprazole** is a proton pump inhibitor and a highly effective suppressor of gastric acid secretion. It is used in the management of peptic ulceration and gastro-oesophageal reflux disease.

14 DRUGS USED IN GASTROENTEROLOGY 2

1 H Proton pump inhibitors such as **lansoprazole** are the most powerful pharmacological agents used to suppress gastric acid production.

2 I **Mesalazine** and other 5-aminosalicylic acid derivatives are used as immuno-modulators in inflammatory bowel disease. The exact mechanism of action is still however unclear.

3 E **Metoclopramide**, a dopamine antagonist, is used as an antiemetic; it also hastens gastric emptying.

4 B **Loperamide** slows intestinal motility, increasing the amount of water reabsorbed, thereby reducing diarrhoea.

5 C Bowel-cleansing solutions such as **sodium picosulfate** are used to clear any solid material from the GI tract before procedures such as colonoscopy.

15 ORAL ULCERATION

1 D **Stevens–Johnson syndrome**, erythema multiforme affecting the mucous membranes, can be a side-effect of penicillin usage.

2 C Infection is unlikely given the history of no new sexual contacts. Oral and genital ulcers occur in **Behçet's syndrome**, an autoimmune condition of unknown aetiology.

3 A **Trauma** to the oral mucosa can cause ulceration. In this case, poorly fitting dentures are the cause of this elderly woman's troubles.

4 I **Squamous cell carcinoma** presents as an irregular lesion within the oral cavity. Smoking is strongly associated.

5 E **Idiopathic**, or aphthous, ulceration is a common problem in the general population. Treatment is usually supportive; in difficult cases topical steroids may be helpful.

16 RECTAL BLEEDING

1 H The most common cause of isolated fresh rectal bleeding is **haemorrhoids**, especially in a young patient in whom an insidious aetiology would be most unusual. Physical examination is typically unremarkable; proctoscopy usually reveals the offending vessels.

2 J The long history of bloody diarrhoea and abdominal pain in a young person point towards inflammatory bowel disease, most probably **ulcerative colitis**.

3 B **Anal fissures**, longitudinal tears in the anal sphincter, are exceptionally painful. Patients often comment that they feel like they are passing razor blades, and delay defecation for as long as possible to avoid pain. Treatment with laxatives and topical glyceryl trinitrate ointment is usually successful.

4 C **Dysentery**, infectious bloody diarrhoea, is common throughout the developing world and is transmitted through contaminated water. The causative organisms are usually *Shigella* or amoeba.

5 G **Intussusception**, the telescoping of one part of bowel into the next, affects children and typically causes bowel obstruction with characteristic redcurrant jelly stools.

17 INVESTIGATION OF RECTAL BLEEDING

1 B **Rigid sigmoidoscopy** can easily and safely visualize the terminal 20 cm of the gastro-intestinal tract, the territory where solitary rectal ulcers are found.

2 A Microcytic anaemia in the elderly is presumed to be colonic carcinoma until proven otherwise. The usual method of investigating a patient would be colonoscopy which can be both diagnostic and therapeutic. However, in the very frail, **CT colography** is a reasonable, and much less invasive, alternative.

3 I Meckel's diverticulum is usually diagnosed at laparotomy. Pre-operatively though a **technetium nuclear medicine scan** can be used to detect the ectopic gastric cells in a Meckel's diverticulum by attaching the radioactive isotope to a compound which binds to gastric mucosa; the lesion is too proximal to be reached with a colonoscope.

4 G Massive rectal bleeding is often found to be secondary to a significant upper gastro-intestinal bleed. In this alcoholic patient, oesophageal varices are the most likely cause of haemorrhage. **Upper GI endoscopy** in this setting can be diagnostic and therapeutic, with either sclerosing injections or banding possible.

5 F Pinpointing the source of gastrointestinal bleeding secondary to angiodysplasia can be challenging. **Visceral angiography** can sometimes identify ectatic vessels where endoscopy has failed.

18 PERIANAL CONDITIONS

1 C **A pilonidal sinus** is an infected tract at the top of the natal cleft caused by ingrowing hairs. Patients with predominantly sedentary occupations, such as lorry drivers are predisposed to this condition. Treatment is by excision of the hair network.

2 A The unpleasant sensation being described by this patient is tenesmus. This can be due to the presence of a mass in the rectum which leads to the urge to defecate while the rectum is empty of faeces. The underlying diagnosis here is probably **rectal cancer**.

3 F A **perianal haematoma**, due to a thrombosed external pile, can be particularly un-comfortable. It appears as a small purple lump, often at the anal verge. If indicated for pain relief, treatment is by incision and drainage.

4 B A **fistula-in-ano** is a common complication of perianal abscesses. An abnormal communication forms between the rectum and the skin, leading to a chronic discharge. Treatment is notoriously difficult and may require further surgery.

5 D **Anal warts** are a sexually transmitted infection, caused by the human papillomavirus. They present as small soft growths occurring around the anus or external genitalia in both men and women. There is no cure, but the lesions may be amenable to cryo-therapy with liquid nitrogen.

X-RAY ANSWERS

1   The barium meal shows a grossly dilated oesophagus, with a smooth narrowing at its lower end. This appearance is consistent with achalasia, failure of relaxation of the lower oesophageal sphincter. The long history makes malignancy much less likely.

2   a) The abdominal X-ray shows multiple air-filled dilated loops of small bowel (note the valvulae conniventes crossing the entire width). The diagnosis is small bowel obstruction.
    b) The most common cause of small bowel obstruction is adhesions after previous abdominal surgery, in this case an appendicectomy.

3   There is free air under both hemidiaphragms indicating the perforation of an intra-abdominal viscus, such as bowel. Common causes of a pneumoperitoneum include perforated peptic ulcer, diverticulum or appendix. Air under the diaphragm may also be seen for a few days after laparotomy or laparoscopy.

4   a) The nasogastric tube lies in the right main bronchus instead of the stomach – it is imperative that this is removed as soon as possible and resited correctly.
    b) A metallic oesophageal stent is visible – this is a palliative treatment for dysphagia in patients with unresectable disease or those unfit for surgery.

5   There is an irregular narrowing of the ascending colon, which is likely to be a colonic carcinoma. These often present insidiously with weight loss and anaemia, rather than a change in bowel habit. There are also some left-sided colonic diverticula.

6   a) There is a grossly dilated loop of bowel arising from the pelvis. This is caused by a sigmoid volvulus, which has the characteristic appearance of a coffee bean on abdominal X-ray.
    b) Decompression of the volvulus with a flatus tube is often successful, and leads to a rush of faeces per rectum. For refractory cases, laparotomy is required.

CHAPTER 6

The liver, pancreas and biliary tree

MULTIPLE CHOICE QUESTIONS

1   The following laboratory results are consistent with excessive alcohol consumption:
   a) Reduced prothrombin time (PT)
   b) High potassium
   c) Reduced mean red blood cell volume (MCV)
   d) Raised γ-glutamyl transferase (γ-GT)
   e) Raised thyroxine

2   The following statements are true of primary biliary cirrhosis:
   a) The sex distribution of the disease is equal
   b) It is caused by excessive alcohol intake
   c) The most useful diagnostic blood test is anti-nuclear antibody levels
   d) It is not a fatal disease
   e) Colestyramine provides symptomatic relief

3   Regarding blood tests in the investigation of liver disease:
   a) A raised alpha-fetoprotein level is suggestive of hepatocellular carcinoma
   b) Microcytosis without anaemia is a common finding in patients who abuse alcohol
   c) Alcoholic cirrhosis gives rise to low α_1-antitrypsin levels
   d) Serum copper is normally raised in Wilson's disease
   e) Serum ferritin is raised in hereditary haemochromatosis

4   The following statements are true with regard to liver function tests:
   a) A high serum albumin indicates acute liver damage
   b) A short PT may be due to vitamin K deficiency
   c) Haemolytic jaundice will produce a conjugated hyperbilirubinaemia
   d) Cholestasis produces a raised alkaline phosphatase level
   e) Alcohol consumption reduces GGT (gamma-glutamyl transferase) levels

5 Hepatomegaly may be caused by:
 a) Malaria
 b) Chronic renal failure
 c) Leukaemia
 d) Right heart failure
 e) Hepatic encephalopathy

6 Clinical features of chronic pancreatitis include:
 a) Steatorrhoea
 b) Haematemesis
 c) Weight loss
 d) Melaena
 e) Epigastric pain

7 The following investigations are recognized to be useful in identifying gallstones in the common bile duct:
 a) Magnetic resonance cholangiopancreatography
 b) Plain abdominal radiograph
 c) Abdominal ultrasound
 d) Mesenteric angiogram
 e) Endoscopic retrograde cholangiopancreatography

8 The following should be treated with antibiotics:
 a) Chronic cholecystitis
 b) Biliary colic
 c) Cholangitis
 d) Asymptomatic gallstones
 e) Acute cholecystitis

9 The following measures are of use in the management of hepatic encephalopathy:
 a) Lactulose
 b) Diazepam
 c) High-protein diet
 d) Neomycin
 e) Furosemide

10 Risk factors for pancreatic carcinoma include the following:
 a) Gallstones
 b) Angiodysplasia
 c) Chronic pancreatitis
 d) *Helicobacter pylori*
 e) Alcohol

11 The following are achievable by endoscopic retrograde cholangiopancreatography:
 a) Biliary stenting
 b) Cholecystectomy
 c) Sphincterotomy
 d) Removal of stones from the common bile duct
 e) Biopsy

12 The following statements are true of pancreatic carcinoma:
- a) Carcinoma of the ampulla of Vater carries the worst prognosis
- b) Carcinomas of the tail usually presents with painless jaundice
- c) The majority are squamous cell carcinomas
- d) Painless jaundice and a palpable gallbladder is more likely to be due to gallstones than to a pancreatic carcinoma
- e) Mean survival is 3 years

13 The following are signs of chronic liver disease:
- a) Spider naevi
- b) Erythema nodosum
- c) Parotid enlargement
- d) Scratch marks
- e) Gynaecomastia

14 The following statements are true of hepatitis C infection:
- a) The infection is acquired from consuming contaminated food
- b) Immunization is offered to high-risk groups in the UK
- c) Screening for the infection is by an anti-hepatitis C virus antibody test
- d) In most cases the infection is cleared spontaneously
- e) Cirrhosis is a complication

15 The following statements are true of liver tumours:
- a) Primary tumours are more common than secondary tumours
- b) CA 19-9 is the most useful tumour marker for hepatocellular carcinoma
- c) Cirrhosis is a risk factor for hepatocellular carcinoma
- d) The average life expectancy after diagnosis of hepatocellular carcinoma is 4 years
- e) Cholangiocarcinomas should not be stented for palliation

16 The following are recognized complications of fulminant hepatic failure:
- a) Hypoglycaemia
- b) Polycythaemia
- c) Hypercalcaemia
- d) Coagulopathy
- e) Cerebral oedema

17 Consequences of alcoholism include:
- a) Cardiomyopathy
- b) Deep vein thrombosis (DVT)
- c) Peptic ulceration
- d) Korsakoff's syndrome
- e) Acute pancreatitis

18 The following are contraindications for liver transplantation:
- a) Alcoholic liver disease
- b) Acute liver failure
- c) Primary biliary cirrhosis
- d) Metastatic liver disease
- e) Chronic hepatitis C infection

19 The following can cause jaundice:
   a) Lymph nodes at the porta hepatis
   b) Diabetes mellitus
   c) Sickle cell anaemia
   d) Simvastatin
   e) Gallstone ileus

20 Complications of gallstones include:
   a) Empyema
   b) Small bowel obstruction
   c) Hypercholesterolaemia
   d) Urinary tract infection
   e) Pancreatitis

21 The following statements are true of primary sclerosing cholangitis:
   a) The disease only affects the common bile duct
   b) There is an association with inflammatory bowel disease
   c) Cholangiocarcinoma is a complication
   d) The condition is diagnosed by positive anti-mitochondrial antibodies (AMA)
   e) Endoscopic retrograde cholangiopancreatography (ERCP) is a useful investigation

22 Causes of chronic pancreatitis include:
   a) Cystic fibrosis
   b) Hereditary haemochromatosis
   c) Diabetes mellitus
   d) Splenectomy
   e) Alcohol

23 The following are potential precipitants of hepatic encephalopathy:
   a) Constipation
   b) Morphine
   c) Variceal haemorrhage
   d) Urinary tract infection
   e) Transjugular intrahepatic portosystemic shunt

24 The following are useful in the management of chronic pancreatitis:
   a) Lifelong metronidazole
   b) Partial pancreatectomy
   c) Pancreatin
   d) Reduction in calorie intake
   e) Coeliac axis nerve block

25 The following statements are true of hereditary haemochromatosis:
   a) It is an autosomal dominant genetic disease
   b) Heart failure is a feature
   c) Diabetes mellitus is a feature
   d) Serum ferritin is low
   e) Penicillamine improves survival

26 The following statements are true with regards to gallstones:
   a) Any cause of haemolysis is a risk factor for cholesterol gallstones
   b) Females are at greater risk of developing cholesterol gallstones
   c) Pigment stones are large and solitary
   d) Approximately 50 per cent are radio-opaque and visible on plain abdominal radiograph
   e) The majority of stones are pigment stones

27 The following statements are true of hepatic encephalopathy:
   a) The condition is irreversible
   b) Ammonia is implicated in the aetiology
   c) Constructional apraxia is a feature
   d) It is best managed with haloperidol
   e) An electroencephalogram may be useful in the diagnosis

28 The following are known causes of liver cirrhosis:
   a) Gallstone ileus
   b) α_1-antitrypsin deficiency
   c) Zollinger–Ellison syndrome
   d) Chronic hepatitis B infection
   e) Wilson's disease

29 The following can cause jaundice:
   a) Sheehan's syndrome
   b) Hereditary haemochromatosis
   c) The oral contraceptive pill
   d) Gilbert's syndrome
   e) Anabolic steroids

30 The following statements are true of Wilson's disease:
   a) It is a sex-linked recessive genetic disease
   b) It may present with Parkinsonian features
   c) Ophthalmoscopy reveals Kayser–Fleischer rings around the retinas
   d) 24-h urinary copper is low
   e) The treatment of choice is plasma exchange

31 The following are causes of ascites:
   a) Peritoneal carcinomatosis
   b) Nephrotic syndrome
   c) Budd–Chiari syndrome
   d) Pancreatitis
   e) Ovarian tumour

32 The following statements are true of endoscopic retrograde cholangiopancreatography (ERCP):
   a) There is no risk of radiation from the procedure
   b) Pancreatitis is a complication
   c) Clotting function must be checked beforehand
   d) Sedation is not required
   e) The procedure is of little use if biliary duct stent insertion is required

33 The following are signs of chronic liver disease:
    a) Goitre
    b) Flapping tremor
    c) Cullen's sign
    d) Testicular atrophy
    e) Loss of body hair

34 In the investigation of jaundice, an abdominal ultrasound is useful for assessing:
    a) Dilatation of the bile ducts
    b) Fatty infiltration of the liver in alcoholics
    c) The presence of ascites
    d) The presence of hepatic metastases
    e) The presence of a liver abscess

35 The following statements are true of hepatitis A infection:
    a) The commonest mode of transmission is between intravenous drug users
    b) The infection is more common in developing countries
    c) In 50 per cent of cases, fulminant hepatitis ensues
    d) 10 per cent of cases become chronic carriers of hepatitis A infection
    e) Universal immunization against the disease is routine in the UK

36 Regarding the management of variceal haemorrhage:
    a) Transjugular intrahepatic portosystemic shunting (TIPS) is reserved for encephalo-
       pathic patients
    b) Emergency oesophageal transection is an option for acute uncontrollable rebleeds
    c) Rebleeding occurs in 10 per cent of patients within the first 2 weeks of the initial
       haemorrhage
    d) A beta-blocker is of use in long-term prevention of variceal rebleeding
    e) Repeated variceal banding is of little use in recurrent variceal bleeding

37 The following are signs of chronic liver disease that may be found in the hands:
    a) Splinter haemorrhages
    b) Leukonychia
    c) Onycholysis
    d) Clubbing
    e) Palmar erythema

38 The following statements are true of ascites:
    a) A fluid thrill indicates cardiac involvement
    b) Aspiration of ascitic fluid is required to differentiate between transudate and exudate
    c) Dietary protein restriction is useful in the management of ascites
    d) Bendroflumethiazide is the diuretic of choice for ascites
    e) A maximum of 1 litre of fluid should be drawn off during ascitic paracentesis

39 The following statements are true of hepatitis B infection:
    a) Sexual intercourse is an important mode of transmission
    b) The presence of hepatitis B e antigen (HBeAg) in the blood indicates high infectivity
    c) In the UK only medical students and doctors are routinely immunized
    d) There is currently no treatment available for chronic carriers
    e) Hepatocellular carcinoma is a complication

40 The following are recognized causes of portal vein hypertension:
   a) Acromegaly
   b) Budd–Chiari syndrome
   c) Chronic renal failure
   d) Right heart failure
   e) Phaeochromocytoma

41 The following are sequelae of decompensated liver cirrhosis:
   a) Renal failure
   b) Encephalopathy
   c) Spontaneous bacterial peritonitis
   d) Lung fibrosis
   e) Hepatocellular carcinoma

42 The following can cause liver cirrhosis:
   a) Cushing's syndrome
   b) Cystic fibrosis
   c) Hereditary haemochromatosis
   d) Phenylketonuria
   e) Methotrexate

43 The following statements are true of autoimmune hepatitis:
   a) Males are more commonly affected than females
   b) The disease may present with liver cirrhosis
   c) Anti-smooth muscle antibodies may be a positive finding
   d) Liver transplantation is first-line therapy
   e) Anti-liver/kidney antibodies may be a positive finding

Answers: see pages 169–175

EXTENDED MATCHING QUESTIONS

1 HEPATITIS

Each of the patients below has been diagnosed with hepatitis. Choose the most likely cause from the options given

A   Hepatitis A
B   Hepatitis B
C   Hepatitis C
D   Hepatitis D
E   Hepatitis E

F   Iatrogenic
G   Autoimmune hepatitis
H   Alcoholic hepatitis
I   Cytomegalovirus hepatitis
J   Infectious mononucleosis

1   A 27-year-old aid worker returns from West Africa as she is 26 weeks pregnant, and her husband is insistent that she have the baby in the UK. Three weeks later she becomes jaundiced and confused. Her husband takes her to the local hospital where she is diagnosed with fulminant hepatic failure. She dies on the intensive therapy unit (ITU) 11 days later.

2   A 56-year-old homeless man comes to the emergency department as he is feeling unwell. On examination, he smells of alcohol, is tender in the right upper quadrant and has an enlarged liver with ascites. His blood tests show haemoglobin (Hb) 10.1 g/dL, white cell count (WCC) 15×10^9/L, platelets 83×10^9/L, aspartate transaminase (AST) 928 IU/L, alanine transaminase (ALT) 402 IU/L, international normalized ratio (INR) 1.3 and ferritin 804 µg/L.

3   A 19-year-old student returns from his gap year backpacking in Asia. A week later he turns yellow and his mother is insistent that he go to the general practitioner (GP) for a diagnosis.

4   A 26-year-old computer programmer goes to her GP as she feels unwell. She has generalized lymphadenopathy and enlarged tonsils. He tells her she has a viral infection and advises bedrest and fluids. Two weeks later she returns still feeling very tired, and is now icteric. Blood tests show AST 122 IU/L, ALT 92 IU/L, and bilirubin 32 µmol/L.

5   A 32-year-old intravenous drug user is known to have hepatitis B and C from using dirty needles, but has never had any symptoms. He goes to the local walk-in centre having turned yellow. He has not been overseas at any point in his life. The doctor performs a liver screen and tells him he has yet another form of hepatitis from injecting drugs.

2 TESTS USED IN THE DIAGNOSIS OF LIVER DISEASE

Choose the most useful test used to help in the diagnosis of each of the conditions below

A   Antimitochondrial antibody
B   Antinuclear antibody
C   Antineutrophil cytoplasmic antibody
D   Anti-smooth muscle antibody
E   Caeruloplasmin

F α_1-antitrypsin
G   Haematinics
H α-fetoprotein
I   Hepatitis B surface antigen
J   Hepatitis B e antigen

1   Hereditary haemochromatosis
2   Primary biliary cirrhosis
3   Autoimmune hepatitis
4   Hepatocellular carcinoma
5   Wilson's disease

3 CAUSES OF LIVER DISEASE

All of the patients below have liver disease. Select the most likely aetiology from the options given

A   Budd–Chiari syndrome
B   Primary biliary cirrhosis
C   Cystic fibrosis
D   Alcohol
E   Hepatitis B

F   Wilson's disease
G   Hereditary haemochromatosis
H   Iatrogenic
I   Hepatitis C
J   Autoimmune hepatitis

1   A 21-year-old secretary presents to her GP with a tremor which is preventing her doing her job. On examination, she has peripheral stigmata of chronic liver disease, dyskinesia, and ataxia. During the consultation she keeps making involuntary movements, which she says have developed over the past month.

2   A 57-year-old milkman goes to his GP for a life assurance check-up, as he is a known diabetic. On examination, he looks well with a tan, but has signs of chronic liver disease and hepatomegaly. He denies drinking alcohol. He is embarrassed to admit that he lives alone because his wife left him as he was impotent.

3   A 67-year-old man goes to his GP complaining of vague abdominal pain and distension. He has known polycythaemia rubra vera, and is awaiting treatment for this. On examination, he has hepatomegaly, shifting dullness in the abdomen, and dilated veins around his umbilicus. He denies drinking alcohol or intravenous drug use.

4   A 71-year-old woman is seen by her rheumatologist as a routine follow-up for her severe rheumatoid arthritis, for which she takes methotrexate. When he sees her she has signs of chronic liver disease, with deranged liver biochemistry. A liver biopsy shows widespread fibrotic change with cirrhosis.

5   A 49-year-old woman is seen by her rheumatologist as a routine follow-up for her Sjögren's syndrome, for which she takes replacement tear solutions. When he sees her, she has signs of chronic liver disease, with deranged liver biochemistry. Anti-smooth muscle antibodies are positive.

4 HEPATOMEGALY

Choose the most likely cause of hepatomegaly for each of the clinical scenarios below

A Lymphoma
B Thalassaemia
C Pyogenic abscess
D Fatty liver
E Alcoholism

F Hydatid disease
G Hepatocellular carcinoma
H Amoebic abscess
I   Reye's syndrome
J Metastases

1 A 72-year-old man with severe chronic obstructive pulmonary disease (COPD) presents with jaundice. On examination, he has a hard irregular liver edge, 4 cm below the costal margin.

2 A 32-year-old Welsh sheep farmer presents to his GP as he has noticed that he has turned yellow. He has a dull ache in the right hypochondrium, with hepatomegaly 3 cm below the costal margin. An X-ray of the abdomen shows a round calcified structure within the liver.

3 A 73-year-old woman goes to her GP for her annual diabetic check-up. He examines her eyes and feet, and then proceeds to feel her abdomen, where he finds a smoothly enlarged liver, 4 cm below the costal margin. He asks her about her alcohol intake, and learns she has not drunk since she was in her 20s.

4 A 23-year-old medical student goes to the university health centre after returning from holiday in Pakistan. She complains of general malaise, fever and abdominal pain. On examination, she has tender hepatomegaly 6 cm below the costal margin. An ultrasound shows a large fluid-filled structure, from which the radiologist aspirates fluid, which he remarks looks like anchovy sauce.

5 A 51-year-old man goes to his GP with abdominal discomfort. He is known to have hereditary haemochromatosis. On examination, he has a significantly enlarged liver which has developed over the course of the past 3 months.

5 ASCITES

Choose the most likely cause of ascites for each of the clinical scenarios below

A   Malignancy
B   Hypoalbuminaemia
C   Cardiac failure
D   Meigs' syndrome
E   Ruptured ectopic pregnancy

F   Tuberculosis
G   Budd–Chiari syndrome
H   Trauma
I   Hypothyroidism
J   Acute pancreatitis

1   A 58-year-old teacher complains of increasing abdominal distension, having previously been fit and well. When she goes to visit the GP, she is found to have ascites and a right-sided pleural effusion. She undergoes surgery a week later and is pleased to find that a benign ovarian tumour was the cause of her symptoms.

2   A 78-year-old woman presents to the emergency department with abdominal pain and distension. The doctor is able to elicit shifting dullness and performs a diagnostic tap. The ascites is an exudate with an amylase of 1200 U/L.

3   A 34-year-old man returns from West Africa and is diagnosed with malaria. Three weeks later he notices his feet swelling up and goes to see his doctor, who also finds clinical evidence of ascites. Urinalysis reveals blood +, protein +++ and leucocytes +.

4   A 68-year-old retired welder is taken to see his GP by his wife. He has lost 5 kg of weight in the past 3 months, but has noticed his abdomen increasing in girth. Blood tests reveal Hb 10.2g/dL, mean corpuscular volume (MCV) 83 fL, WCC 9.1 × 10^9/L, platelets 351 × 10^9/L, CA 19 9 390 U/mL.

5   A 46-year-old Algerian immigrant goes to the local health centre with non-specific complaints of lethargy and fatigue. The doctor detects ascites, and performs a diagnostic tap, which is positive for acid-fast bacilli (AFB).

6 JAUNDICE

Choose the most likely cause of jaundice for each of the clinical scenarios below

A   Haemolysis
B   Carcinoma of the head of the pancreas
C   Dubin–Johnson syndrome
D   Iatrogenic
E   Hepatocellular carcinoma

F   Viral hepatitis
G   Gilbert's syndrome
H   Primary sclerosing cholangitis
I   Gallstones
J   Primary biliary cirrhosis

1 A 31-year-old woman registers as a new patient at her local surgery and tells the doctor that she has an inherited form of jaundice. She cannot remember the name but does recall her hepatologist telling her she suffers from conjugated jaundice.

2 A 26-year-old prisoner is transferred to the local hospital for the treatment of his tuberculosis. Three weeks later his sputum is devoid of tubercle bacilli and he is discharged from hospital. Two days later he returns, complaining he has turned yellow.

3 A 47-year-old actuary, who suffers from occasional flares of ulcerative colitis, makes an appointment to see his gastroenterologist, who performs some blood tests. Three days later she finds that pANCA (antineutrophil cytoplasmic antibody) is positive.

4 A 24-year-old doctor, who is usually fit and well, is told at work that she appears jaundiced. She has not eaten for the past 2 days because she is suffering from influenza.

5 A 79-year-old woman is well known to her GP with vague symptoms of right upper quadrant pain, which he has treated with paracetamol. She says that she finds eating fatty foods difficult. She returns to her GP one afternoon with jaundice and right upper quadrant pain.

7 COMPLICATIONS OF GALLSTONES

Each of the patients below is known to have gallstones. For each of the clinical scenarios below select the most likely complication from the options given

A Acute cholecystitis
B Chronic cholecystitis
C Acute pancreatitis
D Gallstone ileus
E Mucocele

F Empyema
G Ascending cholangitis
H Adenomyomatosis
I Cholecystoduodenal fistula
J Emphysematous cholecystitis

1 A 59-year-old woman is seen in clinic after her GP referred her with a right upper quadrant mass. Her only complaint is persistent nausea. The consultant confirms the presence of the mass, which is non tender, and asks for an ultrasound which shows a distended gallbladder with an impacted stone in the cystic duct.

2 A 69-year-old diabetic man is brought to the emergency department by ambulance. He is pyrexial, tachycardic and hypotensive. On examination of the abdomen, he is tender in the right upper quadrant with a positive Murphy's sign. The doctor is surprised as she can see the gallbladder filled with gas on the plain abdominal X-ray.

3 A 47-year-old woman presents to the emergency department with abdominal pain and vomiting. She is known to have gallstones but has never experienced any symptoms like this before. An abdominal X-ray reveals dilated loops of bowel.

4 A 36-year-old woman presents to hospital with severe epigastric pain. The serum amylase is 1543 IU/mL.

5 A 51-year-old man is admitted with acute cholecystitis. The surgeon decides to treat the patient conservatively, but there is no clinical improvement. The patient is taken to theatre where the surgeon has great difficulty removing the gallbladder through a laparoscopy port, as it is distended with pus.

Answers: see pages 175–177

X-RAY QUESTIONS

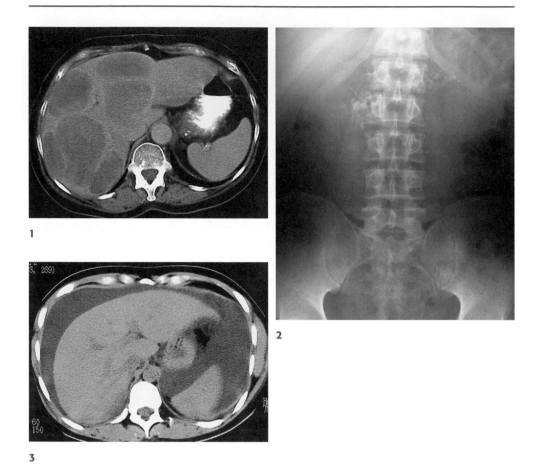

1

2

3

To answer the questions below, please refer to the corresponding numbered X-ray images above.

1   An 89-year-old woman goes to see her GP with a 3-month history of malaise and weight loss. On examination, he finds an enlarged liver and refers her to hospital for further investigation.
    a) What type of scan is this?
    b) What is the most likely cause for these appearances?

2   A 37-year-old man is well known to the doctors in the emergency department, as he attends frequently with alcohol misuse. One day, he tells the doctor that he has been suffering from abdominal pain for the last 3 months. She requests an abdominal X-ray. What is the cause of this patient's abdominal pain?

3   A 53-year-old man, with known alcoholic liver disease, attends outpatients complaining of increasing abdominal distension. The consultant requests a CT scan of his abdomen. What is the cause of the abdominal distension?

Answers: see page 177

ANSWERS

MCQ ANSWERS

1   a) False. This may be increased, due to impairment of clotting factor production.
     b) False.
     c) False. Raised MCV is the typical finding.
     d) True. This is an indication of hepatic damage.
     e) False.

2   a) False. It predominantly affects females.
     b) False. An autoimmune aetiology is suspected.
     c) False. Antimitochondrial antibodies are positive in over 95 per cent of cases.
     d) False. Death ultimately occurs from chronic liver failure or its complications.
     e) True. This relieves pruritus.

3   a) True.
     b) False. Alcohol typically causes macrocytosis.
     c) False. α_1-antitrypsin deficiency causes cirrhosis and emphysema.
     d) False. It is low or normal.
     e) True.

4   a) False. Albumin is a marker of synthetic function, and falls in chronic liver disease.
     b) False. Vitamin K deficiency will produce a raised prothrombin time and international normalized ratio (INR).
     c) False. This causes an unconjugated hyperbilirubinaemia.
     d) True.
     e) False. GGT rises with alcohol consumption.

5   a) True.
     b) False.
     c) True. There is increased turnover of white blood cells in the reticulo-endothelial system.
     d) True.
     e) False. This is a consequence of decompensated liver disease.

6   a) True. This is a symptom of gastrointestinal malabsorption.
     b) False.
     c) True. Anorexia and weight loss may be profound.
     d) False.
     e) True. Pain often radiates through to the back.

7   a) True. This is a useful non-invasive procedure.
     b) False. Few gallstones are radio-opaque.
     c) True. This is the initial investigation of choice.
     d) False. This is used to image the mesenteric blood vessels in gastrointestinal bleeding.
     e) True. This is additionally useful as a therapeutic measure to remove gallstones from the common bile duct.

8 a) False. This is chronic inflammation of the gallbladder caused by gallstones.
   b) False. This is pain arising from obstruction of the cystic or common bile duct by a gallstone.
   c) True. This is inflammation or infection of the bile ducts.
   d) False. A large proportion of the elderly population have asymptomatic stones that require no treatment.
   e) True. This presents similarly to biliary colic but with a greater inflammatory component. Infection may supervene.

9 a) True. Laxatives prevent bacterial breakdown of intestinal matter, thereby reducing ammonia release.
   b) False. Sedatives exacerbate hepatic encephalopathy.
   c) False. This will worsen encephalopathy.
   d) True. This antibiotic sterilizes bowel bacteria.
   e) False. This may cause electrolyte disturbances, thereby exacerbating encephalopathy.

10 a) False.
   b) False.
   c) True. This is recognized as a precancerous lesion.
   d) False.
   e) True.

11 a) True. This relieves biliary obstruction and jaundice.
   b) False. Cholecystectomy is usually performed laparoscopically; sometimes an open operation is required.
   c) True. This refers to the sphincter of Oddi. The procedure allows smaller gallstones to pass into the small bowel.
   d) True. This is a common indication.
   e) True.

12 a) False. This tends to present early with jaundice, facilitating early detection.
   b) False. Carcinoma of the body or tail presents with epigastric pain, anorexia, weight loss. Painless jaundice is a feature of tumours of the pancreatic head.
   c) False. Ductal adenocarcinoma is the most frequent variety.
   d) False. Courvoisier's law states that painless jaundice with a palpable gallbladder is not due to gallstones.
   e) False. The prognosis is extremely poor, with a mean survival of less than 6 months.

13 a) True. These are telangiectasia in the distribution of the superior vena cava.
   b) False.
   c) True.
   d) True. These occur from pruritus.
   e) True.

14 a) False. It is transmitted via the intravenous or sexual route.
   b) False. There is no vaccine currently available.
   c) True. This may take at least a month to be detected.
   d) False. Eighty-five per cent become chronic carriers.
   e) True.

15 a) False. Metastatic liver disease is more frequent.
    b) False. α-Fetoprotein is most useful.
    c) True.
    d) False. It is usually less than 6 months.
    e) False. Stenting is useful to relieve jaundice.

16 a) True. This should be treated with intravenous (i.v.) dextrose solution.
    b) False.
    c) False.
    d) True. The liver's production of clotting factors is impaired. This is managed with vitamin K and fresh-frozen plasma.
    e) True. This is treated with i.v. mannitol 20 per cent.

17 a) True.
    b) False. Alcohol is not a risk factor for DVT.
    c) True. Bleeding peptic ulcers are a cause of haematemesis in alcoholics.
    d) True. This is thiamine deficiency causing memory impairment and confabulation.
    e) True. Alcohol and gallstones are the commonest causes of acute pancreatitis.

18 a) False. This is an indication for the procedure, provided the patient has given up drinking alcohol.
    b) False. Fulminant hepatic failure is an indication for transplantation.
    c) False.
    d) True.
    e) False.

19 a) True. This causes an obstructive jaundice.
    b) False.
    c) True. This can cause a haemolytic jaundice.
    d) True. Jaundice and hepatitis are side-effects of the statins.
    e) False. This is perforation of a gallstone into the small bowel, causing obstruction.

20 a) True. The obstructed gallbladder becomes filled with pus.
    b) True. Gallstone ileus occurs when a gallstone perforates through the gallbladder into the duodenum.
    c) False.
    d) False.
    e) True. This may occur if a gallstone occludes the pancreatic duct.

21 a) False. Intrahepatic and extrahepatic ducts are involved.
    b) True. Ulcerative colitis is associated with the disease.
    c) True.
    d) False. It is AMA negative. Antineutrophil cytoplasmic antibodies (ANCA) are usually present.
    e) True. This reveals multiple strictures in the biliary tree.

22 a) True. The pancreatic ducts become blocked with mucus.
    b) True. There is iron deposition in the pancreas.
    c) False.
    d) False.
    e) True. This is the commonest cause in the Western world.

23 a) True. This encourages intestinal protein breakdown, releasing ammonia into the bloodstream.
   b) True. Central nervous system (CNS) depressants precipitate encephalopathy.
   c) True. The blood in the intestine acts as a protein load, releasing ammonia on breakdown.
   d) True. Sepsis is a precipitant.
   e) True. Ammonia in the portal venous system bypasses the liver and passes to the brain unmetabolized.

24 a) False.
   b) True. This is indicated in those with intolerable pain.
   c) True. Pancreatic enzyme supplements are helpful to replace those enzymes lost by damaged pancreatic tissue.
   d) False. Anorexia and weight loss are common problems. Nutrition should be optimized.
   e) True. This may be useful in patients unresponsive to oral analgesia.

25 a) False. It is autosomal recessive.
   b) True. There is iron deposition in cardiac tissue.
   c) True. There is iron deposition in pancreatic tissue.
   d) False. It is raised.
   e) False. Desferrioxamine chelates iron and is used in those cases where venesection is inappropriate.

26 a) False. It is a risk factor for pigment stones.
   b) True.
   c) False. Pigment stones are small and usually multiple; cholesterol stones are larger and often solitary.
   d) False. Approximately 10 per cent are radio-opaque.
   e) False. Eighty per cent are cholesterol stones.

27 a) False.
   b) True. Intestinal bacteria release ammonia from protein breakdown; the compound is then absorbed and bypasses hepatic metabolism.
   c) True. Patients are asked to draw, for example, a five-pointed star.
   d) False. CNS depressants exacerbate the condition.
   e) True.

28 a) False. This occurs when a gallstone perforates through the gallbladder into the small bowel, causing obstruction.
   b) True. This is a rare genetic disorder, also causing emphysema.
   c) False. This involves hypersecretion of gastrin from a pancreatic gastrinoma, causing peptic ulceration.
   d) True. Hepatitis B and C are among the commonest causes.
   e) True. Toxic accumulation of copper in the liver gives rise to cirrhosis.

29 a) False. This is post-partum pituitary necrosis following circulatory collapse.
    b) True. Iron overload causes liver cirrhosis.
    c) True.
    d) True. An unconjugated hyperbilirubinaemia due to uridine diphospho (UDP)-glucuronyl transferase deficiency.
    e) True. These cause cholestasis.

30 a) False. It is an autosomal recessive disorder.
    b) True. Copper deposition in the basal ganglia causes tremor, dyskinesia and dementia.
    c) False. The rings are seen around the cornea, often with the aid of slit-lamp examination.
    d) False. It is raised.
    e) False. Treatment is with lifelong penicillamine.

31 a) True. This is widespread dissemination of carcinoma throughout the peritoneal cavity.
    b) True. Hypoalbuminaemia is a feature.
    c) True. This is hepatic vein thrombosis, causing portal vein hypertension.
    d) True.
    e) True. An ovarian fibroma, associated with ascites and a right-sided pleural effusion, is known as Meigs' syndrome.

32 a) False. It is performed with the aid of radiological screening.
    b) True.
    c) True. There is a risk of severe haemorrhage from the procedure.
    d) False. This is an uncomfortable procedure and sedation is given.
    e) False. This is one of the indications of ERCP.

33 a) False. This occurs in thyroid disorders.
    b) True.
    c) False. This is peri-umbilical discolouration in acute pancreatitis.
    d) True.
    e) True.

34 a) True.
    b) True.
    c) True.
    d) True.
    e) True.

35 a) False. Transmission is faecal-oral.
    b) True. This reflects the poorer standards of hygiene.
    c) False. This is a rare complication.
    d) False. There is no chronic carrier state.
    e) False. It is usually offered to people travelling to affected regions of the world.

36 a) False. This procedure is used if continued rebleeding occurs. It exacerbates encephalopathy in the long-term.
    b) True. This procedure is combined with ligation of the blood vessels that supply the bleeding varices.
    c) False. Approximately 50 per cent rebleed within this time period.
    d) True. Oral propranolol reduces primary bleeding, secondary bleeding, and mortality.
    e) False. Rebleeding rates are substantially reduced.

37 a) False. They are a sign of infective endocarditis.
    b) True.
    c) False. This is destruction of the nails, as occurs in psoriasis.
    d) True.
    e) True. This is a sign of a hyperdynamic circulation.

38 a) False. This is a clinical sign of ascites, indicating the presence of fluid in the abdomen.
    b) True. The diagnosis is made based on the protein content of the fluid.
    c) False. Low protein is a contributory cause of ascites.
    d) False. Spironolactone is the preferred diuretic.
    e) False. Several litres may be drawn off. Albumin is given beforehand to prevent fluid leaving the intravascular space.

39 a) True. Vertical transmission and intravenous transmission are also important.
    b) True.
    c) False. At-risk groups are vaccinated, including all healthcare personnel, children in high-risk areas, i.v. drug users, homosexuals and prostitutes.
    d) False. Interferon-alpha, lamivudine and adefovir are all treatment options.
    e) True. This may complicate chronic infection.

40 a) False. This is an excess of growth hormone secretion from a pituitary tumour. Systemic hypertension is a feature.
    b) True. This is hepatic vein thrombosis.
    c) False. This is a cause of systemic hypertension.
    d) True.
    e) False. This is a catecholamine-producing tumour, causing systemic hypertension.

41 a) True. This is the hepatorenal syndrome.
    b) True. Ammonia compounds absorbed from the bowel are responsible.
    c) True. This is a complication of ascites.
    d) False.
    e) True. This complication should be screened for regularly with ultrasound and α-fetoprotein measurements.

42 a) False.
    b) True.
    c) True. This is an inherited disorder of iron metabolism.
    d) False. This is an inborn error of metabolism, causing mental retardation in infants.
    e) True. Liver function tests must be monitored in patients on methotrexate therapy.

43 a) False. Females are affected more frequently.
    b) True. Presentation may occur with acute hepatitis, features of autoimmune disease, or chronic liver disease.
    c) True.
    d) False. Patients are first managed medically with corticosteroids or azathioprine. Transplantation is a last resort.
    e) True.

EMQ ANSWERS

1 HEPATITIS

1 E **Hepatitis E** causes a benign clinical syndrome very similar to hepatitis A, both being RNA viruses, transmitted via the faecal-oral route. Its consequences in pregnancy can be devastating however, with a mortality of up to 20 per cent from fulminant hepatic failure in the third trimester.

2 H The presentation of **alcoholic hepatitis** can be quite variable. In this case, the patient has decompensated liver disease: this warrants urgent admission.

3 A **Hepatitis A** is the most common cause of jaundice in travellers. The incubation period is 2–6 weeks; treatment is usually supportive.

4 J The prodromal period before the development of jaundice is consistent with **infectious mononucleosis**. The Epstein–Barr virus can cause a mild hepatitis that usually resolves spontaneously.

5 D **Hepatitis D** can only cause disease in those already infected with hepatitis B. This patient has acquired the virus through intravenous drug abuse, and has now developed an acute hepatitis.

2 TESTS USED IN THE DIAGNOSIS OF LIVER DISEASE

1 G **Haematinics** can be useful to aid in the diagnosis of hereditary haemochromatosis. Patients typically have a raised ferritin and high transferrin saturation. Care needs to be taken though as ferritin is an acute-phase protein. Definitive diagnosis is via HFE genotyping.

2 A Ninety-five per cent of cases of primary biliary cirrhosis are **antimitochondrial antibody** (AMA) positive.

3 D **Anti-smooth muscle antibodies** occur in three-quarters of all cases of autoimmune hepatitis.

4 H **α-fetoprotein** is used as a tumour marker in hepatocellular carcinoma. Most patients with a primary liver malignancy have elevated levels detectable in the blood.

5 E Levels of **caeruloplasmin**, a copper-transporting protein, are low in Wilson's disease.

3 CAUSES OF LIVER DISEASE

1 F **Wilson's disease** is caused by copper deposition in the liver, CNS, cornea, kidneys and other organs. Hepatic involvement leads to chronic liver disease and cirrhosis; deposition of copper in the basal ganglia results in movement disorders.

2 G Deposition of iron in **hereditary haemochromatosis** leads to liver disease, diabetes, hypogonadism and pigmentation of the skin. This patient has features of all of these.

3 A **Budd–Chiari syndrome**, hepatic vein thrombosis, occurs in hypercoagulable states like polycythaemia. The presentation is often insidious: this patient has signs of chronic liver disease and has now developed ascites.

4 H **Iatrogenic**. Methotrexate causes both acute and chronic hepatotoxicity, which may sometimes lead to cirrhosis.

5 J Anti-smooth muscle antibodies are found in most cases of **autoimmune hepatitis**. Sjögren's syndrome is sometimes associated with this disease.

4 HEPATOMEGALY

1 J A hard irregular liver signifies malignant involvement. The information given suggests a long history of smoking: the best answer is therefore liver **metastases** secondary to a lung primary.

2 F **Hydatid disease** is caused by infection with the tapeworm *Echinococcus granulosus*, which occurs in areas where sheep are farmed. The most common site of involvement is the liver, followed by the lung. Cysts may calcify with time.

3 D Non-alcoholic steatohepatitis (NASH) is usually a benign condition, sometimes referred to as **fatty liver**. There is often a preceding history of diabetes or obesity.

4 H Anchovy sauce is the characteristic description of fluid aspirated from an **amoebic abscess**. This medical student has been infected with *Entamoeba histolytica*, while on holiday in Pakistan.

5 G A rapidly enlarging liver on a background of hereditary haemochromatosis should raise the suspicion of **hepatocellular carcinoma**.

5 ASCITES

1 A **Meigs' syndrome** is an uncommon cause of ascites and right-sided pleural effusion in association with a benign ovarian neoplasm. Most women who present with abdominal distension and ascites unfortunately have peritoneal carcinomatosis from ovarian carcinoma.

2 J The elevated amylase points to **acute pancreatitis** as the cause of ascites and abdominal pain.

3 B This gentleman has oedema, significant proteinuria and probably **hypo-albuminaemia**. The underlying diagnosis is nephrotic syndrome secondary to membranous glomerulonephritis caused by malaria.

4 A The insidious history of weight loss and abdominal distension suggests **malignancy**. The elevated CA 19-9 makes pancreatic carcinoma most likely.

5 F This immigrant has constitutional symptoms and AFB in his ascites. Intra-abdominal **tuberculosis** would give rise to both of these.

6 JAUNDICE

1 **C** The inherited conjugated hyperbilirubinaemias are **Dubin–Johnson** and Rotor syndromes.

2 **D** **Iatrogenic.** Hepatotoxicity is common with antituberculous drugs. Significant elevations of liver enzymes mandate stopping therapy and reintroducing drugs individually.

3 **H** **Primary sclerosing cholangitis** is strongly associated with ulcerative colitis. pANCA is often positive, though definitive diagnosis is made via ERCP or magnetic resonance cholangiopancreatography (MRCP).

4 **G** **Gilbert's syndrome**, an inherited unconjugated hyperbilirubinaemia, is a very common condition in which sufferers become mildly icteric when subjected to stress – often illness or fasting. Reassurance is all that is required.

5 **I** A history of difficulty eating fatty foods points towards biliary disease. The sudden onset of jaundice and right upper quadrant pain in this patient suggests obstruction of the biliary tree from **gallstones**.

7 COMPLICATIONS OF GALLSTONES

1 **E** A **mucocele** forms when a gallstone impacts in the cystic duct and the gallbladder epithelium continues to secrete mucus, resulting in distension. If there is no infection the condition is usually painless.

2 **J** This patient is extremely unwell and septic. Gas within the lumen or the wall of the gallbladder is pathognomonic of **emphysematous cholecystitis**, a rare but life threatening condition. Emergency cholecystectomy is indicated.

3 **D** The features described are consistent with small bowel obstruction secondary to **gallstone ileus**. Occasionally gallstones can pass into the intestine and cause bowel obstruction by blocking the lumen; the usual site of impaction is at the ileocaecal valve.

4 **C** The two most common causes of **acute pancreatitis** are gallstones and alcohol. An elevated serum amylase is diagnostic.

5 **F** An **empyema** is defined as pus within a cavity – in this case within the gallbladder. It should be suspected in patients who fail to improve with conservative therapy.

X-RAY ANSWERS

1 a) A computed tomography (CT) scan of the abdomen has been performed.
  b) The liver parenchyma is normally homogenous in density. This scan shows multiple low density lesions, which most probably are metastases from an unknown primary.

2 The plain abdominal X-ray shows diffuse calcification throughout the pancreas, a sign of chronic pancreatitis. This is often related to alcohol misuse and can cause pain refractory to standard analgesics.

3 There is a large volume of ascites within the abdomen. This is shown on the CT scan as a dark rim of fluid surrounding the liver and spleen.

Dermatology

MULTIPLE CHOICE QUESTIONS

1　Causes of genital ulceration include:
   a) Herpes simplex
   b) Giardiasis
   c) Bacterial vaginosis
   d) Syphilis
   e) Lymphogranuloma venereum

2　Systemic causes of pruritus include:
   a) Uraemia
   b) Hypoxia
   c) Iron-deficiency anaemia
   d) Hypocalcaemia
   e) Cholestasis

3　Causes of hair loss include:
   a) Warfarin
   b) Trichotillomania
   c) Iron-deficiency
   d) Rheumatoid arthritis
   e) Hypothyroidism

4　Topical treatment options for acne vulgaris include:
   a) Azelaic acid
   b) Silver nitrate
   c) Benzoyl peroxide
   d) Clotrimazole
   e) Tretinoin

5　Common clinical features of a basal cell carcinoma include:
   a) Telangiectasia
   b) Black pigmentation
   c) Rolled edge
   d) Pustule formation
   e) Pearly appearance

6   The following are usually caused by staphylococcal infection:
    a) Furuncle
    b) Erysipelas
    c) Impetigo
    d) Tinea cruris
    e) Molluscum contagiosum

7   Causes of hypopigmentation include:
    a) Pityriasis versicolor
    b) Chloasma
    c) Pityriasis rosea
    d) Vitiligo
    e) Leprosy

8   Topical treatments for psoriasis include:
    a) Coal tar
    b) Malathion
    c) Imiquimod
    d) Dithranol
    e) Salicylic acid

9   Regarding scabies:
    a) It is caused by *Malassezia furfur*
    b) It is contagious
    c) Oral treatment is usually necessary
    d) Pruritus is worse at night
    e) Erythroderma is a complication

10   The following skin conditions are caused by viruses:
    a) Pemphigus
    b) Molluscum contagiosum
    c) Condylomata acuminata
    d) Shingles
    e) Tinea pedis

11   Causes of general hyperpigmentation include:
    a) Oxygen therapy
    b) Addison's disease
    c) Thyrotoxicosis
    d) Chronic renal failure
    e) Haemochromatosis

12   Causes of erythema multiforme include:
    a) Hypothyroidism
    b) *Mycoplasma pneumoniae*
    c) *Candida albicans*
    d) Herpes simplex
    e) Cushing's disease

13 Causes of erythema nodosum include:
   a) Streptococcal infection
   b) Sarcoidosis
   c) Diabetes mellitus
   d) Crohn's disease
   e) Chronic renal failure

14 The following are malignant skin tumours:
   a) Dermatofibroma
   b) Bowen's disease
   c) Kaposi's sarcoma
   d) Keratoacanthoma
   e) Mycosis fungoides

15 Causes of palmar erythema include:
   a) Anaemia
   b) Thyrotoxicosis
   c) Pregnancy
   d) Carpal tunnel syndrome
   e) Rheumatoid arthritis

Answers: see pages 185–186

EXTENDED MATCHING QUESTIONS

1 TERMS USED IN DERMATOLOGY

Match the descriptions of skin lesions below with their medical names

A   Macule
B   Papule
C   Nodule
D   Ulcer
E   Vesicle

F   Purpura
G   Petechiae
H   Telangiectasia
I   Plaque
J   Bulla

1   A small fluid-filled elevation on the skin.
2   Visible dilatation of small blood vessels under the skin.
3   A 3 mm solid elevated skin lesion.
4   A 1.2 cm solid elevated skin lesion.
5   A large area of bleeding into the skin, which does not blanch on pressure.

2 CUTANEOUS MANIFESTATIONS OF SYSTEMIC DISEASE 1

Match the descriptions of skin lesions below with their medical names

A   Necrobiosis lipoidica
B   Paget's disease
C   Acanthosis nigricans
D   Erythema multiforme
E   Dermatitis herpetiformis

F   Necrolytic migratory erythema
G   Erythema nodosum
H   Erythema gyratum repens
I   Thrombophlebitis migrans
J   Pyoderma gangrenosum

1   An eczematous pruritic rash over the nipple and areola.
2   Red painful nodules over the shins.
3   Concentric, itchy bands of red skin, which move over the skin with time.
4   Hyperpigmented, thickened skin in the armpits.
5   An itchy vesicular rash over the extensor surfaces.

3 CUTANEOUS MANIFESTATIONS OF SYSTEMIC DISEASE 2

Match the conditions below with the most likely associated skin lesion

A   Necrobiosis lipoidica
B   Paget's disease
C   Acanthosis nigricans
D   Erythema multiforme
E   Dermatitis herpetiformis

F   Necrolytic migratory erythema
G   Erythema chronicum migrans
H   Erythema gyratum repens
I   Thrombophlebitis migrans
J   Pyoderma gangrenosum

1   Insulin resistance.
2   Coeliac disease.
3   Lyme disease.
4   Ulcerative colitis.
5   Pancreatic cancer.

4 DISORDERS AFFECTING THE NAILS 1

Match the descriptions of nail lesions below with their medical names

A   Leuconychia
B   Nail pitting
C   Onycholysis
D   Clubbing
E   Paronychia

F   Beau's lines
G   Koilonychia
H   Splinter haemorrhage
I   Onychogryphosis
J   Subungual melanoma

1   Separation of the distal part of the nail from the nail bed.
2   A spoon-shaped nail.
3   Loss of the angle between the nail fold and nail plate.
4   Thickened, distorted nail growth, often of the big toe.
5   Transverse solitary linear depressions in the nails.

5 DISORDERS AFFECTING THE NAILS 2

Match the conditions below with the most likely associated nail lesion

A   Leuconychia
B   Nail pitting
C   Onycholysis
D   Clubbing
E   Paronychia

F   Beau's lines
G   Koilonychia
H   Splinter haemorrhage
I   Onychogryphosis
J   Subungual melanoma

1   Hypoalbuminaemia.
2   Bronchiectasis.
3   Severe illness.
4   Hyperthyroidism.
5   Infective endocarditis.

6 INFECTIONS AFFECTING THE SKIN

All the patients below have signs of infections affecting the skin. Select the most likely diagnosis from the options given

A   Leprosy
B   Erythema infectiosum
C   Tinea capitis
D   Tinea cruris
E   Scabies

F   Molluscum contagiosum
G   Cellulitis
H   Onychomycosis
I   Shingles
J   Pityriasis versicolor

1   A 21-year-old man complains of pain and redness in his groin. On examination, he has large plaques on the medial aspects of both his thighs, with some areas of normal skin within them.
2   A 3-year-old girl is brought to hospital with a temperature of 38.2°C. Examination is unremarkable apart from her cheeks looking bright red, as if they had been slapped hard.
3   A 34-year-old woman goes to see her general practitioner (GP) with her four children. They are all experiencing severe pruritus. On examination, there are red excoriated papules present between the web spaces of the fingers.
4   A 60-year-old man goes to his GP with a thickened, deformed nail that he has had for some months. The GP is sure that an infection is causing his problem
5   A 19-year-old man goes to see his doctor as he has noticed patches of hypopigmentation on his trunk. His doctor says he has seen this before, and takes some scrapings to confirm the diagnosis of a fungal infection.

7 TREATMENT OF INFECTIONS AFFECTING THE SKIN

Select the most appropriate treatment for each of the skin conditions listed below

A   Flucloxacillin
B   Vancomycin
C   Malathion
D   Nystatin
E   Penicillin V

F   Amoxicillin
G   Oral terbinafine
H   Topical terbinafine
I   Oral aciclovir
J   Topical aciclovir

1   Scabies.
2   Shingles.
3   Onychomycosis.
4   Impetigo.
5   Oral candidiasis.

8 PRESENTATION OF SKIN DISEASE

All the patients below have skin disease. Select the most likely diagnosis from the options given

A   Leprosy
B   Psoriasis
C   Pemphigus
D   Kaposi's sarcoma
E   Furuncle

F   Erythema multiforme
G   Eczema
H   Cellulitis
I   Basal cell carcinoma
J   Malignant melanoma

1   A 15-year-old boy presents with small, circular plaques on his trunk. His only past medical history of note has been a sore throat about 2 weeks ago. One of the medical students in the clinic remarks that the plaques look like little raindrops.
2   A 34-year-old taxi driver develops a pleomorphic skin eruption with wheals, bullae and some target lesions. She is taking amoxicillin for a chest infection.
3   A 71-year-old man comes to see his GP concerned about his face. He has a 2 cm well-demarcated lesion on his left cheek, which the GP notes has a rolled, pearly edge.
4   A 66-year-old woman goes to see her GP for a repeat prescription. The GP notices that she has a 3 cm dark lesion on her right calf, with an irregular edge. The patient says it has enlarged recently.
5   A 3-year-old boy is taken to his GP by his parents. They are concerned as he has developed an itchy rash behind his knees. On examination, the area is erythematous and excoriated.

9 ALOPECIA

All the patients below complain of hair loss. Select the most likely diagnosis from the options given

A   Tinea capitis
B   Telogen effluvium
C   Systemic lupus erythematosus
D   Alopecia areata
E   Anagen effluvium

F   Syphilis
G   Radiotherapy
H   Bacterial folliculitis
I   Trichotillomania
J   Androgenic alopecia

1   A 27-year-old pharmacist goes to see her GP, concerned that all her hair has fallen out. He can find nothing wrong on clinical examination, but notes with interest that she was admitted to the intensive therapy unit (ITU) 3 months previously with severe pneumonia.
2   A 61-year-old woman on cytotoxic chemotherapy for non-Hodgkin's lymphoma complains that all her hair has fallen out.
3   A 36-year-old man goes to see his GP complaining of hair loss. He is known to have a personality disorder, but has never been hospitalized. On examination, there is patchy thinning of the hair on the scalp, with multiple different lengths of hair, some of which are twisted together.
4   A 43-year-old woman seeks medical attention as she is suffering from hair loss over her temples and her crown. She is otherwise entirely well.
5   An 8-year-old girl is brought to see her GP by her father. She is suffering from a flaking scalp and hair loss in patches. The GP takes scrapings, which are positive for *Microsporum canis*.

Answers: see pages 187–189

ANSWERS

MCQ ANSWERS

1 a) True. The type II virus usually causes genital ulcers, while type I causes cold sores.
   b) False. This is a gastrointestinal protozoan infection causing diarrhoea.
   c) False. Bacterial vaginosis causes a fishy-smelling discharge.
   d) True. Ulceration is painless.
   e) True. This is a chlamydial infection causing ulceration and lymphadenopathy.

2 a) True. For example, in chronic renal failure.
   b) False.
   c) True. Interestingly, iron-deficiency and polycythaemia can both cause pruritus.
   d) False.
   e) True. Jaundice is a common cause of itching.

3 a) True.
   b) True. This is an obsession with pulling one's own hair out.
   c) True.
   d) False.
   e) True.

4 a) True.
   b) False. Silver nitrate is used for removal of warts.
   c) True.
   d) False. Clotrimazole is an antifungal.
   e) True. Tretinoin is a retinoid.

5 a) True.
   b) False. Black pigmentation is more a feature of melanoma.
   c) True.
   d) False.
   e) True.

6 a) True. This is a hair follicle infection.
   b) False. This is a dermal infection caused by *Streptococcus pyogenes*.
   c) True. This is a superficial skin infection that is common in children. There is a yellow crusting exudate.
   d) False. This is a dermatophyte fungal infection of the groin.
   e) False. This is a viral infection producing pink papules.

7 a) True. This is a skin infection caused by *Malassezia furfur*. Patches appear hypo-pigmented in darker skin and hyperpigmented in fair skin.
   b) False. This is hyperpigmentation of the face occurring in pregnancy and women taking oral contraceptives.
   c) False. This is a rash with pink, oval, scaly patches.
   d) True. Vitiligo is an idiopathic hypopigmentation disorder, with possible auto-immune aetiology.
   e) True. There are anaesthetic patches of hypopigmentation.

8 a) True.
   b) False. Malathion is a treatment for scabies.
   c) False. It is used for anogenital warts.
   d) True. A side-effect of this is staining of the skin and clothes.
   e) True. This is a keratolytic that may be useful for removing scale.

9 a) False. This organism causes pityriasis versicolor. *Sarcoptes scabiei* is the mite responsible for scabies.
   b) True.
   c) False. Topical permethrin or malathion is the standard treatment.
   d) True.
   e) False. Erythroderma is a generalized skin inflammation, usually caused by eczema or psoriasis, covering the majority of the skin. It may occasionally be life-threatening.

10 a) False. This is an autoimmune blistering disease.
    b) True. This is a childhood condition characterized by papules with a central punctum.
    c) True. These are genital warts caused by human papillomavirus (HPV).
    d) True. Herpes zoster causes a vesicular rash in a dermatomal distribution.
    e) False. Otherwise known as 'athlete's foot', this is a fungal dermatophyte infection.

11 a) False.
    b) True. High adrenocorticotrophic hormone (ACTH) levels are responsible.
    c) False.
    d) True.
    e) True. The skin takes on a bronzed appearance.

12 a) False.
    b) True.
    c) False.
    d) True.
    e) False.

13 a) True.
    b) True.
    c) False.
    d) True.
    e) False.

14 a) False. This is a benign dermal nodule.
    b) True. This is a squamous cell carcinoma-in-situ.
    c) True. This is a vascular tumour associated with AIDS.
    d) False. This is a rapidly growing epidermal tumour with a central keratin plug.
    e) True. This is a cutaneous T-cell lymphoma.

15 a) False. Pallor is a feature of anaemia.
    b) True. Palmar erythema is a sign of a hyperdynamic circulation.
    c) True.
    d) False.
    e) True.

EMQ ANSWERS

1 TERMS USED IN DERMATOLOGY

1 E **Vesicle.** Large vesicles are referred to as bullae.
2 H **Telangiectasia.**
3 B **Papule.** Macules are small flat skin lesions.
4 C **Nodules** refer to large papules.
5 F **Purpura.**

2 CUTANEOUS MANIFESTATIONS OF SYSTEMIC DISEASE 1

1 B **Paget's disease** of the nipple indicates an underlying breast cancer.
2 G **Erythema nodosum** occurs in many diseases including sarcoidosis, inflammatory bowel disease, streptococcal infection and tuberculosis.
3 H **Erythema gyratum repens** is an uncommon sign of malignancy, including bronchial and colonic carcinoma.
4 C **Acanthosis nigricans** may be a sign of insulin resistance or underlying gastric malignancy.
5 E **Dermatitis herpetiformis** occurs in association with coeliac disease; treatment is with topical dapsone.

3 CUTANEOUS MANIFESTATIONS OF SYSTEMIC DISEASE 2

1 C **Acanthosis nigricans**, thickened velvety skin under the armpits, is associated with insulin resistance.
2 E **Dermatitis herpetiformis**, a vesicular rash which often occurs over the elbows, is associated with coeliac disease.
3 G **Erythema chronicum migrans**, a red papule that expands over time, is found in most cases of Lyme disease.
4 J **Pyoderma gangrenosum**, an ulcerating lesion which typically affects the lower limbs, can occur in association with inflammatory bowel disease.
5 I **Thrombophlebitis migrans** is a non-metastatic manifestation of pancreatic carcinoma.

4 DISORDERS AFFECTING THE NAILS 1

1 C **Onycholysis** occurs in onychomycosis, psoriasis and hyperthyroidism (Plummer's nails).
2 G **Koilonychia** is a sign of iron-deficiency anaemia.
3 D **Clubbing** has many cardiac, respiratory and gastrointestinal causes.
4 I **Onychogryphosis**, a disease which often affects the elderly, typically causes distortion of the nail of the hallux.
5 F **Beau's lines** indicate periods of systemic illness that affected nail growth.

5 DISORDERS AFFECTING THE NAILS 2

1 A **Leuconychia**, white nails, are sometimes seen in association with cirrhosis.
2 D Suppurative lung diseases such as bronchiectasis and empyema are causes of **clubbing**.
3 F **Beau's lines**, transverse grooves in the nails, can be seen after periods of severe illness. They indicate periods of nail growth arrest.
4 C Plummer's nails or **onycholysis** occur in hyperthyroidism.
5 H **Splinter haemorrhages** occur in both trauma and infective endocarditis.

6 INFECTIONS AFFECTING THE SKIN

1 D The clinical sign being described is central clearing: normal skin within large lesions. This typically occurs in Tinea infections. **Tinea cruris** affects the groin.

2 B **Erythema infectiosum**, or fifth disease, is a viral illness caused by parvovirus B19. The characteristic sign is the appearance of bright red cheeks that look like they have been slapped, with circumoral pallor.

3 E This household is suffering from **scabies** infection. The mite *Sarcoptes scabiei* causes an intensely pruritic rash, classically between the web spaces of the fingers.

4 H **Onychomycosis** is a common cause of nail deformity, resulting from dermatophyte infection.

5 J **Pityriasis versicolor** is a fungal infection caused by *Malassezia furfur*. It presents with macules on the trunks which are often hypopigmented.

7 TREATMENT OF INFECTIONS AFFECTING THE SKIN

1 C Topical **malathion** is the first-line therapy for scabies. All patients and close contacts should be treated.

2 I **Oral aciclovir** is used to shorten the course of herpes zoster infection.

3 G Onychomycosis requires systemic antifungal treatment with **oral terbinafine.**

4 A **Flucloxacillin** is effective against staphylococcal skin infections such as impetigo.

5 D Oral candidiasis often occurs in those receiving antibiotics. It usually responds to treatment with **nystatin.**

8 PRESENTATION OF SKIN DISEASE

1 B Guttate **psoriasis** (from the Latin *gutta*, a drop) causes small lesions, often over the whole body. Its onset is sometimes preceded by an upper respiratory tract infection.

2 F **Erythema multiforme** is, as its name implies, a highly variable rash. Treatment with penicillins is sometimes implicated.

3 I The rolled, pearly edge is the hallmark of a **basal cell carcinoma.** Telangiectasia are also frequently seen over the surface of the lesion.

4 J The irregular edge and history of enlargement are highly suspicious for **malignant melanoma.** Urgent investigation is required.

5 G **Eczema** often affects the flexor surfaces in children. It is extremely pruritic and signs of excoriation are frequently seen.

9 ALOPECIA

1 B **Telogen effluvium.** If normal hair growth is interrupted by severe illness, the usual cycle of continuous shedding is reset, and all hair growth ceases. When new hairs grow, often about 3 months after the insult, they push out all the old hair at once, giving rise to temporary global hair loss. The prognosis is excellent.

2 E **Anagen effluvium** is caused by a sudden insult to the hair follicle, often due to chemotherapy or radiotherapy, resulting in immediate hair loss. Recovery of normal hair growth is expected.

3 I **Trichotillomania** (hair pulling) is more common in children, but may occur in those with psychiatric disease. Clinical features include patchy hair loss with twisted hairs of varying lengths, as the hair is broken irregularly.

4 J **Androgenic alopecia**, or male pattern baldness, is extremely common among men but considerably less so in women, in whom it may cause great distress. Treatment is generally unsatisfactory.

5 A **Tinea capitis**, a fungal infection of the scalp, typically occurs in children. The causative organism, *Microsporum canis*, is usually transmitted from a dog or a cat. The diagnosis is confirmed by scrapings; treatment is with systemic antifungals.

Haematology

MULTIPLE CHOICE QUESTIONS

1   Indications for splenectomy include:
    a) Hereditary spherocytosis
    b) Pernicious anaemia
    c) Idiopathic thrombocytopenic purpura
    d) Abdominal trauma
    e) Alcoholic hepatitis

2   Causes of thrombocytopenia include:
    a) Haemolytic-uraemic syndrome
    b) Rotor syndrome
    c) Viral infection
    d) Heparin
    e) Aplastic anaemia

3   The following statements are true of haemophilia A:
    a) It is due to deficiency of factor VII
    b) It is an autosomal dominant inherited condition
    c) Arthropathy is a complication
    d) Desmopressin is a useful treatment
    e) In severe cases, the disease can progress to haemophilia B

4   Causes of disseminated intravascular coagulation (DIC) include:
    a) Prostate cancer
    b) Cystic fibrosis
    c) Septicaemia
    d) Burns
    e) Placental abruption

5   The following statements are true of leukaemias:
  a) Intrathecal vincristine is useful in the treatment of acute lymphoblastic leukaemia (ALL)
  b) The Philadelphia chromosome is strongly linked with chronic lymphocytic leukaemia (CLL)
  c) Massive splenomegaly occurs in chronic myeloid leukaemia (CML)
  d) Anaemia is a feature
  e) Acute myeloid leukaemia (AML) is generally a disease of young children

6   Consequences of splenectomy may include:
  a) Coeliac disease
  b) Thrombocytopenia
  c) Leukaemia
  d) Howell–Jolly bodies
  e) Meningococcal infection

7   Markers of haemolytic anaemia include:
  a) Conjugated hyperbilirubinaemia
  b) Hypokalaemia
  c) Reticulocytosis
  d) Raised alkaline phosphatase
  e) Low plasma haptoglobin

8   Clinical features of iron-deficiency anaemia include:
  a) Splinter haemorrhages
  b) Oral hairy leukoplakia
  c) Koilonychia
  d) Angular stomatitis
  e) Paterson–Brown-Kelly syndrome

9   The following statements are true of sickle cell anaemia:
  a) It is inherited as a sex-linked recessive condition
  b) Sickle cell trait progresses to sickle cell disease within the first 20 years of life
  c) Parvovirus can precipitate an aplastic crisis
  d) Hydroxycarbamide has no role in the management of sickle cell anaemia
  e) The heterozygous carrier state has no protection against malaria

10   Risk factors for venous thrombosis include:
  a) Homocysteinaemia
  b) Female gender
  c) Malignancy
  d) Blood transfusion
  e) Inflammatory bowel disease

11   The following statements are true of thalassaemia:
  a) It is an acquired disorder of haemoglobin synthesis
  b) Urinary Bence–Jones proteins are diagnostic of the disease
  c) The mean red cell volume is reduced
  d) It is most prevalent in sub-Saharan Africa
  e) Splenectomy may be useful

12 Causes of a massive spleen include:
   a) Kala-azar
   b) Dysentery
   c) Pernicious anaemia
   d) Myeloma
   e) Malaria

13 Consequences of sickle cell disease include:
   a) Gallstones
   b) Peptic ulceration
   c) Leukaemia
   d) Osteomyelitis
   e) Leg ulcers

14 Causes of pancytopenia include:
   a) Systemic lupus erythematosus
   b) Protein C deficiency
   c) Ramipril
   d) Hypersplenism
   e) Aplastic anaemia

15 Causes of microcytic anaemia include:
   a) Pernicious anaemia
   b) Thalassaemia
   c) Vitamin C deficiency
   d) Hyperthyroidism
   e) Sideroblastic anaemia

16 Causes of inherited thrombophilia include:
   a) von Willebrand's disease
   b) Factor V Leiden
   c) Eosinophilia
   d) Protein C excess
   e) Antithrombin III deficiency

17 Complications of blood transfusion include:
   a) Pulmonary oedema
   b) Hyperkalaemia
   c) Anaphylaxis
   d) Cytomegalovirus (CMV) infection
   e) Haemoglobinuria

18 The following statements are true of pernicious anaemia:
   a) The anaemia is typically microcytic
   b) Spastic paraparesis may be a consequence
   c) It is treated with folic acid
   d) It is associated with gastric carcinoma
   e) Genetic screening should be offered to family members

19 Causes of a macrocytic anaemia include:
   a) Spironolactone
   b) Hypothyroidism
   c) Ischaemic heart disease
   d) Methotrexate
   e) Alcohol excess

20 The following is true of low-molecular weight heparins (LMWHs), when compared with unfractionated heparin:
   a) The anticoagulation is easier to reverse
   b) Anticoagulation monitoring is not required
   c) Thrombocytopenia is more of a risk
   d) Duration of action is shorter
   e) They can be given orally

21 Deficiencies of the following enzymes are known causes of red cell metabolic disorders:
   a) Angiotensin-converting enzyme
   b) Pyruvate kinase
   c) Alkaline phosphatase
   d) Creatine kinase
   e) Glucose-6-phosphatase

22 Inherited causes of haemolytic anaemia include:
   a) von Willebrand's disease
   b) Spherocytosis
   c) Phenylketonuria
   d) Thalassaemia
   e) Pyruvate kinase deficiency

23 The following investigations are useful in multiple myeloma:
   a) Lymph node biopsy
   b) Serum electrophoresis
   c) Skull X-ray
   d) 24-h urine collection
   e) Serum calcium

24 The following statements are true of lymphomas:
   a) Prognosis for Hodgkin's lymphoma is worse than that for non-Hodgkin's lymphoma
   b) Staging of Hodgkin's lymphoma takes symptoms into account
   c) Non-Hodgkin's lymphoma is characterized by the presence of Reed–Sternberg cells
   d) High-grade non-Hodgkin's lymphoma has a better prognosis than low-grade
   e) Burkitt's lymphoma is associated with Epstein–Barr virus

25 The following statements are true of polycythaemia rubra vera:
   a) It occurs as a consequence of chronic renal failure
   b) Gout is a complication
   c) Splenomegaly is a feature
   d) Erythropoietin injections are the treatment of choice
   e) Symptoms are more pronounced in low temperatures

Answers: see pages 201–204

EXTENDED MATCHING QUESTIONS

1 MICROCYTIC ANAEMIA

1 Select the most likely cause of microcytic anaemia for each of the scenarios below

A   Lead poisoning
B   Colonic carcinoma
C   Hookworm infestation
D   Anaemia of chronic disease
E   Dietary insufficiency

F   Malabsorption
G   Thalassaemia
H   Sideroblastic anaemia
I   Meckel's diverticulum
J   Aluminium toxicity

1   Some final year medical students have a tutorial on haematology. The professor asks what the most common cause of iron-deficiency anaemia is worldwide.

2   A 75-year-old woman presents to her general practitioner (GP) feeling tired. Routine blood tests show haemoglobin (Hb) 9.2 g/dL, mean corpuscular volume (MCV) 72 fL, and a raised iron and ferritin. The GP is unsure of the diagnosis and refers her to a haematologist, who performs a bone marrow biopsy, which shows rings of iron granules in the cells.

3   An 83-year-old retired dairy farmer goes to his GP with constipation and weight loss. Blood tests show Hb 10.1 g/dL, MCV 74 fL, and reduced serum iron and ferritin.

4   A 71-year-old woman visits her GP for a prescription for some diclofenac for her rheumatoid arthritis. She is clinically anaemic, and blood tests show Hb 9.3 g/dL, MCV 78 fL and low serum iron with a raised ferritin.

5   An 18-year-old student goes to hospital after falling down some stairs having drunk too many cocktails. She has a displaced Colles' fracture and some routine bloods are done before she goes to theatre. Her Hb is 10.1 g/dL, MCV 61 fL, with normal serum iron and ferritin.

2 HAEMOLYTIC ANAEMIA

Match the most likely cause of haemolytic anaemia to the clinical scenarios below

A   Glucose-6-phosphate dehydrogenase
    (G6PD) deficiency
B   Autoimmune
C   Malaria
D   Sickle cell disease
E   Cardiac valve replacement

F   Haemolytic disease of the newborn
G   Transfusion reaction
H   Hereditary spherocytosis
I   Thalassaemia
J   Iatrogenic

1 A newborn baby has prolonged jaundice and anaemia of unknown aetiology. A blood
   film shows a reticulocytosis with round red cells. A direct Coombs' test is negative, but an
   osmotic fragility test is positive.

2 An 8-year-old Cypriot boy attends his GP surgery with fatigue. His haemoglobin is
   8.2 g/dL. On examination, the frontal bones of his skull are especially prominent; a skull
   X-ray is reported as having a 'hair on end' appearance.

3 A 22-year-old student presents extremely unwell to his GP as he is concerned that he has
   fever, headache and is passing black urine. He has returned two weeks previously from a
   safari in Kenya. A full blood count shows Hb 9.2g/dL.

4 A 26-year-old police officer goes to his GP with a cough and fever. She has crackles at her
   right lung base and erythema multiforme. The GP prescribes some erythromycin and
   sends off some bloods. He recalls the patient when he finds Hb 9.6g/dL, bilirubin 29,
   reduced haptoglobin and positive direct Coombs' test.

5 A Sudanese woman presents to her GP with dysuria and frequency. He prescribes a short
   course of nitrofurantoin. She returns two days later complaining of jaundice and fatigue.
   Blood tests reveal Hb 8.2g/dL, bilirubin 39, and negative direct Coombs' test.

3 MACROCYTOSIS

Select the most likely cause of macrocytosis for each of the scenarios below

A   Pernicious anaemia
B   Pregnancy
C   Reticulocytosis
D   Crohn's disease
E   Aplastic anaemia

F   Iatrogenic
G   Alcohol excess
H   Folate deficiency
I   Hypothyroidism
J   Myelodysplasia

1   A 37-year-old photographer goes to her GP complaining of fatigue and diarrhoea for the past year. Blood tests reveal Hb 9.8g/dL and MCV 103 fL. He refers her to hospital where a colonoscopy is performed. A biopsy reveals granulomas in the terminal ileum.

2   A 59-year-old woman presents at her GP surgery with glossitis, angular stomatitis and paraesthesiae in her feet. She had last been to see him a year earlier to ask for more steroids for her Addison's disease. Examination reveals a peripheral neuropathy with loss of proprioception and vibration sense.

3   A 32-year-old motorcycle courier is hit by a car travelling at 42 mph and taken to hospital after being extricated from the wreckage some hours later. The house officer sends off a full blood count in the emergency department and is puzzled to find Hb 7.3 g/dL and MCV 104 fL.

4   A 69-year-old woman sees her GP complaining of increasing fatigue and weight gain. Her skin is dry; she has also noticed that she is losing her hair. Blood tests reveal a normal haemoglobin, but an MCV of 102 fL.

5   A 42-year-old social worker comes to see her GP for her regular review. Her epilepsy is well controlled with phenytoin. Some routine bloods reveal Hb 10.2 g/dL, MCV 104 fL.

4 SPLENOMEGALY

The patients below are all found to have splenomegaly. Match the most likely cause of this with the clinical scenarios

A   Hodgkin's disease
B   Infective endocarditis
C   Chronic myeloid leukaemia
D   Sarcoidosis
E   Malaria

F   Amyloidosis
G   Thalassaemia
H   Infectious mononucleosis
I   Haemolytic anaemia
J   Felty's syndrome

1   An 18-year-old student goes to the emergency department feeling unwell. She complains of odynophagia and general malaise. On examination, she has tonsillitis with cervical lymph-adenopathy and splenomegaly. The junior doctor gives her some amoxicillin for the tonsillitis. He is surprised to see her return 2 days later complaining of a maculopapular rash.

2   A 61-year-old woman with severe rheumatoid arthritis tells her rheumatologist she is bruising easily. She has obvious deformities of rheumatoid disease and palpable splenomegaly. A full blood count reveals Hb 8.0g/dL, MCV 84 fL, platelets 96×10^9/L and neutrophils 1.5×10^9/L.

3   A 7-year-old boy presents to paediatric outpatients with anaemia. His mother does not speak much English as she has just emigrated from Naples. The consultant finds splenomegaly and orders some blood tests which show Hb 9.2g/dL, MCV 62 fL and normal haematinics. A direct Coombs' test is negative.

4   A 32-year-old dressmaker goes to her GP with a chronic cough. He examines her and finds splenomegaly and some tender nodules on her shins, which she says have been there for 2 months. A chest X-ray shows bilateral hilar lymphadenopathy.

5   A 68-year-old man has a routine health check-up and is found to be anaemic with splenomegaly. He is in generally good health but has had an aortic valve replacement 4 years ago, for which he takes warfarin. There are no murmurs. Blood tests reveal Hb 10.6 g/dL, MCV 86 fL and unconjugated bilirubin 32 μmol/L. Liver function is otherwise normal.

5 DISORDERS OF COAGULATION

The patients below all complain of easy bruising. Match the most likely cause of this with the clinical scenarios

A von Willebrand's disease
B Alcoholism
C Disseminated intravascular coagulation
D Haemophilia A
E Scurvy

F Haemolytic uraemic syndrome
G Haemophilia B
H Idiopathic thrombocytopenic purpura
I Iatrogenic
J Aplastic anaemia

1 A 6-year-old girl presents to the emergency department and is found to have widespread petechiae and haemorrhagic bullae on her buccal mucosa. She is usually well but has had a cold about 2 weeks ago. Bloods show Hb 12.3g/dL, white cell count (WCC) 6.7×10^9/L with normal prothrombin time (PT) and activated partial thromboplastin time (APTT).

2 A 26-year-old social worker finds that he bruises easily playing football. Blood tests reveal that he has a prolonged APTT, with normal PT and bleeding time. Levels of Factor VIII:C are 6 per cent of normal.

3 A 47-year-old solicitor sees his GP after his employer asks for a health check due to excessive sick leave. On examination, he has purpura over his arms and shins and marked hepatomegaly. He admits that he does not eat well. His PT and APTT are prolonged, but the bleeding time is normal.

4 A 12-year-old boy is seen in haematology clinic for easy bruising. Blood tests reveal a prolonged APTT, with normal PT and bleeding time. Factor IX cannot be detected.

5 A 27-year-old librarian is having her first child. During childbirth she becomes acutely short of breath and then develops significant epistaxis and vaginal bleeding. Blood tests show a prolonged PT, APTT with a very low level of fibrinogen. She is transferred to the intensive care unit for further management.

6 DRUGS USED TO TREAT THROMBOSIS

Choose the most likely drug to be used for each of the scenarios below

A Aspirin
B Clopidogrel
C Unfractionated heparin
D Dipyridamole
E Abciximab

F Warfarin
G Streptokinase
H Enoxaparin
I Tissue plasminogen activator
J Hirudin

1 An anterior myocardial infarction in a patient who has received thrombolysis 6 months previously. The registrar wants to thrombolyse the patient again.

2 An acutely ischaemic lower limb with suspected arterial thrombosis.

3 Prophylaxis against deep venous thrombosis in a patient undergoing hip replacement.

4 Atrial fibrillation in a 68-year-old patient with diabetes.

5 Oral medication used as an adjunct to aspirin in the treatment of acute coronary syndrome.

7 POLYCYTHAEMIA

Match the clinical histories below with the most likely cause of polycythaemia

A   Dehydration
B   High altitude
C   Smoking
D   Wilms' tumour
E   Stress polycythaemia

F   Polycythaemia rubra vera
G   Renal cell carcinoma
H   Right to left cardiac shunt
I   Cerebellar haemangioblastoma
J   Hepatocellular carcinoma

1   A 4-year-old boy presents to his GP with haematuria. The GP finds that he has a mass in his abdomen and orders some blood tests which reveal Hb 17.2g/dL.

2   A 67-year-old man goes to see his doctor with non-specific symptoms of tiredness and malaise. The GP finds him to have splenomegaly and thinks he looks plethoric, and so takes some blood, which shows Hb 19.3g/dL, WCC 14×10^9/L and platelets 890×10^9/L.

3   A 43-year-old homeless man with hepatitis C presents to the emergency department with increasing abdominal distension. Examination reveals tense ascites. The registrar performs a full set of blood tests, which reveal Hb 20.1g/dL, WCC 7×10^9/L, platelets 160 $\times 10^9$/L and alpha-fetoprotein 3000 ng/mL.

4   A 19-year-old athlete preparing for the Olympic Games comes to the emergency department with a twisted ankle. He has just returned from a 4-month period training overseas. Some routine bloods show Hb 19.8g/dL, WCC 4×10^9/L and platelets 340×10^9/L.

5   A 78-year-old woman is brought in to hospital by ambulance after having been found lying on the floor of her sheltered housing where she had been for 14 h. She has a broken right neck of femur and is consented for theatre. The surgeons are puzzled however when the Hb is found to be 18.1g/dL.

8 ANTICOAGULATION

Choose the most appropriate target for the international normalized ratio (INR) for each of the stems below

A   1
B   1.5
C   2
D   2.5
E   3

F   3.5
G   4
H   4.5
I   5
J   5.5

1   Atrial fibrillation.
2   Deep venous thrombosis.
3   Coronary artery bypass grafting.
4   Pulmonary embolism.
5   Deep venous thrombosis while on warfarin.

9 CERVICAL LYMPHADENOPATHY

The patients below all present to their GP with cervical lymphadenopathy. Select the most likely diagnosis from the options below

A Hodgkin's disease
B Tuberculosis
C Gastric carcinoma
D HIV
E Streptococcal infection

F Infectious mononucleosis
G Sarcoidosis
H Thyroid carcinoma
I Non-Hodgkin's lymphoma
J Acute lymphoblastic leukaemia

1 A 71-year-old alcoholic man, who is being investigated for iron-deficiency anaemia, is found to have a hard supraclavicular lymph node on the left side of his neck.
2 A 19-year-old ballet dancer complains of lumps in her neck that are increasing in size. She complains of intermittent fever, night sweats and weight loss. The GP arranges for a lymph node biopsy which shows cells which the pathologist describes as looking like 'owl eyes'.
3 A 21-year-old struggling artist complains of lumps in her neck which are increasing in size. She also remarks on intermittent fever, night sweats and weight loss. The GP arranges for a lymph node biopsy which shows caseating granulomas.
4 A 4-year-old boy tells his mother he feels tired and weak. She has taken him to the doctor five times in the past 2 months for a variety of infections. On this visit, the GP finds he has cervical lymphadenopathy, but no fever, and takes some blood. The lab calls him two days later to tell him the Hb is 9.5g/dL, WCC 60×10^9/L (70 per cent blasts).
5 A 3-year-old girl goes to her GP with a 24-h history of sore throat and fever. On examination, there is evident pharyngitis with exudate and tender cervical lymphadenopathy.

Answers: see pages 205–207

ANSWERS

MCQ ANSWERS

1 a) True. This is a form of inherited red cell membrane defect, causing haemolytic anaemia.
   b) False.
   c) True. Splenectomy is indicated if steroid treatment is unsuccessful.
   d) True. If left untreated, haemorrhage from a ruptured spleen may be fatal.
   e) False.

2 a) True. This is thrombocytopenia, microangiopathic haemolytic anaemia (MAHA) and renal failure. It is related to thrombotic thrombocytopenic purpura.
   b) False. This is a genetic disorder causing a conjugated hyperbilirubinaemia.
   c) True.
   d) True. This is known as heparin-induced thrombocytopenia, or HIT.
   e) True. There is a lack of platelet production in the bone marrow.

3 a) False. Factor VIII deficiency is responsible.
   b) False. It is sex-linked recessive.
   c) True. Recurrent haemarthroses give rise to a disabling arthropathy.
   d) True. This increases factor VIII levels and is useful in mild cases.
   e) False. Haemophilia B is a deficiency of factor IX.

4 a) True. DIC can occur in any malignancy.
   b) False.
   c) True. This is especially true of Gram-negative septicaemia – such as meningococcal infection.
   d) True.
   e) True. Other obstetric causes include amniotic fluid embolus, retained placenta or dead foetus, pre-eclampsia, and septic abortion.

5 a) False. It must never be given via this route, as it is neurotoxic. Methotrexate is given intrathecally in ALL.
   b) False. It is found in over 95 per cent of chronic myeloid leukaemia cases.
   c) True.
   d) True. Anaemia occurs as a result of bone marrow failure.
   e) False. It is rare in children.

6 a) False.
   b) False. Thrombocytosis occurs for a few weeks after splenectomy, but may persist in about one-third of cases.
   c) False.
   d) True. Nuclear remnants are seen inside red cells after splenectomy.
   e) True. There is increased vulnerability to infection from encapsulated bacteria – pneumococcus, meningococcus and haemophilus.

7 a) False. Bilirubin is released from the excess breakdown of red cells – this is in the unconjugated form.
   b) False.
   c) True. This is an indicator of increased red cell production to compensate for the haemolysis.
   d) False. Alkaline phosphatase is increased in obstructive liver disease and bone disease.
   e) True.

8 a) False. These are a feature of infective endocarditis.
   b) False. This is a tongue lesion caused by Epstein–Barr virus in immunocompromised patients.
   c) True. This describes spoon-shaped nails.
   d) True. Fissures and inflammation occur at the corner of the mouth.
   e) True. This is an oesophageal web occurring in iron-deficient patients, causing dysphagia.

9 a) False. It is an autosomal recessive condition.
   b) False.
   c) True. There is reduced blood cell formation. Transfusion is required.
   d) False. Hydroxycarbamide is a useful drug; it increases fetal haemoglobin production.
   e) False. There is some protection against *Plasmodium falciparum* malaria.

10 a) True.
   b) False. However, there is an increased risk during pregnancy.
   c) True. This is a hypercoagulable state.
   d) False. Massive transfusion can lead to a bleeding tendency due to depletion of platelets and coagulation factors.
   e) True. There is a threefold increased risk of thrombosis.

11 a) False. It is a genetic disorder.
   b) False. They are a feature of multiple myeloma.
   c) True.
   d) False. The distribution extends from the Mediterranean to South East Asia.
   e) True. If splenomegaly is present, splenectomy is useful. Prophylaxis against infection is required.

12 a) True. This is visceral leishmaniasis
   b) False.
   c) False.
   d) False.
   e) True. Other causes are myelofibrosis, and chronic myeloid leukaemia.

13 a) True. Gallstones occur as a result of increased bilirubin production from haemolysis.
   b) False.
   c) False.
   d) True. Sickle disease causes bone necrosis. Infection (osteomyelitis) is commonly due to *Salmonella*.
   e) True. These occur secondary to lower limb ischaemia.

14 a) True.
    b) False. This is a cause of thrombophilia.
    c) False.
    d) True. Blood cells become trapped and destroyed in the spleen.
    e) True. There is a pancytopenia with hypocellular bone marrow.

15 a) False. Lack of intrinsic factor causes vitamin B_{12} deficiency, resulting in a macrocytic, megaloblastic anaemia.
    b) True. This is an inherited anaemia involving defective synthesis of the globin portion of the haemoglobin molecule.
    c) False.
    d) False.
    e) True. This is a form of microcytic anaemia characterized by sideroblasts in the bone marrow.

16 a) False. This is a bleeding disorder involving deficient or abnormal von Willebrand factor, which is needed for normal platelet function.
    b) True. There is a mutation in the factor V gene, causing resistance to activated protein C.
    c) False.
    d) False. Deficiency of protein C or S causes thrombophilia.
    e) True. This is inherited as autosomal dominant.

17 a) True. Blood must be transfused cautiously with furosemide in patients with heart failure.
    b) True. This may occur with massive transfusion.
    c) True. Severe reactions must be managed immediately by stopping the transfusion and administering adrenaline.
    d) True. Immunocompromised patients should receive blood from CMV-negative donors.
    e) True. This is a feature of acute haemolytic transfusion reaction.

18 a) False. The lack of vitamin B_{12} causes a macrocytic, megaloblastic anaemia.
    b) True. Severe vitamin B_{12} deficiency causes subacute combined degeneration of the cord.
    c) False. Pernicious anaemia causes vitamin B_{12} deficiency; hydroxocobalamin is therefore used in its treatment.
    d) True. There is also an association with other autoimmune diseases.
    e) False. It is not a genetic disease.

19 a) False.
    b) True.
    c) False.
    d) True. Methotrexate is an antifolate drug.
    e) True. This may also be a cause of macrocytosis without anaemia.

20 a) False. The action of unfractionated heparin ceases soon after stopping the infusion. LMWH's action is more difficult to terminate.
    b) True. The response to LMWH is more predictable; monitoring is generally not needed.
    c) False. There is a reduced risk of thrombocytopenia as compared with unfractionated heparin.
    d) False. The duration is longer, and is normally given as a subcutaneous injection once or twice a day.
    e) False. Administration is by subcutaneous injection. Unfractionated heparin is given in the same way or as an intravenous infusion.

21 a) False. This enzyme catalyses the conversion of angiotensin I to II; it is most abundant in the lungs.
    b) True. This is an autosomal recessive inherited deficiency: it causes haemolytic anaemia and splenic enlargement.
    c) False. This is an enzyme found in bone and the liver.
    d) False. This is a widespread enzyme found in skeletal and cardiac muscle, and a range of other organs.
    e) True. Glucose-6-phosphatase deficiency is an X-linked inherited haemolytic anaemia. Oxidative crises may be precipitated by ingestion of drugs or fava beans.

22 a) False. This is a bleeding disorder involving defective or deficient von Willebrand's factor.
    b) True. This is a red cell membrane defect, with autosomal dominant inheritance.
    c) False. This is an inherited deficiency in phenylalanine hydroxylase, which can cause cognitive impairment.
    d) True. There is defective production of the globin chain component of haemoglobin.
    e) True. This is an autosomal recessive defect in red cell metabolism. Splenomegaly is a feature.

23 a) False.
    b) True. This reveals a monoclonal band, indicating paraproteinaemia.
    c) True. This may demonstrate lytic lesions.
    d) True. This is to look for Bence–Jones protein.
    e) True. Serum calcium is typically raised.

24 a) False.
    b) True. B symptoms confer a worse prognosis.
    c) False. These are large multinucleate cells that are classically seen in Hodgkin's lymphoma.
    d) True. High-grade lymphomas are potentially curable.
    e) True. It occurs in West African children, commonly presenting with a jaw tumour.

25 a) False. In polycythaemia rubra vera, failure of apoptosis leads to proliferation of red cells.
    b) True. This is due to increased cell turnover.
    c) True.
    d) False. Venesection is often successful.
    e) False. The classic history is of pruritus developing on having a hot bath.

EMQ ANSWERS

1 MICROCYTIC ANAEMIA

1 C The most common cause of iron-deficiency anaemia worldwide is chronic intestinal blood loss through **hookworm infestation.**

2 H The raised iron and ferritin are not consistent with a diagnosis of iron-deficiency anaemia. The presence of ringed cells in the marrow provides the clue that this is **sideroblastic anaemia.**

3 B Iron-deficiency anaemia in the elderly is **colonic carcinoma** until proven otherwise. The weight loss is in keeping with this diagnosis.

4 D There are two possible diagnoses here: iron-deficiency anaemia secondary to diclofenac, and **anaemia of chronic disease** secondary to rheumatoid arthritis. The high ferritin (due to the inflammatory process) indicates that the latter is more likely.

5 G This student has a profound microcytosis and a mild anaemia. The degree of microcytosis for the level of haemoglobin is not consistent with iron-deficiency anaemia, and this is confirmed by the normal haematinics. The most likely cause of this picture is **thalassaemia** trait.

2 HAEMOLYTIC ANAEMIA

1 H **Hereditary spherocytosis** is a congenital haemolytic anaemia in which the red cells cannot pass through the microcirculation. Diagnosis is via blood film and the osmotic fragility test (the cells are more susceptible to haemolysis in dilute saline solutions than normal red cells).

2 I The ethnic origin of this child, anaemia, and frontal bossing all suggest **thalassaemia.** The characteristic hair on end appearance of the skull is due to expansion of the diploic marrow.

3 C This student has developed a haemolytic anaemia secondary to **malaria.** The term 'blackwater fever' is sometimes used to describe falciparum malaria when it presents in this way.

4 B This patient has been treated for pneumonia. The most likely organism is *Mycoplasma pneumoniae*, given the presence of erythema multiforme. A well-recognized complication of this is the development of cold **autoimmune** haemolytic anaemia, resulting in a positive direct antiglobulin test (direct Coombs' test) and unconjugated hyperbilirubinaemia.

5 A This patient is suffering from acute haemolysis, probably precipitated by the nitrofurantoin. Patients with **G6PD deficiency** are highly susceptible to developing haemolysis when given this drug; other drugs that should be avoided include quinolones and sulphonamides.

3 MACROCYTOSIS

1 D **Crohn's disease** has a predilection for the terminal ileum. In this patient, malabsorption of vitamin B_{12} at this site is the most likely cause of the macrocytosis.

2 A Addison's disease is strongly associated with other autoimmune diseases. **Pernicious anaemia** has developed in this patient, resulting in a neuropathy affecting the dorsal columns of the spinal cord.

3 C The low haemoglobin indicates severe blood loss: as a compensatory mechanism the bone marrow releases **reticulocytes**, immature red blood cells, into the peripheral circulation. These are larger than normal red blood cells, and therefore can cause an apparent macrocytosis on the full blood count.

4 I This woman describes symptoms of **hypothyroidism**, which is a cause of non-megalo-blastic macrocytosis.

5 F **Iatrogenic.** Macrocytic anaemia is an important complication of phenytoin therapy.

4 SPLENOMEGALY

1 H The combination of tonsillitis and splenomegaly should raise the suspicion of **infectious mononucleosis.** Amoxicillin should never be used to treat tonsillitis because of the complication of a rash, should the tonsillitis be caused by the Epstein–Barr virus.

2 J This patient has the characteristic triad of **Felty's syndrome**: rheumatoid arthritis, splenomegaly and neutropenia.

3 G **Thalassaemia** causes a profound microcytosis and anaemia in susceptible populations, such as those from the borders of the Mediterranean. Splenomegaly is found when haemopoiesis begins to occur outside the bone marrow.

4 D The combination of bilateral hilar lymphadenopathy and erythema nodosum are pathognomonic of **sarcoidosis.** Splenomegaly can be a feature of this disease.

5 I Haemolysis is the most common cause of unconjugated hyperbilirubinaemia. This patient probably has a degree of chronic mechanical **haemolytic anaemia** from his prosthetic aortic valve replacement (he would not take warfarin if it were a biological valve).

5 DISORDERS OF COAGULATION

1 H The sudden onset of bleeding in a young child after a trivial viral illness is a good history for **idiopathic thrombocytopenic purpura** (ITP). Treatment is usually with steroids or immunoglobulin, and the prognosis is generally good.

2 D **Haemophilia A** is an X-linked condition in which there are reduced levels of factor VIII. The APTT is prolonged. The severity and clinical presentation of the illness depend on the percentage activity of factor VIII.

3 B **Alcoholism** is a common cause of deranged clotting. This patient has several features: absenteeism from work, easy bruising and hepatomegaly. The PT and APTT are prolonged due to a decrease in synthetic function by the liver, which may be partially reversed by the administration of vitamin K.

4 G **Haemophilia B**, or Christmas disease, is a genetic condition where there is deficiency of factor IX. Presentation is similar to that of haemophilia A.

5 C The very low level of fibrinogen and derangement of clotting suggest **disseminated intravascular coagulation**, where clotting factors are consumed throughout the vascular tree. Amniotic fluid embolism during childbirth is a well-recognized cause.

6 DRUGS USED TO TREAT THROMBOSIS

1 I The only thrombolytic drugs are streptokinase and **tissue plasminogen activator.** Of these, streptokinase is contraindicated as antibodies form after administration, precluding its use again as a thrombolytic agent.

2 C **Unfractionated heparin** is used in the management of acute arterial thrombosis, as it can be reversed quickly should the need for surgery arise.

3 H Low-molecular weight heparins such as **enoxaparin** are preferred over unfractionated heparin in the prophylaxis of deep venous thrombosis, as they are easier to administer and more effective. There is no need to monitor the APTT.

4 F   **Warfarin** is the oral drug of choice for all non-pregnant patients who need long-term anticoagulation.

5 B   **Clopidogrel**, an oral platelet adenosine diphosphate (ADP) antagonist, is used with aspirin and parenteral heparin in the management of acute coronary syndromes.

7 POLYCYTHAEMIA

1 D   **Wilms' tumour** (nephroblastoma) is the most common abdominal tumour in children. The characteristic presentation is with a loin mass and haematuria; polycythaemia may be a feature.

2 F   This gentleman has **polycythaemia rubra vera**, as evidenced by the splenomegaly, which is not a feature of the secondary polycythaemias. Note the increase in number of all cell types.

3 J   An alpha-fetoprotein this high with ascites is effectively diagnostic of a **hepatocellular carcinoma**. These typically occur in cirrhotic livers, which in this patient would most likely be due to either alcohol or viral hepatitis.

4 B   It is common for athletes to undertake **high altitude** training, in an effort to increase their haemoglobin and consequently oxygen-carrying capacity.

5 A   **Dehydration** is probably the cause of the apparent polycythaemia in this patient: lying on the floor for a prolonged period of time results in significant fluid losses, particularly in the elderly.

8 ANTICOAGULATION

1 D   2.5.

2 D   2.5.

3 A   1.

4 D   2.5.

5 F   3.5.

Current target INR recommendations for anticoagulation include:

- INR 2.5 for treatment of deep vein thrombosis/pulmonary embolism (DVT/PE), atrial fibrillation
- INR 3.5 for recurrent DVT and PE (in patients already on warfarin)
- INR 2.5–3.5 for prosthetic valves, depending on valve type and location.

9 CERVICAL LYMPHADENOPATHY

1 C   The lymph node is Virchow's node (Troisier's sign), which is associated with **gastric malignancy**.

2 A   Owl eyes or binucleate cells are pathognomonic of **Hodgkin's disease**. In this case, the patient also has constitutional 'B' symptoms, which are associated with a worse prognosis.

3 B   Caseating granulomas are characteristic of **tuberculosis** (TB); the constitutional symptoms are also in keeping with this diagnosis. TB is associated with overcrowding, poor housing and inadequate nutrition.

4 J   Recurrent infections often occur in **acute lymphoblastic leukaemia** (ALL). The grossly elevated white cell count, with a predominance of blast cells, makes ALL the best answer.

5 E   This is a common presentation in primary care. The most likely bacterial cause of these symptoms is **streptococcal infection**, often by *Streptococcus pyogenes*.

Endocrinology

MULTIPLE CHOICE QUESTIONS

1 The following signs are associated with hypocalcaemia:
   a) Tinel's sign
   b) Brudzinski's sign
   c) Chvostek's sign
   d) Quincke's sign
   e) Trousseau's sign

2 Causes of hypercalcaemia include:
   a) Multiple myeloma
   b) Osteoporosis
   c) Parathyroidectomy
   d) Paget's disease
   e) Sarcoidosis

3 Clinical features of Cushing's syndrome include:
   a) Corrigan's sign
   b) Weight loss
   c) Erythema nodosum
   d) Proximal myopathy
   e) Thin skin

4 The following tests are of use in the diagnosis of acromegaly:
   a) Plasma adrenocorticotrophic hormone (ACTH)
   b) Water deprivation test
   c) Synacthen test
   d) Oral glucose tolerance test
   e) Insulin-like growth factor-1 level

5 A pituitary adenoma may present with the following:
   a) IIIrd nerve palsy
   b) Amnesia
   c) Hemisensory loss
   d) Visual field loss
   e) Cerebrospinal fluid (CSF) rhinorrhoea

6   Causes of secondary diabetes mellitus include:
   a) Hereditary haemochromatosis
   b) Lung adenocarcinoma
   c) Chronic renal failure
   d) Acromegaly
   e) Sarcoidosis

7   The following statements are true of the treatment of diabetes type 2:
   a) Gliclazide is the treatment of choice in obese patients
   b) Oral antidiabetic drugs should be started immediately in a newly diagnosed type 2 diabetic
   c) Hypoglycaemia is a common side-effect of metformin
   d) Oral antidiabetic drugs should be stopped 7 days before major surgery
   e) Insulin should be considered for poorly controlled diabetics already on oral anti-diabetic agents

8   The following are neurological complications of diabetes mellitus:
   a) Impotence
   b) Cerebellar syndrome
   c) Postural hypotension
   d) Charcot's joints
   e) Subacute combined degeneration of the cord

9   Causes of hypoglycaemia include:
   a) Glucagonoma
   b) Smoking
   c) Cushing's disease
   d) Alcohol
   e) Insulinoma

10 Symptoms of hyperprolactinaemia in females include:
   a) Oligomenorrhoea
   b) Psychosis
   c) Hyperpigmentation
   d) Galactorrhoea
   e) Heightened libido

11 The following statements are true of diabetes insipidus:
   a) Urine osmolality is low
   b) Hysterical drinking is a cause
   c) A Synacthen test is diagnostic
   d) Desmopressin must be administered intravenously
   e) Treatment is with fluid restriction to 1 L/day

12 Clinical features of hyperthyroidism include:
   a) Dysdiadochokinesis
   b) Diminished appetite
   c) Irritability
   d) Atrial fibrillation
   e) Weight gain

13 Causes of hyperthyroidism include:
   a) Hashimoto's thyroiditis
   b) Hypopituitarism
   c) Propylthiouracil
   d) De Quervain's thyroiditis
   e) Amiodarone

14 The following statements are true of the management of hyperthyroidism:
   a) Carbimazole must be started in conjunction with propylthiouracil
   b) The major side-effect of carbimazole is anaphylaxis
   c) Radio-iodine is safe in the third trimester of pregnancy
   d) Hypothyroidism is a risk of radio-iodine therapy
   e) Propranolol is of little benefit

15 Signs of hypothyroidism include:
   a) Dementia
   b) Hirsutism
   c) Bradycardia
   d) Hyper-reflexia
   e) Carpal tunnel syndrome

16 Ocular features of Graves' disease include:
   a) Cataract
   b) Iritis
   c) Exophthalmos
   d) Proliferative retinopathy
   e) Ophthalmoplegia

17 Causes of male hypogonadism include:
   a) Cirrhosis
   b) Turner's syndrome
   c) Kallmann's syndrome
   d) Hyperprolactinaemia
   e) Klinefelter's syndrome

18 The following statements are true of thyroid carcinoma:
   a) Medullary carcinoma is the commonest type
   b) They do not metastasize to bone
   c) Papillary carcinoma has the worst prognosis
   d) It is the third leading cause of death from cancer in males in the UK
   e) Radio-iodine is useful in the treatment of papillary carcinomas

19 Clinical features of Cushing's syndrome include:
   a) Vertebral fracture
   b) Hypotension
   c) Spade-like hands
   d) Psychosis
   e) Abdominal striae

20 Complications of acromegaly include:
  a) Colon cancer
  b) Cushing's disease
  c) Cardiomyopathy
  d) Phaeochromocytoma
  e) Diabetes mellitus

21 The following can cause Cushing's syndrome:
  a) Diabetes mellitus
  b) Adrenalectomy
  c) Pituitary adenoma
  d) Adrenal carcinoma
  e) Small cell lung cancer

22 Anterior pituitary hormones include:
  a) Antidiuretic hormone (ADH)
  b) Thyrotrophin-releasing hormone (TRH)
  c) Follicle-stimulating hormone (FSH)
  d) Prolactin
  e) Corticotrophin-releasing hormone (CRH)

23 Diabetes mellitus is a risk factor for the following:
  a) Charcot arthropathy
  b) Stroke
  c) Fibrosing alveolitis
  d) Peripheral neuropathy
  e) Nephrotic syndrome

24 Complications of subtotal thyroidectomy include:
  a) Mallory–Weiss tear
  b) Laryngeal nerve palsy
  c) Boerhaave's syndrome
  d) Hypocalcaemia
  e) Thyrotoxic crisis

25 Complications of polycystic ovarian syndrome include:
  a) Ectopic pregnancy
  b) Endometrial cancer
  c) Infertility
  d) Hyperthyroidism
  e) Diabetes mellitus

26 Causes of hypopituitarism include:
  a) Diabetes mellitus
  b) Craniopharyngioma
  c) Anorexia nervosa
  d) Wilson's disease
  e) Sheehan's syndrome

27 Use of the combined oral contraceptive pill confers an increased risk of:
   a) Endometrial cancer
   b) Breast cancer
   c) Venous thromboembolism
   d) Ovarian cancer
   e) Gallstones

28 The following biochemical findings are consistent with a diagnosis of Addison's disease:
   a) Low potassium
   b) Low sodium
   c) High glucose
   d) Low adrenocorticotrophic hormone (ACTH)
   e) High renin

29 Causes of amenorrhoea include:
   a) Endometrial carcinoma
   b) Anorexia nervosa
   c) Fallopian tubal ligation
   d) Prolactinoma
   e) Polycystic ovarian syndrome

30 Causes of hyperprolactinaemia include:
   a) Salbutamol
   b) Pregnancy
   c) Oophorectomy
   d) Epilepsy
   e) Metoclopramide

31 Clinical features of Addison's disease include:
   a) Hirsutism
   b) Hyperpigmentation
   c) Weight gain
   d) Spider naevi
   e) Postural hypotension

32 Sequelae of menopause include:
   a) Breast hypertrophy
   b) Urinary incontinence
   c) Hirsutism
   d) Osteoporosis
   e) Reduced ischaemic heart disease risk

33 Features of acromegaly include:
   a) Abdominal striae
   b) Prognathism
   c) Carpal tunnel syndrome
   d) Dental caries
   e) Tongue fasciculation

34 Clinical features of acromegaly include:
   a) Thinned skin
   b) Arthropathy
   c) Hair loss
   d) Pruritus
   e) Proximal myopathy

35 The following are causes of syndrome of inappropriate antidiuretic hormone secretion (SIADH):
   a) Head injury
   b) Community-acquired pneumonia
   c) Diabetes insipidus
   d) Meningitis
   e) Lung cancer

36 Causes of primary hypothyroidism include:
   a) Graves' disease
   b) Post-partum thyroiditis
   c) Hypopituitarism
   d) Dietary insufficiency
   e) Hashimoto's thyroiditis

37 Features of hypercalcaemia include:
   a) Skull thickening
   b) Depression
   c) Constipation
   d) Dental loss
   e) Polyuria

38 Secondary causes of hypertension include:
   a) Conn's syndrome
   b) Acromegaly
   c) Addison's disease
   d) Phaeochromocytoma
   e) Cushing's syndrome

39 Symptoms of hypothyroidism include:
   a) Palpitations
   b) Weight gain
   c) Diarrhoea
   d) Low mood
   e) Hot flushes

40 Post-menopausal hormone replacement therapy (HRT) reduces the risk of:
   a) Endometrial cancer
   b) Osteoporosis
   c) Breast cancer
   d) Venous thromboembolism
   e) Coronary artery disease

Answers: see pages 221–226

EXTENDED MATCHING QUESTIONS

1 HYPERGLYCAEMIA

Choose the most likely cause of hyperglycaemia for each of the clinical scenarios below

A Cushing's syndrome
B Phaeochromocytoma
C Iatrogenic
D Cushing's disease
E Glucagonoma

F Thyrotoxicosis
G Haemochromatosis
H Acromegaly
I Cystic fibrosis
J Chronic pancreatitis

1 A 68-year-old woman presents to her general practitioner (GP) with recurrent skin infections. Fasting blood glucose is 14.2 mmol/L. The GP looks at her medical records and sees that she has had her parathyroids removed for hyperparathyroidism and has also been treated surgically for a prolactinoma.

2 A 39-year-old woman goes to see her doctor about her inexorable weight gain. She has put on 8 kg in the past 4 months, despite not having changed her diet. On examination, she has an interscapular fat pad, proximal myopathy, centripetal obesity and bitemporal hemianopia.

3 A 59-year-old woman goes to see her doctor as she is feeling tired. Her blood pressure is 180/106 mmHg and blood glucose 13.1 mmol/L. The GP notices that there are small gaps between each of her teeth.

4 A 32-year-old diabetic man is admitted to hospital with acute asthma. On the ward round the consultant looks at the blood glucose chart and sees that his glycaemic control is much worse than usual.

5 A 42-year-old homeless man is well known to the gastroenterology team, with frequent admissions for spontaneous bacterial peritonitis. On one admission, his fasting blood sugar is found to be 9.3 mmol/L.

2 INVESTIGATION OF ENDOCRINE DISEASE

Choose the best diagnostic test for each of the endocrine conditions below

A Water-deprivation test
B Low-dose dexamethasone suppression test
C Urinary metanephrines
D Glucose tolerance test
E Urine and plasma osmolality

F Perimetry
G Short Synacthen (tetracosactide) test
H Serum androgens
I Thyroglobulin
J Serum prolactin

1 Addison's disease.
2 Acromegaly.
3 Congenital adrenal hyperplasia.
4 Diabetes insipidus.
5 Phaeochromocytoma.

3 MEDICAL TREATMENT OF ENDOCRINE DISEASE

Choose the drug most likely to be used to treat each of the conditions below

A   Insulin
B   Fludrocortisone
C   Spironolactone
D   Oestrogens
E   Bromocriptine

F   Levothyroxine sodium
G   Gliclazide
H   Carbimazole
I   Phenoxybenzamine/metoprolol
J   Metformin

1   Phaeochromocytoma.
2   Conn's syndrome.
3   Graves' disease.
4   Addison's disease.
5   Prolactinoma.

4 COMPLICATIONS OF DRUGS USED TO TREAT ENDOCRINE DISEASE

Choose the drug most likely to cause each of the complications listed below

A   Insulin
B   Fludrocortisone
C   Spironolactone
D   Alendronate
E   Bromocriptine

F   Levothyroxine sodium
G   Gliclazide
H   Carbimazole
I   Phenoxybenzamine/metoprolol
J   Metformin

1   Agranulocytosis.
2   Hyperkalaemia.
3   Lactic acidosis when given with radiological contrast.
4   Fat hypertrophy.
5   Gynaecomastia.

5 DISORDERS OF CALCIUM METABOLISM

Each of the clinical scenarios below involves a patient with a disorder of calcium metabolism. Choose the most likely cause of this from the options given

A   Primary hyperparathyroidism
B   Secondary hyperparathyroidism
C   Tertiary hyperparathyroidism
D   Hypercalcaemia of malignancy
E   Hypoparathyroidism

F   Pseudohypoparathyroidism
G   Pseudopseudohypoparathyroidism
H   Iatrogenic
I   Sarcoidosis
J   Myeloma

1   A 49-year-old woman attends the local renal unit for dialysis three times per week. She goes to her GP with paraesthesiae. Blood tests reveal elevated urea and creatinine, low calcium, high parathyroid hormone (PTH) and high phosphate.

2   An 81-year-old man is walking out of the supermarket when his leg suddenly gives way underneath him causing him to hit his head. He is taken to the emergency department where blood tests show hypercalcaemia and an erythrocyte sedimentation rate (ESR) of 90 mm/h. X-rays of his hip show a fractured neck of femur; his skull X-ray shows multiple lytic lesions.

3   A 31-year-old woman presents to her GP with fatigue and depression. A routine set of bloods shows a normal calcium, low phosphate and elevated levels of PTH.

4   A 72-year-old man on renal dialysis goes to see his nephrologists. He has been on renal dialysis for 8 years. His nephrologist is concerned as he has elevated urea and creatinine, high calcium, high PTH and high phosphate.

5   An 82-year-old man goes to his GP as he is feeling constipated. He takes atenolol and bendroflumethiazide for his hypertension, but is otherwise well. The GP takes the opportunity to perform some blood tests, which show a mildly elevated calcium level.

6 PRESENTATIONS OF ENDOCRINE DISEASE

Choose the most likely diagnosis from the options given for each of the clinical scenarios below

A   Graves' disease
B   Acromegaly
C   Addison's disease
D   Conn's syndrome
E   Nelson's syndrome
F   Gigantism
G   Cushing's disease
H   Diabetes mellitus
I   Hypothyroidism
J   Diabetes insipidus

1   A 68-year-old retired security guard registers with a new GP. His GP remarks that he appears well tanned. The patient says that he has had the tan ever since he was treated for a problem with his steroid levels.

2   A 35-year-old chemist presents to the emergency department with vomiting. Her abdomen is soft, and she has noticed no change in her bowel habit. She has never been in hospital before. On examination, she has postural hypotension and pigmented palmar creases and gums.

3   A 79-year-old woman goes to her GP as she is feeling weak. She is on medication for diabetes and high blood pressure, which have both been difficult to control. Examination reveals a proximal myopathy, bitemporal hemianopia and a large tongue.

4   A 56-year-old banker goes to his GP as his wife has been nagging him to have his cholesterol checked. He has a blood pressure of 160/110 mmHg. Blood tests show Na$^+$ 148 mmol/L, K$^+$ 3.2 mmol/L, with normal lipid profile.

5   A 63-year-old obese man goes to his GP as he is feeling weak. He is on medication for diabetes and high blood pressure, which have both been difficult to control. Examination reveals a proximal myopathy, bitemporal hemianopia and striae.

7 MEDICATION USED TO TREAT DIABETES MELLITUS

Choose the most appropriate drug from the options given for each of the patients below

A   Metformin
B   Gliclazide
C   Acarbose
D   Glucagon
E   Rosiglitazone
F   50 per cent dextrose solution
G   Sliding-scale intravenous insulin
H   Insulin glargine
I   Insulin lispro
J   Porcine insulin

1   An overweight 55-year-old lorry driver presents to his GP with frequent skin infections. His GP diagnoses diabetes mellitus and starts him on an oral hypoglycaemic agent.

2   A 21-year-old student presents to the emergency department with vomiting. Arterial blood gas analysis shows an elevated glucose, metabolic acidosis and increased anion gap. The foundation doctor asks his registrar what drug he should give the patient.

3   A 37-year-old man with type 1 diabetes is found by his wife to be completely unresponsive in the middle of the night. She calls an ambulance, and then remembers that he has some medication for this eventuality in the bedside cupboard.

4   A newly diagnosed patient with type 1 diabetes goes to her GP for a medication review. She is having trouble with her regimen and suffering from frequent hypoglycaemic episodes. He tells her he is going to give her a new long-acting insulin that she should take once a day.

5   A 63-year-old patient with type 2 diabetes, with a history of poor glycaemic control, returns to her GP saying the new drug he gave her has made her exceptionally flatulent, and that she risks losing her job at the local library if this continues.

8 COMPLICATIONS OF DIABETES MELLITUS

Choose the most likely complications of diabetes from the options given for each of the clinical scenarios below

A   Diabetic ketoacidosis
B   Hyperosmolar non-ketotic state
C   Lactic acidosis
D   Hypoglycaemia
E   Microalbuminuria

F   Background retinopathy
G   Pre-proliferative retinopathy
H   Proliferative retinopathy
I   Autonomic neuropathy
J   Peripheral neuropathy

1   A 68-year-old man goes for a private medical check-up. The physician diligently dilates his pupils and notices cotton wool spots and venous beading.

2   A 57-year-old interpreter has had type 2 diabetes for 20 years. She develops an ulcer under her second toe, and goes to see her doctor. On examination, the foot is warm and well perfused, and surprisingly painless given the severity of the ulcer.

3   A 71-year-old man goes to see his GP with his wife. The GP has looked after his diabetes for the past 30 years. The patient is embarrassed to admit that he is impotent; his wife is insistent that the GP make a diagnosis as to the cause.

4   A 43-year-old man presents to the emergency department feeling unwell. He is known to have type 2 diabetes, and is on oral hypoglycaemics. On examination, he is tachycardic and is hyperventilating. Blood tests reveal Na^+ 136 mmol/L, K^+ 4.0 mmol/L, urea 5.5 mmol/L and glucose 9.5 mmol/L; arterial blood gas analysis shows pH 7.27, Po_2 11.3 kPa, Pco_2 4.8 kPa, with an anion gap of 24. His urine is negative for ketones.

5   A 43-year-old financial advisor complains of blurred vision on a visit to his GP. He is diagnosed as having type 2 diabetes. Fundoscopy reveals blood vessels within the vitreous humour.

9 HYPOGLYCAEMIA

All the patients below have hypoglycaemia. Select the most likely cause of this from the options given

A   Factitious
B   Dumping syndrome
C   Addison's disease
D   Liver failure
E   Sarcoma

F   Alcohol
G   Insulinoma
H   Chronic renal failure
I   Iatrogenic
J   Malnutrition

1   A 67-year-old man presents to his GP complaining of feeling pale, sweaty, nauseated and anxious after meals. He is usually fit and well. On examination of his abdomen, there is a midline laparotomy scar from where he had a partial gastrectomy 5 years ago. The GP arranges to have his blood glucose measured during these attacks, and finds that it is 2.6 mmol/L.

2   A 45-year-old, previously healthy, shop assistant goes to her GP saying that she has started suffering from bouts of sweating and collapse. These episodes can be brought on by fasting. During her last collapse, an ambulance was called and her blood glucose was found to be 2.1 mmol/L. She recovered instantly on administration of intravenous (i.v.) dextrose.

3   A 19-year-old fashion student attends the endocrinology outpatient clinic because of recurrent episodes of hypoglycaemia. Her blood glucose measured during these attacks has been as low as 1.2 mmol/L. Other blood tests have shown normal renal and liver function. C-peptide levels are also normal.

4   A 31-year-old travel agent returns from holiday in Senegal and presents to the emergency department 24 h later with confusion and fever. Blood films show *P. falciparum* parasites and he is started on i.v. quinine. Two days later he feels much better, but the nurses on the ward detect a blood glucose of 2.3 mmol/L.

5   A 46-year-old pop star takes a paracetamol overdose after a long period of depression. He presents to the emergency department 24 h later, regretting his actions. Three days later his blood tests reveal prothrombin time (PT) 58 s, activated partial thromboplastin time (APTT) 102 s, and glucose 2.1 mmol/L.

10 DRUGS USED TO MANIPULATE HORMONES

Select the most appropriate drug for each of the indications below

A   Finasteride
B   Hydrocortisone
C   Danazol
D   Fludrocortisone
E   Calcitonin

F   Clomifene
G   Tamoxifen
H   Goserelin
I   Octreotide
J   Levothyroxine sodium

1   Stimulation of ovulation in a woman trying to conceive by *in vitro* fertilization (IVF).
2   A daily treatment for breast cancer.
3   Treatment of anaphylaxis.
4   A drug used to improve urinary flow in men with benign prostatic hyperplasia.
5   A drug with significant mineralocorticoid activity.

11 DISORDERS OF THE THYROID GLAND

Each of the patients below seeks medical attention for a thyroid disorder. Choose the most likely diagnosis from the options given

A   Graves' disease
B   Papillary carcinoma
C   Thyroglossal cyst
D   de Quervain's thyroiditis
E   Hashimoto's thyroiditis

F   Thyroglossal fistula
G   Medullary carcinoma
H   Lingual thyroid
I   Anaplastic carcinoma
J   Multinodular goitre

1   A 93-year-old judge presents to his doctor with a 4-month history of neck swelling and hoarse voice. Examination reveals a craggy thyroid, fixed to the underlying tissues, with associated lymphadenopathy.

2   A 42-year-old pharmacist presents to her GP with diarrhoea. On examination, she is tachycardic, warm peripherally and has a bounding pulse. The GP also notes that her eyes seem to be bulging.

3   A 27-year-old baker goes to see his doctor because he has noticed a lump in his neck. The lump is in the midline; the GP is interested to see that it moves upwards when the patient protrudes his tongue.

4   A 46-year-old cleaner visits her doctor because she has noticed her neck seems to be getting bigger. She is very concerned as she has recently been in hospital to have a phaeochromocytoma excised. Examination reveals a scar in the neck from a previous operation for hyperparathyroidism and a lump in the thyroid.

5   A 37-year-old nurse sees her doctor with a fever and signs of hyperthyroidism. Blood tests show an elevated C-reactive protein but no autoantibodies. Six weeks later she returns, now complaining of lethargy, fatigue and constipation.

Answers: see pages 227–230

ANSWERS

MCQ ANSWERS

1 a) False. Tapping over the carpal tunnel produces paraesthesiae in the thumb and radial two-and-a-half fingers – a test for carpal tunnel syndrome.
   b) False. This is a sign of meningism: passive flexion of the neck leads to flexion of hips and knees.
   c) True. Tapping over the facial nerve gives rise to twitching of the facial muscles.
   d) False. This is capillary pulsation in the nailbed seen in aortic regurgitation.
   e) True. This is carpopedal spasm seen on inflation of a sphygmomanometer cuff around the arm.

2 a) True.
   b) False.
   c) False. Hyperparathyroidism is an important cause of hypercalcaemia. Parathyroid-ectomy causes hypocalcaemia.
   d) False. Calcium is normal.
   e) True.

3 a) False. This is rapid filling and emptying of the carotid arteries – a sign of aortic regurgitation.
   b) False. Weight gain is a feature.
   c) False. This describes tender erythematous lesions over the shins.
   d) True.
   e) True.

4 a) False. This may be useful in the investigation of Cushing's syndrome.
   b) False. This is a test for diabetes insipidus.
   c) False. This is a useful investigation for Addison's disease.
   d) True. This is the gold standard test for acromegaly. There is failure of suppression of growth hormone after administration of glucose.
   e) True. Typically raised in acromegaly, this serves as an indicator of growth hormone secretion over the previous 24 h.

5 a) True. This is caused by pressure on the oculomotor nerve at the cavernous sinus.
   b) False.
   c) False.
   d) True. This is caused by pressure on the optic chiasm.
   e) True. Erosion through the sphenoid sinus produces CSF rhinorrhoea.

6 a) True. Iron deposition in the pancreas is responsible.
   b) False.
   c) False.
   d) True.
   e) False.

7 **a)** False. Sulphonylureas cause weight gain. Metformin is preferable in obese individuals.
  b) False. Lifestyle and dietary changes should be implemented first.
  c) False. Hypoglycaemia is uncommon. It occurs more frequently with sulphonylureas.
  d) False. They are normally omitted on the morning of surgery.
  e) True. Commonly, tablets eventually fail to maintain glycaemic control, and insulin may then become necessary.

8 **a)** True. Impotence is a common consequence of diabetic autonomic neuropathy.
  b) False.
  c) True. There is loss of peripheral sympathetic tone, due to autonomic neuropathy.
  d) True. These are neuropathic joints.
  e) False. This is a feature of vitamin B_{12} deficiency.

9 **a)** False. This is a pancreatic tumour causing hyperglycaemia.
  b) False.
  c) False. There is a tendency for hyperglycaemia.
  d) True. This is a common cause.
  e) True. This is an insulin-secreting pancreatic tumour which causes fasting hypoglycaemia.

10 **a)** True. Hyperprolactinaemia inhibits gonadotrophin-releasing hormone (GnRH) and gonadotrophin secretion.
  b) False.
  c) False.
  d) True. This may even occur in males.
  e) False. Libido is reduced.

11 **a)** True. Plasma osmolality is concomitantly high or high-normal.
  b) False. It may share biochemical findings and clinical features with diabetes insipidus, but the two are differentiated with a water deprivation test.
  c) False.
  d) False. Cranial diabetes insipidus is treated with desmopressin; this can be given intranasally, orally, or by injection.
  e) False. This is the treatment of the syndrome of inappropriate antidiuretic hormone secretion (SIADH).

12 **a)** False. This is a cerebellar sign.
  b) False. Appetite is heightened.
  c) True.
  d) True. Heart rhythm may reveal sinus tachycardia or atrial fibrillation.
  e) False. Weight loss is a feature.

13 **a)** False. This is a cause of hypothyroidism.
  b) False.
  c) False. This is an antithyroid drug.
  d) True. This is a transient viral cause of hyperthyroidism.
  e) True. This is a cause of hyper- or hypothyroidism.

14 a) False. These drugs are used as single agents. Carbimazole is more widely used in the UK.

   b) False. The major side-effects of carbimazole and propylthiouracil are bone marrow suppression and agranulocytosis.

   c) False. Pregnancy and breast-feeding are contraindications.

   d) True.

   e) False. Beta-blockers do not render patients euthyroid but are useful for symptom control.

15 a) True. Hypothyroidism must be excluded in new-onset dementia.

   b) False. The hair becomes dry and thin, with loss of the outer third of the eyebrows.

   c) True.

   d) False. Reflexes are slow to relax.

   e) True.

16 a) False.

   b) False.

   c) True. This is protrusion of the eyeball when viewed from the side.

   d) False. This is a feature of diabetic eye disease.

   e) True. This is especially found in the superior rectus.

17 a) True. Hypogonadism is a feature of chronic liver disease.

   b) False. This is a female sex chromosomal disorder (karyotype XO).

   c) True. There is isolated GnRH deficiency, associated with anosmia and other features.

   d) True. This causes inhibition of GnRH and gonadotrophin release.

   e) True. This is a male chromosomal disorder (XXY), featuring small testes, androgen deficiency and infertility.

18 a) False. Papillary carcinomas account for approximately 70 per cent.

   b) False. Follicular carcinomas metastasize early to the lungs and bone.

   c) False. Papillary carcinomas have a relatively good prognosis. Anaplastic carcinoma has an appalling prognosis.

   d) False. The order in males is: lung, prostate, colorectal etc. Thyroid carcinoma accounts for about 0.4 per cent of cancer deaths in the total population.

   e) True. It is used to ablate residual thyroid tissue after thyroidectomy.

19 a) True. Osteoporosis is a consequence of Cushing's syndrome.

   b) False. Hypertension is typical.

   c) False. This is a feature of acromegaly.

   d) True.

   e) True.

20 a) True. Premalignant colonic polyposis is more common.

   b) False.

   c) True. Excessive growth hormone causes ventricular hypertrophy and cardio-myopathic heart failure.

   d) False. This is a catecholamine-producing tumour, usually of the adrenal medulla.

   e) True.

21 a) False. But diabetes may be a complication of Cushing's syndrome.
    b) False. This is a cause of Addison's disease.
    c) True. This is Cushing's disease. The adenoma oversecretes ACTH, stimulating excessive endogenous steroid production.
    d) True. Cortisol is overproduced, suppressing ACTH secretion.
    e) True. This is a potential source of ectopic ACTH secretion.

22 a) False. Vasopressin is a posterior pituitary hormone.
    b) False. This is a hypothalamic hormone that stimulates pituitary thyroid-stimulating hormone (TSH) release.
    c) True. FSH is a pituitary gonadotrophin required for follicle development.
    d) True. This is a pituitary hormone that stimulates lactation.
    e) False. CRH is a hormone released by the hypothalamus that stimulates pituitary ACTH release.

23 a) True. This is a neuropathic joint.
    b) True. Diabetics have double the risk of stroke.
    c) False.
    d) True. This is typically a symmetrical, predominantly sensory, distal neuropathy.
    e) True.

24 a) False. This is an oesophageal mucosal tear, caused by vomiting.
    b) True. This may be unilateral or bilateral. Pre-operative laryngoscopy is important to exclude pre-existing vocal cord dysfunction.
    c) False. This is oesophageal rupture, often occurring after heavy alcohol consumption and vomiting.
    d) True. This occurs as a result of the proximity of the parathyroid glands. It is usually transient.
    e) True. This may occur if the patient has not been rendered euthyroid pre-operatively.

25 a) False.
    b) True. The risk of ovarian and endometrial cancers is increased.
    c) True.
    d) False.
    e) True. There is a twofold increased risk. The insulin resistance is linked with hyper-lipidaemia, hypertension and increased risk of stroke.

26 a) False.
    b) True. This is a childhood pituitary tumour.
    c) True. This causes functional disturbance in pituitary hormone secretion.
    d) False.
    e) True. This is pituitary infarction following postpartum haemorrhage.

27 a) False. The pill offers some protection against endometrial and ovarian cancers.
    b) True.
    c) True. The pill should be avoided in those patients who are at high risk from thrombo-embolism.
    d) False.
    e) True. Oral contraceptives predispose to cholestasis.

28 a) False. Classically, potassium levels are high and sodium low; this is due to mineralo-corticoid deficiency.
   b) True.
   c) False. Glucose may be low.
   d) False. ACTH is high due to loss of inhibitory feedback by cortisol on the hypo-thalamic–pituitary axis.
   e) True. Aldosterone is low, with a high renin.

29 a) False. This may result in intermenstrual bleeding, but does not interfere with normal menses.
   b) True. Poor nutrition causes a disruption in the hypothalamic–pituitary axis.
   c) False.
   d) True. High levels of prolactin are responsible.
   e) True. This is the most frequent cause.

30 a) False.
   b) True. Physiological causes include pregnancy, stress, and lactation.
   c) False.
   d) False. Pathological causes include pituitary tumours (especially prolactinoma), low TRH, polycystic ovarian syndrome, acromegaly and renal failure.
   e) True. Drugs are common causes: dopamine antagonists, oestrogens, tricyclic anti-depressants, cimetidine and others.

31 a) False. Hair loss may be a feature.
   b) True. This is due to high levels of ACTH in primary hypoadrenalism.
   c) False. Weight loss is a feature due to the lack of endogenous steroid.
   d) False. This is a sign of chronic liver disease.
   e) True. This is a result of mineralocorticoid deficiency.

32 a) False. Breast atrophy occurs secondary to oestrogen deficiency.
   b) True. Postmenopausal lack of oestrogen decreases intraurethral pressure, predispos-ing to stress incontinence.
   c) False.
   d) True. Bone density falls steeply in postmenopausal women.
   e) False. The lack of oestrogen confers an increased risk of ischaemic heart disease.

33 a) False. These are a sign of steroid excess.
   b) True. This is a large jaw.
   c) True. Soft tissue enlargement causes median nerve compression in the carpal tunnel.
   d) False.
   e) False. The tongue may be enlarged.

34 a) False. The skin becomes coarse and oily.
   b) True. This is due to overgrowth of soft tissue at joints.
   c) False. Mild hirsutism may be a feature in females.
   d) False.
   e) True.

35 a) True.
    b) True. Atypical pneumonia is the commonest pulmonary cause.
    c) False.
    d) True.
    e) True. This is especially true of small cell lung cancer.

36 a) False. This is an autoimmune cause of thyrotoxicosis.
    b) True.
    c) False. This is a rare cause of secondary hypothyroidism.
    d) True. Hypothyroidism can be caused by lack of iodine in, for example, mountainous areas.
    e) True. This is an autoimmune cause of hypothyroidism and goitre.

37 a) False.
    b) True. Lethargy, tiredness and depression may occur.
    c) True. Abdominal pain and constipation are features.
    d) False.
    e) True. Polydipsia, polyuria, renal stones and renal failure are all possible features of hypercalcaemia.

38 a) True. This is primary hyperaldosteronism secondary to an adrenal adenoma. Retention of sodium and water causes hypertension.
    b) True. There is excessive growth hormone from a pituitary adenoma.
    c) False. Postural hypotension is a feature as a result of mineralocorticoid deficiency.
    d) True. This is a rare catecholamine-secreting tumour, usually of the adrenal medulla.
    e) True. There are excessive glucocorticoid levels.

39 a) False.
    b) True.
    c) False. Constipation is a symptom.
    d) True. Depression, slowness of thought, and low libido are all symptoms of hypothyroidism.
    e) False. Cold intolerance is typical.

40 a) False. There is an increased risk, although this risk is less pronounced in combined oestrogen and progesterone HRT.
    b) True. HRT is one form of prevention of osteoporosis, but is not first-line.
    c) False. There is a slight increased risk associated with HRT.
    d) False. There is an increased risk of deep vein thrombosis and pulmonary embolism.
    e) False. Postmenopausal oestrogen deficiency increases coronary artery disease risk, but HRT is not preventative.

EMQ ANSWERS

1 HYPERGLYCAEMIA

1 **E** Parathyroid and pituitary disease in combination raise the suspicion of multiple endocrine neoplasia type 1. This is associated with pancreatic islet cell tumours, such as gastrinoma, insulinoma and **glucagonoma**.

2 **D** The characteristics described are typical of Cushing's syndrome, with muscle wasting and obesity. However, bitemporal hemianopia is associated with lesions at the optic chiasm, suggesting a pituitary origin and therefore **Cushing's disease**.

3 **H** Increased interdental separation, hypertension and hyperglycaemia are all features of **acromegaly**. Other symptoms may include tight rings, prognathism (a prominent jaw) and spade-like hands.

4 **C** **Iatrogenic**. The assumption here is that all patients admitted to hospital with acute asthma are treated with corticosteroids. These have a tendency to worsen glycaemic control: some diabetic patients may need to increase their dose of insulin to compensate.

5 **J** The most likely cause of this man's liver disease is alcohol. **Chronic pancreatitis** is frequently seen with chronic alcohol abuse and may lead to exocrine and endocrine pancreatic dysfunction.

2 INVESTIGATION OF ENDOCRINE DISEASE

1 **G** The **short Synacthen (tetracosactide) test** is used in the investigation of hypo-adrenalism. Cortisol measurements are taken before and after administration: a failure to respond implies adrenal dysfunction.

2 **D** The diagnosis of acromegaly is made on the lack of suppression of growth hormone after a **glucose tolerance test**. Growth hormone (along with glucagon, cortisol, and adrenaline) usually counteracts the effects of insulin.

3 **H** Enzymatic defects in the adrenal cortex lead to failure of production of cortisol, with resultant increase in **serum androgens**.

4 **A** A **water-deprivation test** will show a sustained diuresis in true diabetes insipidus, with no increase in urine osmolality, as would be expected with progressive dehydration.

5 **C** Catecholamines are elevated in phaeochromocytoma; the diagnosis rests on a 24-h collection of **urinary metanephrines**, which are breakdown products of adrenaline and noradrenaline.

3 MEDICAL TREATMENT OF ENDOCRINE DISEASE

1 I α- and β-blockade with **phenoxybenzamine/metoprolol** is essential in phaeochromo-cytoma before surgery. Phenoxybenzamine, an irreversible α-blocker, is always administered first, and then a β-blocker is added some days later.

2 C Conn's syndrome, primary hyperaldosteronism, is caused by excess secretion of aldosterone from the adrenal cortex. **Spironolactone**, an aldosterone antagonist, can be used to counteract these effects.

3 H **Carbimazole** is used as first-line medical therapy for Graves' disease; radio-iodine and surgery are alternatives. For those intolerant of carbimazole, propylthiouracil can be used.

4 B Addison's disease, primary hypoadrenalism, is characterized by deficiencies of gluco-corticoid and mineralocorticoid. Replacement with hydrocortisone (glucocorticoid) and **fludrocortisone** (mineralocorticoid) is needed to treat these deficiencies.

5 E **Bromocriptine**, a dopamine agonist, can be used to treat prolactinomas. Prolactin release is inhibited by dopamine.

4 COMPLICATIONS OF DRUGS USED TO TREAT ENDOCRINE DISEASE

1 H An important side-effect of **carbimazole** is agranulocytosis. Patients who present with symptoms of infection, especially sore throat, should have an urgent full blood count.

2 C **Spironolactone**, a potassium-sparing diuretic, can cause hyperkalaemia and hyponatraemia through its antagonism of the action of aldosterone.

3 J It is important to discontinue **metformin** therapy for 3 days after contrast administration, to prevent the small risk of lactic acidosis.

4 A Lipohypertrophy is a well-recognized complication of subcutaneous **insulin** injection. Patients usually minimize this complication by changing their injection sites.

5 C **Spironolactone** may cause gynaecomastia; other drugs that are also implicated include digoxin and cimetidine.

5 DISORDERS OF CALCIUM METABOLISM

1 B **Secondary hyperparathyroidism** occurs secondary to renal disease. The clinical features are hypocalcaemia with an elevated PTH, reflecting the failing endocrine function of the kidney to activate vitamin D.

2 J The history of a fracture without any trauma is suspicious for a pathological fracture due to malignant involvement. The lytic lesions on skull X-ray and the elevated ESR suggest multiple **myeloma** as the underlying cause.

3 A The PTH level is inappropriately high for the calcium concentration. The diagnosis is therefore **primary hyperparathyroidism**.

4 C **Tertiary hyperparathyroidism** occurs after a prolonged period of secondary hyper-parathyroidism; the parathyroids begin to secrete PTH autonomously, resulting in an elevated calcium and phosphate.

5 H **Iatrogenic.** Thiazide diuretics, such as bendroflumethiazide, can cause hyper-calcaemia. In contrast, loop diuretics, such as furosemide, cause hypocalcaemia.

6 PRESENTATIONS OF ENDOCRINE DISEASE

1 E Hyperpigmentation after bilateral adrenalectomy for Cushing's disease is referred to as **Nelson's syndrome**. It is rare, as most patients with Cushing's disease now undergo pituitary surgery.

2 C This patient has acute hypoadrenalism. The vomiting, postural hypotension and pigmented palmar creases are all in keeping with a diagnosis of **Addison's disease**.

3 B Hypertension, diabetes and macroglossia are all associated with **acromegaly**. The bitemporal hemianopia suggests a pituitary lesion compressing the optic chiasm.

4 D **Conn's syndrome** is a cause of secondary hypertension. The excess aldosterone results in hypernatraemia and hypokalaemia.

5 G The clinical features here are those of **Cushing's disease**. Again, the bitemporal hemianopia suggests a pituitary tumour causing excessive steroid production.

7 MEDICATION USED TO TREAT DIABETES MELLITUS

1 A **Metformin** is the first-line pharmacological treatment for type 2 diabetes in obese individuals.

2 G Diabetic ketoacidosis often presents in this manner. **Sliding-scale intravenous insulin** therapy must be instituted as soon as possible. Note that the increased anion gap is due to the presence of acidic ketones in the blood.

3 D **Glucagon** can be used to treat hypoglycaemia; unlike dextrose it can be administered subcutaneously or intramuscularly.

4 H **Insulin glargine** is long-acting: it only needs to be administered once per day. It has been shown to reduce the number of episodes of hypoglycaemia.

5 C **Acarbose** inhibits intestinal α-glucosidase, delaying the absorption of starch. The major side-effect is flatulence; however this tends to decrease with time.

8 COMPLICATIONS OF DIABETES MELLITUS

1 G Cotton wool spots and venous beading are both features of diabetic **pre-proliferative retinopathy**. Type 2 diabetes can present with complications of the disease.

2 J Neuropathic ulcers are common in patients who have diabetic **peripheral neuropathy**. They are typically painless and occur over pressure points such as the heel and heads of the metatarsals.

3 I **Autonomic neuropathy** may contribute to impotence in diabetics: 50 per cent of diabetic men over 55 years of age suffer from erectile failure.

4 C The anion gap is increased in this patient implying the presence of an acidic particle in the blood. Ketones are excluded given the absence of ketonuria. The most likely diagnosis is **lactic acidosis** secondary to metformin therapy.

5 H **Proliferative retinopathy** is an ophthalmic emergency. New vessel formation within the vitreous humour warrants urgent laser photocoagulation, or vision may be permanently lost.

9 HYPOGLYCAEMIA

1 **B** Rapid gastric emptying in patients who have had a partial gastrectomy leads to **dumping syndrome**, where a large carbohydrate load enters the small intestine and causes hypersecretion of insulin.

2 **G** Spontaneous episodes of symptomatic hypoglycaemia relieved by the administration of glucose suggest the presence of an **insulinoma**. These symptoms are often brought on by fasting.

3 **A** **Factitious** hypoglycaemia occurs in patients secretly administering insulin or oral hypoglycaemics. This condition is differentiated from an insulinoma by normal C-peptide levels.

4 **I** **Iatrogenic**. Hypoglycaemia is well-recognized as a side-effect of quinine therapy. Malaria is also a cause of hypoglycaemia but is not listed in the options available.

5 **D** **Liver failure** can cause hypoglycaemia; in this case, this has been induced by paracetamol overdose.

10 DRUGS USED TO MANIPULATE HORMONES

1 **F** **Clomifene** is an anti-oestrogen that stimulates pituitary gonadotrophin release, thereby increasing the chances of ovulation.

2 **G** **Tamoxifen**, an oestrogen antagonist, is used as a daily oral medication in the treatment of breast cancer.

3 **B** **Hydrocortisone** is an important treatment in anaphylaxis. It takes some time to work, so it is important that it is given early in the treatment of any patient with this condition.

4 **A** **Finasteride** is a 5α-reductase inhibitor which inhibits the conversion of testosterone to dihydrotestosterone. It reduces prostatic size and hence improves urinary flow rates.

5 **D** **Fludrocortisone** is the treatment of choice for mineralocorticoid replacement in Addison's disease.

11 DISORDERS OF THE THYROID GLAND

1 **I** **Anaplastic carcinoma** affects the elderly and has an extremely poor prognosis. In this patient the cancer has invaded the recurrent laryngeal nerve (giving rise to hoarseness) and subcutaneous tissues. Palliative radiotherapy is sometimes given.

2 **A** This middle-aged woman is clinically hyperthyroid. The exophthalmos picked up by the GP is a sign of **Graves' disease** and does not occur in other forms of hyperthyroidism.

3 **C** A **thyroglossal cyst** is an embryological remnant of the migration of the thyroid gland caudally from the base of the tongue via the thyroglossal duct. As they are still attached to the tongue, they characteristically move upwards on tongue protrusion.

4 **G** A neck lump in a patient with a past medical history of phaeochromocytoma and hyperparathyroidism raises the possibility of multiple endocrine neoplasia (MEN) type 2, which is associated with **medullary carcinoma** of the thyroid.

5 **D** The history of a febrile illness causing hyperthyroidism with subsequent hypothyroidism is consistent with **de Quervain's thyroiditis**.

CHAPTER 10

The urinary tract

MULTIPLE CHOICE QUESTIONS

1   The following statements are true of prostatic cancer:
   a) The tumour is a squamous cell carcinoma
   b) There is a national prostate-specific antigen (PSA) screening programme for men over 65 years of age
   c) Diagnosis is aided by trans-urethral ultrasound and biopsy
   d) Radical prostatectomy is a treatment option
   e) Spinal cord compression is a complication

2   Causes of haematuria include:
   a) Pyelonephritis
   b) Diabetes insipidus
   c) Glomerulonephritis
   d) Diabetic ketoacidosis
   e) Prostatic carcinoma

3   Indications for haemodialysis in acute renal failure include:
   a) Pulmonary oedema
   b) Hypokalaemia
   c) Hyponatraemia
   d) Metabolic acidosis
   e) Hypercalcaemia

4   Risk factors for urinary tract infection include:
   a) Polydipsia
   b) Male gender
   c) Diabetes mellitus
   d) Faecal incontinence
   e) Sexual intercourse

5 The following statements are true of urinary tract infection:
   a) The commonest offending organism in community-acquired infection is *Enterococcus faecalis*
   b) Diagnosis relies on a bacterial count of >10 000 organisms per mL of urine
   c) Proteus infection predisposes to renal tract calculi
   d) Acute pyelonephritis is usually asymptomatic
   e) Asymptomatic bacteriuria of pregnancy requires no treatment

6 The following are useful in the prevention of renal stone disease:
   a) Dietary change
   b) Good diabetic control
   c) Meticulous blood pressure control
   d) High fluid intake
   e) Reduction in alcohol consumption

7 Causes of urinary tract obstruction include:
   a) Pelviureteric neuromuscular dysfunction
   b) Renal artery stenosis
   c) Vesical calculus
   d) Cystitis
   e) Urethral stricture

8 Glomerulonephritis may present in the following ways:
   a) Nephritic syndrome
   b) Prostatism
   c) Chronic renal failure
   d) Felty syndrome
   e) Nephrotic syndrome

9 Complications of trans-urethral resection of the prostate include:
   a) Retrograde ejaculation
   b) Pneumaturia
   c) Haematospermia
   d) Hypogonadism
   e) Impotence

10 Regarding acute urinary retention:
   a) It is not as painful as chronic retention
   b) Retention arising from urethral trauma should be treated by urethral catheterization
   c) Uraemia may result
   d) It may be caused by a urethral ulcer
   e) Opioid analgesics may be responsible

11 Causes of bilateral hydronephrosis include:
   a) Retroperitoneal fibrosis
   b) Renal calculus
   c) Urethral stricture
   d) Gentamicin
   e) Prostatic cancer

12 The following have a role in the management of chronic renal failure:
   a) Sodium restriction
   b) Bisphosphonates
   c) Antihypertensives
   d) Erythropoietin
   e) Spironolactone

13 Complications of male urethral catheterization include:
   a) Cystitis
   b) Hydrocele
   c) Urethral stricture
   d) Haematuria
   e) Paraphimosis

14 Causes of urethral stricture include:
   a) Diabetes mellitus
   b) Pyelonephritis
   c) Catheterization
   d) Smoking
   e) Chlamydia infection

15 Features of uraemia include:
   a) Pericarditis
   b) Lymphadenopathy
   c) Pleural effusion
   d) Pruritus
   e) Encephalopathy

16 Causes of haematuria include:
   a) Rifampicin
   b) Schistosomiasis
   c) Candidiasis
   d) Catheterization
   e) Warfarin

17 Causes of proteinuria include:
   a) Starvation
   b) Fever
   c) Jaundice
   d) Diabetes mellitus
   e) Hypertension

18 The following investigations of the renal tract involve ionizing radiation:
   a) Dimercaptosuccinic acid (DMSA) scan
   b) Micturating cystourethrography
   c) Intravenous urography (IVU)
   d) Renal ultrasound
   e) Diethylenetriamine penta-acetic acid (DTPA) scan

19 Causes of impotence include:
   a) Leriche's syndrome
   b) Trans-urethral prostatectomy
   c) Candidiasis
   d) Diabetes mellitus
   e) Propranolol

20 Causes of glomerulonephritis include:
   a) Immunoglobulin A (IgA) nephropathy
   b) Henoch–Schönlein purpura
   c) Streptococcal infection
   d) Tietze's syndrome
   e) Goodpasture's syndrome

21 Nephritic syndrome is characterized by:
   a) Glycosuria
   b) Proteinuria
   c) Oliguria
   d) Ketonuria
   e) Haematuria

22 Causes of a palpable renal mass include:
   a) Reflux nephropathy
   b) Polycystic kidney disease
   c) Hydronephrosis
   d) Nephrotic syndrome
   e) Horseshoe kidney

23 Benign prostatic hypertrophy may be treated with the following:
   a) Cystectomy
   b) Finasteride
   c) Tolterodine
   d) Tamsulosin
   e) Trans-urethral prostatic resection

24 The following conditions are recognized causes of renal failure:
   a) Multiple myeloma
   b) Amyloidosis
   c) Bowen's disease
   d) Aspergillosis
   e) Haemolytic uraemic syndrome

25 Risk factors for bladder cancer include:
   a) Diabetes mellitus
   b) Schistosomiasis
   c) Alcohol consumption
   d) Industrial dyes
   e) Cigarette smoking

26 Features of nephrotic syndrome are:
   a) Peripheral oedema
   b) Hypercholesterolaemia
   c) Hypocalcaemia
   d) Hypoalbuminaemia
   e) Hypernatraemia

27 Associated features of polycystic kidney disease include:
   a) Mitral valve prolapse
   b) Subarachnoid haemorrhage
   c) Pancreatic cancer
   d) Hepatic cysts
   e) Hypertension

28 Complications of renal transplantation include:
   a) Neuropathic bladder
   b) Cytomegalovirus infection
   c) Malignancy
   d) Renovascular occlusion
   e) Hypertension

29 Causes of polyuria include:
   a) Hypercalcaemia
   b) Diabetes mellitus
   c) Urinary tract infection
   d) Diabetes insipidus
   e) Prostatism

30 The following are endogenous nephrotoxins:
   a) Albumin
   b) Urate
   c) Dopamine
   d) Myoglobin
   e) Light immunoglobulin chains

31 Causes of renal stones include:
   a) Hypocalcaemia
   b) Urinary tract infection
   c) Hyperoxaluria
   d) Polydipsia
   e) Hyperuricaemia

32 The following are useful investigations in renal stone disease:
   a) Renal angiogram
   b) Renal ultrasound
   c) Renal biopsy
   d) Abdominal plain film
   e) Intravenous urogram

33 The following are complications of renal stone disease:
a) Phimosis
b) Renal obstruction
c) Vesico-cutaneous fistula
d) Neuropathic bladder
e) Urinary tract infection

34 Causes of urinary tract obstruction include:
a) Sloughed papilla
b) Retroperitoneal fibrosis
c) Glomerulonephritis
d) Diabetes insipidus
e) Prostatic hypertrophy

35 Complications of chronic renal failure include:
a) Liver failure
b) Hypertension
c) Osteodystrophy
d) Parkinsonism
e) Anaemia

36 Causes of pre-renal acute renal failure include:
a) Vancomycin toxicity
b) Acute haemorrhage
c) Radiocontrast
d) Left ventricular failure
e) Renal artery stenosis

Answers: see pages 243–248

EXTENDED MATCHING QUESTIONS

1 RENAL FAILURE

Each of the patients below presents with renal failure. Choose the most likely cause from the options given

A   Nephrotic syndrome
B   Retroperitoneal fibrosis
C   Glomerulonephritis
D   Benign prostatic hyperplasia
E   Chronic pyelonephritis

F   Hepatorenal syndrome
G   Rhabdomyolysis
H   Interstitial nephritis
I   Polycystic kidney disease
J   Acute tubular necrosis

1   A 38-year-old woman with a history of severe migraine for the past 20 years, treated with sumatriptan and methysergide, goes to hospital with abdominal pain. Blood tests show acute renal failure; an ultrasound shows bilateral hydronephrosis.

2   A 37-year-old Turkish man is rescued after being trapped under a collapsed building for 36 h after an earthquake. Despite this, he is well hydrated. A urine dipstick shows blood ++++.

3   A 19-year-old student goes to see her general practitioner (GP) feeling tired. She is well known to him as she has suffered from multiple urinary tract infections. He looks on his computer and finds a micturating cystogram result from 5 years ago which showed bilateral vesico-ureteric reflux.

4   A 33-year-old man is found to have bilateral loin masses and renal failure. He says his father is currently on haemodialysis.

5   A 41-year-old woman, with severe osteoarthritis, takes paracetamol, ibuprofen and codeine to control her pain. A routine blood test by her GP reveals a degree of renal failure: the GP says her medication may well be to blame.

2 INVESTIGATION OF RENAL DISEASE

Choose the most appropriate next investigation from the options given for each of the patients below

A   DTPA nuclear medicine scan
B   DMSA nuclear medicine scan
C   Renal biopsy
D   Micturating cystogram
E   Abdominal X-ray
F   Renal angiogram

G   Computed tomography (CT) scan of the abdomen/pelvis
H   Renal ultrasound
I   Magnetic resonance imaging (MRI) of the abdomen
J   Intravenous urogram

1 A 32-year-old policeman presents to the emergency department at 3 am with loin pain radiating to his groin. He cannot stop writhing round in pain. Urinalysis shows blood ++.

2 A 79-year-old man is brought to hospital confused. There is no medical history. Blood tests reveal an elevated urea and creatinine. The consultant wants to know if the renal failure is acute or chronic.

3 A 12-year-old girl suffers from recurrent kidney infections. An ultrasound scan shows no abnormality. The consultant wonders whether she has vesico-ureteric reflux.

4 A 45-year-old woman with systemic lupus erythematosus is seen in clinic with worsening renal function. The registrar says she may well need treatment.

5 A previously healthy 25-year-old is seen in the emergency department on a Sunday afternoon and is diagnosed with a renal stone. The doctor tries to refer him to urology, but is told to find out if the patient is obstructed first.

3 POLYURIA

Each of the patients below presents with polyuria. Choose the most likely underlying diagnosis from the options given

A   Cranial diabetes insipidus
B   Nephrogenic diabetes insipidus
C   Diabetes mellitus
D   Hypercalcaemia
E   Psychogenic polydipsia

F   Hypokalaemia
G   Chronic renal failure
H   Hyperaldosteronism
I   Urinary tract infection
J   Alcohol

1 A 62-year-old man visits his doctor, complaining he has to get up two to three times at night to pass water. His GP looks back on his computer, and notes that this patient has been to see him three times in the last 6 months with soft tissue infections.

2 A 29-year-old woman with bipolar disorder goes to see her doctor complaining of polyuria. She is producing 6 L of urine per day. Blood tests reveal a plasma osmolality of 295 mosmol/kg and urine osmolality of 250 mosmol/kg. The urine output does not change after administration of desmopressin.

3 A 32-year-old motorcycle courier develops polyuria after an accident in which he came off his motorcycle at 35 mph. His GP offers him some desmopressin, which he says helps.

4 An 18-year-old youth staggers into the emergency department at 0300 on Saturday morning with ataxia and a GCS of 14. He wanders off to the bathroom every half an hour to pass large volumes of dilute urine.

5 A 79-year-old woman with multiple myeloma goes to see her GP, saying that she has to pass urine every hour, including at night. A urine dipstick shows blood + and trace protein.

4 PRESENTATION OF RENAL DISEASE

Choose the most likely diagnosis for each of the patients below

A   Nephrotic syndrome
B   Acute pyelonephritis
C   Glomerulonephritis
D   Interstitial nephritis
E   Cystitis

F   Acute renal failure
G   Chronic renal failure
H   Renal artery stenosis
I   Nephrocalcinosis
J   Polycystic kidney disease

1   A 43-year-old woman, with past medical history of primary hyperparathyroidism, presents to the emergency department with abdominal distension, constipation and vomiting. An abdominal X-ray is performed to check for dilated loops of bowel. The doctor is surprised when she sees both kidneys clearly on the X-ray.

2   A 21-year-old medical student presents to the emergency department with fever, right loin tenderness and urinary frequency.

3   A 7-year-old boy is taken to his doctor by his mother as she has noticed that his eyes and scrotum have become swollen. A urine dipstick shows trace blood and protein ++++.

4   A 14-year-old girl sees her doctor for a follow-up appointment after a sore throat 2 weeks ago. She tells him that she has not passed urine for the last day, so he sends her to hospital, where she is found to have a blood pressure of 180/110 mmHg. Urinalysis shows blood +++ and protein +. The registrar asks for urgent urine microscopy, which reveals red cell casts.

5   A 29-year-old woman goes to see her doctor with macroscopic haematuria. He finds a mass in her right loin. While he is examining her, she remarks how her mother died at a similar age from a brain haemorrhage.

5 URINE ABNORMALITIES IN RENAL DISEASE

Each of the patients below has been found to have abnormal urine. Choose the most likely cause of this from the options given

A   Tuberculosis
B   Glomerulonephritis
C   Porphyria
D   Urinary tract infection
E   Malaria

F   Diabetes insipidus
G   Interstitial nephritis
H   Multiple myeloma
I   Diabetes mellitus
J   Gout

1   A 73-year-old man goes to see his GP with back pain. Blood tests reveal a normochromic normocytic anaemia. The urine electrophoresis shows free light chains.

2   A 32-year-old woman is being investigated for the cause of her acute renal failure. The pathologist excitedly rings the renal registrar saying he has found eosinophils in the urine.

3   A 59-year-old man goes to hospital clutching a pot of his urine, which is bright orange. Unfortunately he speaks no English. He has brought a few of his medications with him, including atenolol, bendroflumethiazide, co-dydramol, rifampicin, calcium and isoniazid.

4   A 20-year-old woman is admitted to hospital with a suspected acute abdomen. The doctor asks for a urine sample and takes it away to test it with a dipstick. Unfortunately he is called away urgently, and when he returns half an hour later the urine has turned bright red.

5   Some medical students are taken to the microscope by an enthusiastic nephrologist. He shows them the urine of a young patient with renal failure. He is particularly excited as he has found some red cell casts.

6 URINARY TRACT OBSTRUCTION

Choose the most likely cause of urinary tract obstruction in each of the patients below

A   Renal stones
B   Paraphimosis
C   Blocked catheter
D   Urethral stricture
E   Neurogenic bladder

F   Papillary necrosis
G   Benign prostatic hyperplasia
H   Phimosis
I   Ureteric stricture
J   Prostate cancer

1   A 6-year-old Ghanaian boy is brought to the emergency department by his mother, as he is complaining of severe abdominal pain. Blood tests show him to be in acute renal failure, despite him being well-filled. A renal ultrasound shows right-sided hydronephrosis.
2   A 12-year-old boy is seen by a paediatrician for frequent urinary tract infections. He tells her that his foreskin blows up like a balloon every time he goes to urinate.
3   A 71-year-old man presents to hospital in acute urinary retention. A urinary catheter is passed; the residual volume is 1.9 L.
4   A 63-year-old man is catheterized on the ward by the surgical house officer on call. Unfortunately, she forgets to replace the foreskin. Six hours after the catheter is removed, he goes into acute urinary retention.
5   A 79-year-old man presents to hospital in urinary retention. He says he has not had this problem since he had a trans-urethral resection of the prostate (TURP) 5 years ago. The junior doctor on call attempts to insert a catheter, but neither he nor the urology registrar can insert it more than 3 cm, despite pushing quite hard.

7 PRESENTATIONS OF UROLOGICAL DISEASE

Choose the most likely diagnosis for each of the clinical scenarios below

A   Acute pyelonephritis
B   Renal calculi
C   Prostate cancer
D   Renal cell carcinoma
E   Bladder cancer

F   Bladder calculi
G   Acute bacterial prostatitis
H   Phimosis
I   Benign prostatic hyperplasia
J   Acute cystitis

1   A 68-year-old woman presents with a history of painless macroscopic haematuria that has not resolved after a course of antibiotics from her GP. She is a lifelong smoker.
2   An 80-year-old man sees his GP. He complains of back pain and an unintentional 2-stone weight loss over the last 6 months. He mentions he has suffered urinary hesitancy over the last few months. Examination reveals a palpable bladder and craggy, irregular prostate.
3   A 40-year-old is brought to the emergency department by ambulance with right loin pain radiating to the groin. She is rolling about in agony, screaming in pain. A urine dipstick reveals blood +++.
4   A 28-year-old woman is seen in the emergency department. She is generally unwell with a pyrexia of 39.5°C, rigors, nausea and vomiting. She mentions she has just completed a 3 day course of antibiotics for a urinary tract infection. She has left renal angle pain on examination.
5   A 70-year-old is seen by his GP, as he is concerned that he has urinary frequency and poor urinary stream. He is also tired as he wakes up at least three times each night needing to pass urine. He is otherwise entirely well.

8 SCROTAL SWELLINGS

Each of the patients below has presented with a swollen testicle. Choose the most likely diagnosis from the options given

A   Varicocele
B   Haematocoele
C   Testicular torsion
D   Testicular tumour
E   Epididymo-orchitis

F   Indirect inguinal hernia
G   Hydrocele
H   Epididymal cyst
I   Sperm granuloma
J   Sebaceous cyst

1   An 18-year-old man presents to the emergency department with a 4 h history of an exquisitely tender right testicle accompanied by nausea and vomiting. On examination, his testicle is tender and retracted; the scrotal skin is hot, red and oedematous.

2   A patient sees his GP complaining of several lumps on the scrotal skin. They have been there for some months but he is concerned as one of the lumps is red, tender and discharging.

3   A man sees his doctor complaining of a dragging sensation in his left testicle. On examination, the right testicle is normal but the left feels like a bag of worms.

4   A 25-year-old mechanic is seen in the urology outpatient department with a swelling in the right scrotum accompanied by a sensation of heaviness. On examination, there is a firm, irregular swelling attached to the scrotal skin.

5   An 18-year-old man presents to the emergency department with a tender left testicle. He complains of feeling generally unwell. His scrotal skin is hot, red and oedematous and there is tenderness on epididymal palpation. Urine dipstick shows blood and leucocytes.

Answers: see pages 248–251

X-RAY QUESTIONS

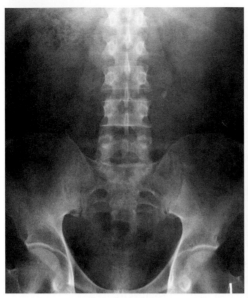

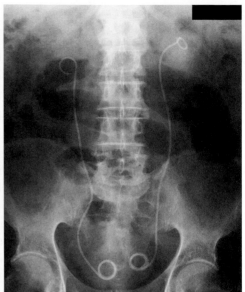

1

2

To answer the questions below, please refer to the corresponding numbered X-ray images above.

1   A 37-year-old police officer goes to hospital, complaining of excruciating left-sided inter-
    mittent abdominal pain. A urine dipstick shows blood +++. The doctor requests a plain
    abdominal film.
    a) What is the cause of this man's abdominal pain?
    b) Is there a need for further imaging?

2   A 43-year-old woman presented to hospital in acute renal failure secondary to her ovarian
    carcinoma. What procedure has been performed?

Answers: see page 251

ANSWERS

MCQ ANSWERS

1   a) False. Histologically it is an adenocarcinoma.
    b) False.
    c) False. These procedures are carried out via the transrectal route.
    d) True. Operative treatment or radiotherapy are options for disease confined to the prostate.
    e) True. Bone metastasis is common.

2   a) True. This is infection of the kidneys; the patient is often acutely unwell.
    b) False. There is impaired renal water resorption due to lack of antidiuretic hormone (ADH), or ineffective response to ADH.
    c) True. Red cell casts are found in the urine.
    d) False. Ketones are found in the urine.
    e) True. This is a cause of painless haematuria.

3   a) True. This is due to insufficient excretion of water.
    b) False. Persistent life-threatening hyperkalaemia is an indication for dialysis.
    c) False.
    d) True.
    e) False. The indications are: hyperkalaemia, pulmonary oedema, acidosis, uraemia.

4   a) False.
    b) False. This is a protective factor and is related to the longer course of the urethra.
    c) True.
    d) True. Urinary tract infection is most often caused by faecal flora.
    e) True. This promotes the transfer of bacteria along the female urethra.

5   a) False. *Escherichia coli* is the most common infecting organism.
    b) False. The typically quoted figure is >100 000 of the same organism per mL.
    c) True.
    d) False. The patient is usually profoundly unwell.
    e) False. It must always be treated to prevent complications such as acute pyelonephritis and premature labour.

6   a) True. For example, reducing calcium, vitamin D or oxalate intake, depending on the composition of the calculi.
    b) False.
    c) False.
    d) True. Remaining well-hydrated protects against calculus formation.
    e) False.

7   a) True. This is a functional defect in the collecting system, which is commoner in males than females.
    b) False. This restricts perfusion of the kidneys but does not obstruct the outflow of urine.
    c) True. A large calculus in the bladder can cause outflow obstruction.
    d) False.
    e) True. Examples are strictures caused by instrumentation or urethritis.

8   a) True. This is characterized by haematuria, proteinuria, hypertension, peripheral oedema, oliguria and uraemia.

   b) False. Symptoms such as hesitancy, poor stream and terminal dribbling occur as a result of outflow obstruction.

   c) True. Glomerulonephritis is the third commonest cause of chronic renal failure in the Western world, after diabetes mellitus and hypertension.

   d) False. This is a syndrome encompassing rheumatoid arthritis, splenomegaly, neutropenia and lymphadenopathy.

   e) True. This is characterized by proteinuria, hypoalbuminaemia, peripheral oedema and hypercholesterolaemia.

9   a) True. This occurs commonly.

   b) False. This is a symptom of a vesico-colic fistula.

   c) True.

   d) False.

   e) True. This occurs in approximately 10 per cent.

10 a) False. It is acutely painful, while chronic retention is usually painless.

   b) False. This would exacerbate the urethral damage. Suprapubic catheterization is useful.

   c) True. Post-renal renal failure will result if the retention is not relieved.

   d) True.

   e) True.

11 a) True.

   b) False. This can cause unilateral hydronephrosis.

   c) True.

   d) False. This is a nephrotoxic drug.

   e) True.

12 a) True. This reduces fluid overload and hypertension.

   b) False. These are used in osteoporosis and Paget's disease.

   c) True. Angiotensin-converting enzyme (ACE) inhibitors have an important role.

   d) True. This is an expensive treatment used for anaemia of chronic renal failure.

   e) False. This predisposes to hyperkalaemia.

13 a) True. The catheter is a source of sepsis.

   b) False. This is a fluid collection in the processus vaginalis.

   c) True. This may occur with repeated traumatic catheterization.

   d) True. This is a common complication.

   e) True. This may occur if the foreskin is not replaced after insertion of a urinary catheter. The retracted foreskin forms a constricting band, leading to swelling of the glans, and difficulty in replacing the foreskin.

14 a) False.

   b) False.

   c) True. Repeated urethral instrumentation can lead to stricture formation.

   d) False.

   e) True. In addition, gonorrhoea is another cause.

15 a) True.
    b) False.
    c) True.
    d) True.
    e) True.

16 a) False. This antituberculous drug stains urine and tears orange.
    b) True. This is a parasitic infection of the bladder.
    c) False.
    d) True. Urethral trauma during the procedure is a common cause of haematuria.
    e) True. Haematuria is a risk of over-anticoagulation.

17 a) False. This may result in ketonuria.
    b) True. This is functional proteinuria.
    c) False. Urinary bilirubin may be detectable in cholestatic jaundice.
    d) True. Proteinuria occurs in diabetic nephropathy.
    e) True. This causes glomerular damage.

18 a) True. A form of static scintigraphy using technetium isotopes, it indicates the relative function provided by each kidney and reveals scarring.
    b) True. This is an unpleasant investigation used to identify vesico-ureteric reflux in children. It involves fluoroscopic screening.
    c) True. IVU outlines the renal tract with contrast. Sequential plain films help identify obstruction.
    d) False. This is useful to identify renal size, hydronephrosis, and renal masses.
    e) True. A form of dynamic scintigraphy (using technetium isotopes), it provides functional information about the renal tract.

19 a) True. Due to aorto-iliac vascular disease preventing sufficient blood flow to the penis, it comprises buttock claudication, impotence and absent femoral pulses.
    b) True. This occurs as a complication in approximately 10 per cent of patients.
    c) False.
    d) True. Diabetic neuropathy gives rise to neurogenic impotence.
    e) True. Beta-blockers are an important cause.

20 a) True. This is the commonest worldwide cause.
    b) True. This is a syndrome involving glomerulonephritis, purpuric rash, polyarthritis and abdominal symptoms.
    c) True. This is the commonest cause of proliferative glomerulonephritis.
    d) False. This is idiopathic costochondritis.
    e) True. Anti-glomerular basement membrane antibodies cause a proliferative glomerulonephritis and haemoptysis.

21 a) False.
    b) True.
    c) True.
    d) False.
    e) True. Features of nephritic syndrome are haematuria, proteinuria, hypertension, oedema, oliguria and uraemia.

22 a) False. Otherwise known as chronic pyelonephritis, this is a cause of shrunken, scarred kidneys.
    b) True. Cysts are present throughout both kidneys. There is an adult form which is inherited as autosomal dominant, and a rarer childhood autosomal recessive form.
    c) True. This may cause renal enlargement.
    d) False.
    e) True. This is a congenital abnormality involving fusion of the kidneys in the midline.

23 a) False.
    b) True. A 5α-reductase inhibitor, it reduces prostatic volume.
    c) False. This is an antimuscarinic drug used to treat urinary incontinence due to detrusor instability.
    d) True. An α-blocker, it decreases smooth muscle tone.
    e) True. This is a common operation.

24 a) True. Light immunoglobulin chains are renally excreted and cause tubular damage.
    b) True. Amyloid causes renal damage.
    c) False. This is intra-epidermal carcinoma-in-situ.
    d) False. This is a fungal pulmonary condition.
    e) True. This is the commonest cause of acute renal failure in children; intravascular haemolysis and thrombocytopenia are additional features.

25 a) False.
    b) True. In developing nations, this is a cause of squamous cell carcinoma of the bladder.
    c) False.
    d) True. Aromatic amines are carcinogens.
    e) True.

26 a) True.
    b) True.
    c) False.
    d) True.
    e) False. The syndrome includes proteinuria, peripheral oedema and hypo-albuminaemia; hypercholesterolaemia is often present.

27 a) True.
    b) True. This is due to berry aneurysm rupture.
    c) False. Pancreatic cyst formation is recognized.
    d) True. Thirty per cent have associated liver cysts.
    e) True. This is a common finding.

28 a) False.
    b) True. Opportunistic infections are more common due to the immunosuppression required.
    c) True. This is likely to be due to immunosuppression and infection by viruses with malignant potential.
    d) True.
    e) True. Hypertension occurs in at least 50 per cent of patients.

29 a) True. It causes thirst and polyuria.
    b) True. This is one of the main presenting clinical features of diabetes mellitus.
    c) False. This may cause frequency, but not polyuria.
    d) True. This is cranial or nephrogenic in origin.
    e) False. Prostatism is a cause of frequency, but not of polyuria.

30 a) False.
    b) True. Cytotoxic drugs cause urate nephropathy in lymphoproliferative or myclo-proliferative disorders.
    c) False.
    d) True. This is released by damaged muscle in rhabdomyolysis.
    e) True. These cause renal damage in multiple myeloma.

31 a) False. Hypercalcaemia and hypercalciuria are risk factors.
    b) True. This is particularly true of Proteus infection; mixed composition stones are formed, often large e.g. staghorn calculi.
    c) True. For example, due to high dietary intake or small bowel disease.
    d) False. Dehydration is a risk factor.
    e) True. This predisposes to urate stones.

32 a) False.
    b) True. This will exclude hydronephrosis or obstruction.
    c) False.
    d) True. Eighty per cent of renal stones are visible on plain radiographic film.
    e) True. This may reveal filling defects along the renal tract.

33 a) False.
    b) True. This should be relieved as soon as possible, especially it there is coexisting infection.
    c) False.
    d) False.
    e) True. Renal tracts damaged by calculi are more prone to infection.

34 a) True. This occurs in diabetes mellitus and analgesic nephropathy.
    b) True. This is an autoimmune condition causing progressive obstruction of the ureters.
    c) False.
    d) False.
    e) True. This is a common cause of obstruction in elderly men.

35 a) False.
    b) True.
    c) True. This is due to defective renal vitamin D metabolism.
    d) False.
    e) True. Anaemia occurs due to failure of erythropoietin production.

36 a) False. Vancomycin is directly nephrotoxic; it is therefore a cause of intrinsic renal failure.
   b) True. Loss of circulating volume causes renal hypoperfusion.
   c) False. This nephrotoxin causes intrinsic renal failure.
   d) True. Poor cardiac output causes hypoperfusion of the kidneys.
   e) True. This restricts renal blood supply.

EMQ ANSWERS

1 RENAL FAILURE

1 B The drug methysergide is a powerful antimigraine agent but does have the unfortunate side-effect of **retroperitoneal fibrosis**. This patient has bilateral hydronephrosis indicating both ureters are involved, causing post-renal renal failure.

2 G **Rhabdomyolysis**, the breakdown of muscle, is a well-recognized complication of crush injuries (and statin treatment). Myoglobin is excreted in the urine but gives a false-positive reading as blood on the dipstick.

3 E **Chronic pyelonephritis**, a condition in which the kidneys are scarred by bilateral vesico-ureteric reflux, is the most likely cause of this patient's renal failure. Note that recurrent acute pyelonephritis does not cause chronic pyelonephritis.

4 I Palpable, enlarged kidneys with renal failure are most likely to be due to autosomal dominant **polycystic kidney disease** (ADPKD). The positive family history supports this.

5 H **Interstitial nephritis** is an underdiagnosed condition which is a common side-effect of drugs such as non-steroidal anti-inflammatory drugs (NSAIDs, e.g. diclofenac) and penicillins. There is often an elevated blood eosinophil count; eosinophiluria may also be a feature.

INVESTIGATION OF RENAL DISEASE

1 E The history of excruciating pain radiating to the groin and microscopic haematuria suggests renal stone disease. As most stones are radio-opaque, an **abdominal X-ray** is the most appropriate first-line test.

2 H The best test to differentiate acute from chronic renal failure is a **renal ultrasound**. Patients with chronic renal failure usually, but not always, have small, shrunken kidneys.

3 D A **micturating cystogram**, where X-rays are taken while a bladder full of contrast is voided, can diagnose vesico-ureteric reflux if contrast travels up the ureters to the kidneys.

4 C A **renal biopsy** is needed here to establish the exact cause of the deterioration in renal function in this patient with systemic lupus erythematosus. Different histological appearances require different treatments.

5 J The best investigations to check for renal tract obstruction are the **intravenous urogram** (IVU) and renal ultrasound. On a Sunday afternoon in the emergency department, an IVU is more practical.

3 POLYURIA

1 **C** Type 2 **diabetes mellitus** often presents insidiously, with constitutional symptoms, polyuria and frequent infections. Doctors have to have a high index of suspicion for this condition.

2 **B** This patient has a high normal plasma osmolality and inappropriately dilute urine, indicating diabetes insipidus. The lack of response to desmopressin suggests **nephrogenic diabetes insipidus**, probably secondary to lithium therapy for bipolar disorder.

3 **A** **Cranial diabetes insipidus** is relatively common after head injury. Exogenous administration of desmopressin may be needed in the short term until the body recovers.

4 **J** This young man is intoxicated with **alcohol**. He is polyuric as alcohol suppresses antidiuretic hormone (ADH) and is likely to be consumed with large volumes of fluid.

5 **D** **Hypercalcaemia** can result in a significant diuresis. In this patient, this is probably secondary to malignancy. Rehydration and bisphosphonates are indicated.

4 PRESENTATION OF RENAL DISEASE

1 **I** The kidneys are usually poorly, if at all, visible on X-ray. **Nephrocalcinosis**, calcification of the renal parenchyma, leads to the finding of prominent kidneys. In this case, it is secondary to primary hyperparathyroidism.

2 **D** This is a typical history for **acute pyelonephritis** – fever is unusual in urinary tract infection confined to the bladder. An intravenous antibiotic, such as cefuroxime, would be appropriate treatment.

3 **A** This young boy has oedema and significant proteinuria, two out of the three criteria necessary to confirm **nephrotic syndrome**. Blood tests would be expected to show hypoalbuminaemia.

4 **C** Post-streptococcal **glomerulonephritis** typically occurs 2–3 weeks after an infection such as otitis media or sore throat. Red cell casts in the urine are pathognomonic of glomerular inflammation.

5 **J** Cerebral aneurysms are associated with autosomal dominant **polycystic kidney disease**. A palpable kidney with macroscopic haematuria in a patient with such a family history would warrant urgent further assessment.

5 URINE ABNORMALITIES IN RENAL DISEASE

1 **H** Back pain may be the first sign of **multiple myeloma**. Most, but not all, patients with this condition have a detectable serum paraprotein. Associated light chains in the urine are known as Bence–Jones protein.

2 **G** Eosinophiluria is suggestive of **interstitial nephritis**, an allergic disease often secondary to drug administration.

3 **A** It is likely that this gentleman is an immigrant as he speaks no English. One of the important side-effects of rifampicin is its ability to stain body secretions red or orange, including urine or tears. The underlying diagnosis is **tuberculosis**, in this case treated with rifampicin and isoniazid.

4 **C** Acute intermittent **porphyria** can mimic an acute abdomen, and many patients have exploratory surgery before the diagnosis is finally made. The urine may change colour on standing to turn red, brown or black. The laboratory measurement of urinary porphyrins is usually diagnostic.

5 **B** Red cell casts are rarely seen but are virtually pathognomonic of **glomerulonephritis**.

6 URINARY TRACT INFECTION

1 F Sickle cell disease can affect the kidney, causing **papillary necrosis**. A sloughed papilla can migrate into the ureter causing obstruction.

2 H **Phimosis** is a common paediatric problem. A tight foreskin around the glans penis can predispose to recurrent infections and urinary tract obstruction. Treatment with topical steroid is usually successful; where this fails formal circumcision is indicated.

3 G **Benign prostatic hyperplasia** is very common. Patients typically have an enlarged bilobed prostate on rectal examination, with symptoms of urgency, hesitancy, frequency, terminal dribbling and poor stream. In this patient this is likely to be long-standing given the grossly enlarged bladder volume.

4 B **Paraphimosis** results from oedema of a retracted foreskin, leading to an inability to replace it to its normal position. Immediate replacement is necessary for pain control and to prevent distal ischaemia.

5 D The fact that the catheter cannot be passed more than 3 cm suggests a **urethral stricture**. This is probably secondary to the introduction of surgical instrumentation when this patient had his TURP.

7 PRESENTATIONS OF UROLOGICAL DISEASE

1 E Macroscopic haematuria always warrants further investigation as there is often a serious underlying cause. Here, the failure to resolve after antibiotics eliminates infection as a potential cause. The history of smoking makes **bladder cancer** much more likely as the two are associated.

2 C The weight loss here is sinister. This patient is the right age for **prostate cancer**: 50 per cent of new cases present with bladder outlet obstruction. The back pain can be attributed to bony metastasis.

3 B This story sounds like ureteric colic from **renal calculi**. A urine dipstick will typically show blood and helps to verify the diagnosis. She will need an intravenous urogram to exclude hydronephrosis.

4 A Occasionally a simple urinary tract infection can ascend and cause **acute pyelo-nephritis**. A urine sample for microscopy, sensitivity and culture is essential to determine the appropriate antibiotic therapy.

5 I This man is describing symptoms of **benign prostatic hyperplasia**. Patients usually present with the typical symptoms of bladder outflow obstruction, or with complications such as retention, infection or stone formation. On rectal examination, the prostate is smooth and symmetrical. A family history is frequently present.

8 SCROTAL SWELLINGS

1 C **Testicular torsion** typically presents around puberty and is rare over 25 years of age. There is sudden onset of pain in the scrotum and groin. There may be a history of vigorous exercise. To be sure of salvage, surgery must be performed within 6–8 h of onset of symptoms.

2 J **Sebaceous cysts** may occur on the scrotal skin as small, tense, spherical swellings. There may be a punctum centrally.

3 A The patient must be standing to fully examine a **varicocele**. The 'bag of worms' effect is due to dilated veins. The left side is most commonly affected.

4 D The tethering suggests a malignant process. Most **testicular tumours** are detected when they are small; it is rare for tethering to have occurred at presentation. Testicular tumours metastasize to the para-aortic and mediastinal nodes.

5 E Symptoms of **epididymo-orchitis** are usually unilateral; the patient often has associated systemic upset. The tenderness is initially confined to the epididymis, but eventually spreads to the testis.

X-RAY ANSWERS

1 a) There is a left-sided ureteric calculus situated at the level of L3/L4. This is responsible for this patient's renal colic.

   b) Further imaging is necessary to ensure that the left kidney is not obstructed. This can most easily be achieved with either an IVU or a renal ultrasound.

2 This patient has undergone bilateral double-J stenting to relieve ureteric obstruction secondary to pelvic malignancy. The top of the stent lies within the renal pelvis and the bottom in the bladder. The stents need to be changed every 6 months to prevent blockage.

CHAPTER 11

Clinical pharmacology

MULTIPLE CHOICE QUESTIONS

1   The following are disease-modifying antirheumatic drugs (DMARDs) used to treat rheumatoid arthritis:
    a) Penicillamine
    b) Colchicine
    c) Tacrolimus
    d) Hydroxychloroquine
    e) Sulfasalazine

2   The following drugs are safe to use routinely for simple constipation:
    a) Ispaghula husk
    b) Co-danthramer
    c) Senna
    d) Loperamide
    e) Sodium picosulfate

3   The following statements are true of steroid therapy:
    a) Prednisolone is more potent than dexamethasone
    b) Steroids should be stopped 2 weeks before major surgery
    c) Topical steroids do not have systemic side-effects
    d) Oral steroids should be taken at night
    e) Doses should be increased during intercurrent illness

4   Drugs used in Parkinson's disease include:
    a) Selegiline
    b) Indinavir
    c) Sumatriptan
    d) Pergolide
    e) Apomorphine

5   The following antibiotics are commonly used to treat simple cystitis:
    a) Nitrofurantoin
    b) Vancomycin
    c) Flucloxacillin
    d) Cefalexin
    e) Amoxicillin

6   The following require a controlled drug prescription:
    a) Codeine
    b) Diazepam
    c) Tramadol
    d) Methadone
    e) Fentanyl

7   Side-effects of the opioid analgesics include:
    a) Confusion
    b) Hypertension
    c) Constipation
    d) Vomiting
    e) Urinary retention

8   The following are used in the treatment of osteoporosis:
    a) Phosphate supplements
    b) Cyproterone
    c) Alendronate
    d) Raloxifene
    e) Calcium supplements

9   The following statements are true of warfarin:
    a) Therapy is monitored using the prothrombin time (PT)
    b) Rifampicin potentiates its effect
    c) It is safe in pregnancy
    d) Its effect is reversed by protamine
    e) Jaundice is a side-effect

10 The following conditions require anticoagulation with warfarin to achieve the stated
    target international normalized ratio (INR) range:
    a) Deep vein thrombosis: 2–3
    b) Pulmonary embolism: 3–4
    c) Atrial fibrillation: 1–2
    d) Mechanical prosthetic heart valve: 2–3
    e) Recurrent deep vein thrombosis on warfarin treatment: 4–5

11 The following drugs can precipitate acute renal failure:
    a) Ramipril
    b) Diclofenac
    c) Nifedipine
    d) Gentamicin
    e) Furosemide

12 The following drugs may be useful in the management of migraine:
    a) Sumatriptan
    b) Propranolol
    c) Ergotamine
    d) Pizotifen
    e) Naproxen

13 Iatrogenic causes of hypothyroidism include:
   a) Ciprofloxacin
   b) Lithium
   c) Amiodarone
   d) Atenolol
   e) Warfarin

14 Drugs that can precipitate parkinsonian symptoms include:
   a) Propranolol
   b) Metoclopramide
   c) Haloperidol
   d) Cimetidine
   e) Prochlorperazine

15 Drugs that can cause gynaecomastia include:
   a) Erythromycin
   b) Cimetidine
   c) Bendroflumethiazide
   d) Digoxin
   e) Spironolactone

16 The following drugs can be used as anti-emetics:
   a) Fluoxetine
   b) Ondansetron
   c) Phenytoin
   d) Domperidone
   e) Haloperidol

17 The following drugs are useful in the treatment of *H. pylori* peptic ulcer disease:
   a) Amoxicillin
   b) Lansoprazole
   c) Bismuth chelate
   d) Clarithromycin
   e) Metronidazole

18 The following drugs can be given for pain relief:
   a) Cyclizine
   b) Carbamazepine
   c) Amitriptyline
   d) Gabapentin
   e) Prochlorperazine

19 Morphine can be given via the following routes:
   a) Intramuscular
   b) Orally
   c) Intravenous
   d) Subcutaneous
   e) Rectal

20 The following drugs are known to cause liver damage:
   a) Halothane
   b) Methotrexate
   c) Oral contraceptive pill
   d) Chlorpromazine
   e) Isoniazid

21 The following drugs are recognized to be useful in gastro-oesophageal reflux disease:
   a) Alginates
   b) Cimetidine
   c) Anti-*H. pylori* triple therapy
   d) Potassium supplements
   e) Metoclopramide

22 The following may be used in the management of hyperkalaemia:
   a) Insulin-dextrose infusion
   b) Salbutamol nebulizers
   c) Calcium gluconate
   d) Magnesium supplementation
   e) Calcium resonium

Answers: see pages 262–265

EXTENDED MATCHING QUESTIONS

1 THERAPEUTIC DRUG MONITORING

All of the drugs below, or their effects, can be monitored in clinical practice. For each of the scenarios below choose the most likely drug responsible for the side-effects described

A Gentamicin
B Amiodarone
C Lithium
D Digoxin
E Ciclosporin

F Aminophylline
G Phenytoin
H Carbamazepine
I Vancomycin
J Warfarin

1 A 37-year-old intravenous drug user with Gram-negative sepsis develops acute renal failure on the ward.

2 A 31-year-old comes to hospital having an acute asthma attack. Her peak flow is 28 per cent of predicted. She is given intravenous medication, and improves but unfortunately develops ventricular tachycardia 3 h later.

3 A 69-year-old woman decides she will get better more quickly if she takes all her tablets in one go. She presents to the emergency department two days later with a massive gastro-intestinal bleed.

4 A 71-year-old man is brought in by his wife because she says he is not quite right. He is suffering from anorexia, nausea, vomiting and comments that objects appear more yellow than usual. An electrocardiogram (ECG) shows no P waves, T wave inversion in V_5–V_6 and ST depression, which looks like a reverse tick.

5 A 21-year-old supermarket assistant is admitted to hospital with vomiting, ataxia, dysarthria, tremor and heart block. She recovers uneventfully, but when better does not communicate or make eye contact with the medical team.

2 ANTIVIRAL AGENTS

For each scenario below, choose the most appropriate antiviral from the options given

A Oseltamivir
B Amantadine
C Interferon-α
D Nelfinavir
E Lamivudine

F Ribavirin
G Aciclovir
H Zidovudine
I Ganciclovir
J Foscarnet

1 A drug used with interferon-α in the treatment of chronic hepatitis B.

2 A drug used to treat herpes simplex encephalitis.

3 The drug of choice for the treatment of avian influenza.

4 First-line therapy for cytomegalovirus retinitis.

5 An antiviral drug also used in the treatment of Parkinson's disease.

3 ANTIBIOTICS 1

Choose the most appropriate antibiotic for each of the clinical scenarios below

A Phenoxymethylpenicillin
B Benzylpenicillin
C Flucloxacillin
D Trimethoprim
E Erythromycin

F Metronidazole
G Vancomycin
H Chloramphenicol
I Isoniazid
J Co-trimoxazole

1 First-line treatment for a urinary tract infection.
2 Treatment of meticillin-resistant *Staphylococcus aureus* (MRSA) pneumonia
3 Part of a cocktail used to treat tuberculosis.
4 Used as first-line oral treatment for streptococcal cellulitis.
5 Used in the treatment of conjunctivitis.

4 SIDE-EFFECTS OF MEDICATION 1

Choose the medication most likely to be responsible for the side-effects illustrated in the scenarios below

A Salbutamol
B Carbimazole
C Metoclopramide
D Amiodarone
E Gentamicin

F Bendroflumethiazide
G Clindamycin
H Codeine
I Metformin
J Ibuprofen

1 A 74-year-old man has a coronary angiogram for exertional chest pain. Eight hours later he is noted to be tachypnoeic; blood gas analysis reveals a pH of 7.26 with an anion gap of 25.
2 A 61-year-old woman complains of tinnitus after having a course of drugs administered intravenously.
3 A 71-year-old man goes back to his general practitioner (GP) saying the medicine he was given has made him constipated.
4 A 23-year-old woman has food poisoning and goes to her GP, who prescribes some anti-emetics. Two hours after the first dose, she returns in severe pain, unable to move her eyes from looking upwards.
5 A 58-year-old man makes an appointment with his doctor, complaining of weight loss, palpitations and diarrhoea. He has a fine tremor and tachycardia on examination. His GP says that his medication is probably to blame.

5 ANTIDOTES 1

Select the most appropriate antidote for overdoses of each of the substances below

A   Pralidoxime
B   Fomepizole
C   *N*-acetylcysteine
D   Protamine
E   Naloxone

F   Dicobalt edetate
G   Dantrolene
H   Glucagon
I   Dimercaprol
J   Flumazenil

1   Codeine phosphate.
2   Metoprolol.
3   Diazepam.
4   Ethylene glycol (antifreeze).
5   Heparin.

6 DRUGS OF ABUSE

Each of the following patients presents to the emergency department, but either refuses or is unable to tell the doctor the name of the drug they have taken. Choose the most likely substance from the options given

A   Cocaine
B   Ketamine
C   Heroin
D   LSD
E   Gamma hydroxybutyric acid (GHB)

F   Ecstasy
G   Cannabis
H   Methadone
I   Amyl nitrite
J   Diazepam

1   A 31-year-old man comes in complaining of central crushing chest pain, with an ECG showing features of ischaemia. His pupils are dilated and he has a tachycardia of 130 beats/min. The doctor suspects an illicit substance may be involved.
2   A 23-year-old woman comes to the emergency department with vomiting, blurred vision and slurred speech. She says that she feels a sense of depersonalization. Her pulse is 125 beats/min. The patient says that she has had some Special K. The junior on-call doctor is suspicious that she is lying, as it is dinnertime.
3   A 27-year-old is brought in by ambulance. He is rushed to resus as he is centrally and peripherally cyanosed. The junior doctor tries to take arterial blood gases five times, but obtains what she thinks is a venous sample every time. Analysis reveals arterial oxygen saturation (Sao_2) 87 per cent on room air, partial pressure of oxygen (Po_2) 13.4 kPa, partial pressure of carbon dioxide (Pco_2) 4.85 kPa, methaemoglobin (metHb) 32 per cent. The patient says that he has taken an aphrodisiac that evening.
4   A 19-year-old student is taken to hospital by his friends. He tells the receptionist that he thinks he can fly; she is so concerned that she asks one of the doctors to come through and see him straight away. Despite his evident agitation, the doctor is able to gather that he took an illicit substance at a nightclub 2 h ago.
5   A 42-year-old man is brought to the emergency department by his wife. He is drowsy and has a respiratory rate of 7 breaths/min. She says that he has no medical problems and only ever sees the GP for insomnia.

7 ANTIBIOTICS 2

Choose the most appropriate antibiotic for each of the clinical scenarios below

A   Metronidazole
B   Benzylpenicillin
C   Cefuroxime
D   Nitrofurantoin
E   Erythromycin

F   Ciprofloxacin
G   Doxycycline
H   Gentamicin
I   Rifampicin
J   Co-trimoxazole

1   A 38-year-old woman with known HIV presents to the emergency department with a history of fever and productive cough. Her last CD4 count was 94 cells/µL. The doctors are a little surprised when the chest X-ray appears normal.

2   A 63-year-old man goes to respiratory outpatients where he is seen regularly for his bronchiectasis. He complains that he is producing thick, viscid, green sputum. The registrar finds that he has been colonized with *Pseudomonas* in the past. She prescribes him an antibiotic and tells him to return in a week if he feels no better.

3   A 19-year old woman goes to hospital with right loin pain, a fever of 38°C, and hypotension. Urine is positive for blood, protein, and nitrites. Along with i.v. fluids, the doctor starts immediate i.v. antibiotics.

4   A 16-year-old boy is taken by his mother to see their GP. She is very concerned as three children at his school have died from meningococcal septicaemia. The GP reassures her and tells her that he will give the boy a short course of antibiotics.

5   A 73-year-old man develops profuse, watery diarrhoea whilst in hospital. The team suspects that this is an adverse reaction. The diarrhoea is positive for *Clostridium difficile* toxin. The house officer institutes immediate antibiotic treatment.

8 SIDE-EFFECTS OF MEDICATION 2

Choose the medication most likely to be responsible for the side-effects illustrated in the scenarios below

A   Furosemide
B   Carbimazole
C   Sando-K
D   Amiodarone
E   Loperamide

F   Heparin
G   Simvastatin
H   Codeine phosphate
I   Metoclopramide
J   Ibuprofen

1   Agranulocytosis.
2   Gout.
3   Rhabdomyolysis.
4   Osteoporosis.
5   Hyperprolactinaemia.

9 IATROGENIC CAUSES OF GASTROINTESTINAL BLEEDING

Each of the drugs listed can cause gastrointestinal bleeding. Choose the most likely drug to cause this complication for each of the clinical scenarios below

A Enoxaparin
B Dipyridamole
C Hirudin
D Abciximab
E Unfractionated heparin

F Warfarin
G Aspirin
H Sando-K
I Alendronate
J Diclofenac

1 A 73-year-old woman is admitted to hospital with an upper gastrointestinal bleed. An endoscopy shows severe oesophagitis which the gastroenterologist comments is probably secondary to the medication she is taking. She replies that she is only taking pills for leg cramps and osteoporosis.

2 A 66-year-old woman is rushed to hospital by her husband when she starts vomiting blood. An urgent endoscopy shows severe gastritis. Her only comorbidity is severe rheumatoid arthritis, which she finds quite debilitating.

3 A 62-year-old management consultant is admitted to hospital with severe pneumonia. Three days after admission he remarks upon the passage of black, tarry stools.

4 A 53-year-old man is seen in the emergency department with central crushing chest pain and ST elevation on his ECG. After initial treatment, he is taken through to the cardiac catheterization laboratory where the cardiology registrar gives him an additional drug before his angioplasty. Some hours later the patient develops gastrointestinal bleeding and remembers the registrar said that this was a well-recognized side-effect.

5 A 54-year-old carpenter is discharged after a 4-day hospital admission for a small myocardial infarction. He is started on several new medications, which he is told he must continue for life. Six months later he returns complaining of melaena.

10 ANTIDOTES 2

Select the most appropriate antidote for overdoses of each of the substances below

A   Pralidoxime
B   Methylthioninium chloride
C   *N*-acetylcysteine
D   Protamine
E   Naloxone

F   Dicobalt edetate
G   Dantrolene
H   Vitamin K
I   Dimercaprol
J   Flumazenil

1   A 76-year-old man tries to commit suicide by taking all his tablets in one go. He regrets his actions and takes the empty bottles to the emergency department. The doctor inspects the bottles and notes that they once contained warfarin and multivitamins; blood tests reveal an INR of 8.3. When the doctor goes back to see the patient, she notices he is having a nose bleed.

2   An elderly couple, who have been living in a Victorian house for decades, go to see their GP because of fatigue. He finds them both to be anaemic and orders a blood film which shows basophilic stippling. He diagnoses lead poisoning and refers them to a specialist for further treatment.

3   A 21-year-old clubber is rushed to hospital after she collapses on the dance floor. On arrival her core temperature is 44°C, and her Glasgow Coma Scale (GCS) is 3/15. A friend who has travelled with her in the ambulance says that she has taken four ecstasy tablets that evening.

4   A 14-year-old teenager takes 8 g of paracetamol after she sees her boyfriend with another girl. She regrets her actions 5 h later and asks her mother to take her to the emergency department. The doctor says that he is keen to begin treatment.

5   A terrorist organization releases a large quantity of insecticide in a crowded building. Many people are brought into hospital with small pupils, bradycardia, and diarrhoea. The consultant recognizes the features of organophosphate poisoning, and asks his juniors to begin treatment while he dons his biohazard suit.

11 PRESCRIPTION DRUGS

Select a drug from the options given for each of the statements below

A   Cannabis
B   Heroin
C   Dexamfetamine
D   Temazepam
E   Diazepam

F   Amoxicillin
G   Esomeprazole
H   Co-codamol
I   Diclofenac
J   Insulin

1   Cannot be prescribed by a doctor.
2   A drug for which the prescription must be written entirely by hand.
3   A controlled drug that can be issued by computer-generated prescription.
4   Available over the counter from a pharmacy without prescription.
5   Can only be prescribed to drug addicts by doctors with a special licence.

Answers: see pages 265–268

ANSWERS

MCQ ANSWERS

1 a) True. It is also used in Wilson's disease.
   b) False. This is a drug used for gout.
   c) False. This is an immunosuppressant drug used by organ transplant recipients.
   d) True. This is an antimalarial drug.
   e) True. This and methotrexate are the DMARDs of choice.

2 a) True. This is a bulk-forming laxative.
   b) False. This is potentially carcinogenic and is only used for terminally ill patients.
   c) True. This is a stimulant laxative.
   d) False. This is an antimotility drug used in the treatment of diarrhoea.
   e) False. This is a powerful stimulant laxative, used for bowel evacuation before radio-logical procedures of the colon.

3 a) False.
   b) False. It is important to maintain steroid cover peri-operatively to avoid an Addisonian crisis.
   c) False. High-dose topical preparations are absorbed systemically from the skin.
   d) False. They should be taken in the morning to coincide with the natural circadian rhythm.
   e) True.

4 a) True. This is a monoamine oxidase (MAO)-B inhibitor, used in conjunction with levodopa to reduce end-of-dose deterioration.
   b) False. This is an antiretroviral drug.
   c) False. This is a 5-hydroxytryptamine ($5\text{-}HT_1$) agonist, used for treatment of migraine.
   d) True. This is a dopamine receptor agonist.
   e) True. This is a dopamine receptor agonist, useful for the on–off syndrome.

5 a) True.
   b) False.
   c) False.
   d) True.
   e) True.

6 a) False.
   b) False.
   c) False.
   d) True.
   e) True.

7 a) True.
   b) False. Hypotension is a side-effect.
   c) True.
   d) True.
   e) True.

8 a) False.
   b) False. This is an anti-androgen drug.
   c) True. This is a bisphosphonate.
   d) True. This is a selective oestrogen receptor modulator useful for postmenopausal osteoporosis.
   e) True. These are important in the elderly, whose dietary intake might be insufficient.

9 a) True. The international normalized ratio (INR) is the ratio of the patient's PT to a control.
   b) False. This drug is a hepatic enzyme inducer, increasing the metabolism of warfarin.
   c) False. It is teratogenic in the first trimester, and may cause placental or fetal haemorrhage towards the end of term.
   d) False. Protamine reverses anticoagulation with heparin. Prothrombin complex concentrate or fresh-frozen plasma provide rapid reversal of anticoagulation with warfarin. Vitamin K reverses warfarin's effects more slowly.
   e) True. This occurs rarely.

10 a) True.
   b) False. The target is the same as for deep vein thrombosis, 2–3.
   c) False. The target should be 2–3.
   d) False. These are highly thrombogenic and require a target of 3–4.
   e) False. Treatment should aim for a range of 3–4.

11 a) True. Angiotensin-converting enzyme (ACE) inhibitors reduce renal perfusion.
   b) True. Non-steroidal anti-inflammatory drugs (NSAIDs) can cause acute tubulo-interstitial nephritis.
   c) False.
   d) True. Aminoglycosides are directly nephrotoxic.
   e) True. This reduces circulating volume and also is a cause of acute tubulointerstitial nephritis.

12 a) True. This is a 5-HT$_1$ agonist, used for treatment of migraine.
   b) True. This is a beta blocker, sometimes used for prophylaxis.
   c) True. This is a 5-HT agonist, used for treatment.
   d) True. This is a 5-HT antagonist and antihistamine, used as a prophylactic agent.
   e) True. This is an NSAID. Simple analgesia and NSAIDs should be tried first before other drugs.

13 a) False.
   b) True. Thyroid function should be checked every 6 to 12 months on stabilized regimes of lithium.
   c) True. This can cause hyper- or hypothyroidism.
   d) False. Beta-blockers can reverse symptoms of thyrotoxicosis but do not cause hypothyroidism.
   e) False.

14 a) False.
    b) True. This is an anti-emetic – it acts as a dopamine antagonist.
    c) True. This is a butyrophenone antipsychotic – a dopamine antagonist.
    d) False.
    e) True. This is a phenothiazine antipsychotic, also an anti-emetic. It is a dopamine antagonist.

15 a) False.
    b) True.
    c) False.
    d) True.
    e) True. Gynaecomastia is caused by an abnormal rise in the oestrogen/androgen ratio.

16 a) False. This is an antidepressant (selective serotonin reuptake inhibitor).
    b) True. This is a 5-HT_3 antagonist.
    c) False. This is an anti-epileptic.
    d) True. This promotes gastric motility.
    e) True. This drug has widespread use in palliative care.

17 a) True.
    b) True. This is a proton pump inhibitor.
    c) True.
    d) True.
    e) True.

18 a) False. This is an antihistamine, used as an anti-emetic.
    b) True. This is an anti-epileptic that can be used for trigeminal neuralgia.
    c) True. This is a tricyclic antidepressant used in neuropathic pain.
    d) True. This is an anti-epileptic that is commonly used for neuropathic pain.
    e) False. This is an antipsychotic and anti-emetic.

19 a) True.
    b) True.
    c) True.
    d) True. However, diamorphine is often preferred via this route.
    e) True.

20 a) True. This is a gaseous anaesthetic agent.
    b) True. This is a DMARD.
    c) True.
    d) True. This is a phenothiazine neuroleptic drug.
    e) True. This is an antituberculous drug.

21 a) True. An example is Gaviscon.
    b) True. This is an H_2-receptor antagonist.
    c) False. This is first-line for peptic ulcer disease.
    d) False.
    e) True. This assists gastric emptying.

22 a) True.
   b) True. The sympathetic effect of salbutamol drives potassium into cells.
   c) True. This does not reduce serum potassium concentration but temporarily stabilizes the myocardium.
   d) False. This may be useful in the treatment of hypokalaemia if hypomagnesaemia is also present.
   e) True. This is an oral ion-exchange resin.

EMQ ANSWERS

1 THERAPEUTIC DRUG MONITORING

1 A Aminoglycosides such as **gentamicin** are frequently used in hospital practice to treat Gram-negative infections. Its principal side-effects are nephrotoxicity and ototoxicity.

2 F **Aminophylline** is only occasionally given for severe asthma; cardiac arrhythmias are an important side-effect, particularly after parenteral therapy.

3 J Over-anticoagulation with **warfarin** is frequently seen. In this case rapid reversal is required with prothrombin complex as the patient is actively bleeding.

4 D This gentleman is suffering from **digoxin** toxicity. Digoxin can cause a varied clinical presentation when levels are too high. Visual disturbance and ECG changes may both be features.

5 C **Lithium** can be dangerous in overdose, sometimes necessitating dialysis. This patient has features of depression and has probably been given lithium for bipolar disorder.

2 ANTIVIRAL AGENTS

1 E A combination of interferon α and **lamivudine** is used to treat chronic hepatitis B; ribavirin and interferon-α are used together to treat hepatitis C.

2 G **Aciclovir**, a nucleoside analogue, is active against herpes simplex and varicella-zoster and can be used to treat encephalitis, chickenpox, shingles and mucocutaneous ulceration.

3 A **Oseltamivir**, commonly known as Tamiflu, is the treatment of choice for bird flu. There have been some reports of resistance to this agent.

4 I Intravenous **ganciclovir** is highly effective against cytomegalovirus but its toxicity precludes its usage outside sight- or life-threatening disease.

5 B **Amantadine**, an antiviral agent that has been used to treat influenza, is sometimes used in the treatment of Parkinson's disease. Its mechanism of action has still not been fully elucidated.

3 ANTIBIOTICS 1

1 D **Trimethoprim**, an antifolate drug, is widely used for the treatment of the community-acquired urinary tract infections. There are, however, increasing reports of resistance.

2 G **Vancomycin** and teicoplanin are both effective against MRSA; teicoplanin has the advantage of not needing therapeutic drug level monitoring.

3 I Drugs commonly used to treat tuberculosis include rifampicin, **isoniazid**, pyrazinamide and ethambutol.

4 A **Phenoxymethylpenicillin** (also known as penicillin V) is orally active against streptococcal infections.

5 H **Chloramphenicol** is a broad-spectrum antibiotic most commonly used topically for the treatment of eye infections. Haematological side-effects, including aplastic anaemia, limit its systemic use apart from in life-threatening infections.

4 SIDE-EFFECTS OF MEDICATION 1

1 I This man has a metabolic acidosis with an increased anion gap, presumably due to increased lactate. **Metformin** can occasionally cause this side-effect in patients exposed to radiological contrast media.

2 E All aminoglycosides, including **gentamicin**, can cause ototoxicity. Care should be taken not to simultaneously administer these drugs with other ototoxic medications such as furosemide.

3 H Opioids, such as **codeine**, morphine and tramadol, frequently cause constipation. Prophylactic prescription of laxatives is often sensible to prevent this.

4 C This unfortunate woman is suffering from an oculogyric crisis, precipitated by **metoclopramide**. This complication can occur, particularly in young females. Treatment with procyclidine or benzatropine is rapidly effective.

5 D This patient is clinically hyperthyroid. Both hypo- and hyperthyroidism are seen with **amiodarone** therapy; treatment can be difficult.

5 ANTIDOTES 1

1 E Opioid toxicity is best treated with **naloxone**, an opioid antagonist. It rapidly reverses the respiratory depression and sedation associated with opiates, but has a short half-life so may need repeated administration.

2 H Overdoses of beta-blockers may be difficult to treat with conventional anticholinergics such as atropine. **Glucagon** is useful in this setting as it stimulates the heart by a mechanism independent of the beta-receptor.

3 J **Flumazenil** is a benzodiazepine antagonist which can be used to reverse the effects of drugs such as diazepam or midazolam. Care must be taken however as it can precipitate fits in susceptible patients.

4 B **Fomepizole** inhibits alcohol dehydrogenase and prevents the metabolism of ethylene glycol into toxic by-products. As it is extremely expensive, it is only used in severe cases.

5 D **Protamine** can be used to reverse the anticoagulant effect of heparin. Paradoxically however, protamine itself can act as an anticoagulant if administered in excess.

6 DRUGS OF ABUSE

1 A **Cocaine** prevents the reuptake of noradrenaline and commonly causes sympatho-mimetic effects such as tachycardia and dilated pupils. Cardiac ischaemia and arrhythmias are well-recognized complications.

2 B Special K is a street name for **ketamine**, a drug used in medicine as an anaesthetic. Feelings of depersonalization and hallucinations are often seen; treatment is usually supportive.

3 I Methaemoglobinaemia occurs when the iron component of haem is oxidized from the ferrous (Fe^{2+}) form to the ferric (Fe^{3+}) form. In adults this is usually caused by drugs such as **amyl nitrite** ('poppers'), antimalarials, and sulfonamides.

4 D **LSD** alters normal consciousness and perception. It may lead to individuals believing that they have special powers. Recovery usually occurs after a few hours, although psychosis may persist for several days.

5 J Benzodiazepines, such as **diazepam**, are some of the most commonly prescribed drugs. They can be useful short-term treatments for anxiety or insomnia, but are frequently abused. Toxicity leads to respiratory depression.

7 ANTIBIOTICS 2

1 J **Co-trimoxazole**, a combination of the antibiotics trimethoprim and sulfamethoxazole, is used to treat *Pneumocystis carinii* pneumonia. Typically this disease presents in the immunocompromised, with signs of respiratory infection but with a normal chest X-ray.

2 F Commonly used antibiotics active against *Pseudomonas* include **ciprofloxacin**, piperacillin, and ceftazidime. Of these, ciprofloxacin is the only drug that may be administered orally.

3 C **Cefuroxime**, a second-generation cephalosporin, is often used as first-line treatment for pyelonephritis; it has both Gram-positive and Gram-negative cover.

4 I The only licensed treatment for the secondary prevention of meningococcal disease is **rifampicin**. Patients should be warned about the reddish discoloration of their secretions.

5 A *Clostridium difficile* is sensitive to both **metronidazole** and oral vancomycin. Infection with this organism after broad-spectrum antibiotic therapy is a common compli-cation, which may be potentially fatal.

8 SIDE-EFFECTS OF MEDICATION 2

1 B A rare but important side-effect of **carbimazole** is agranulocytosis: all patients pre-senting with symptoms of infection, especially sore throat, should have an urgent full blood count.

2 A Both loop diuretics, such as **furosemide**, and thiazide diuretics, such as bendro-flumethiazide, cause hyperuricaemia and may precipitate attacks of acute gout.

3 G **Simvastatin**. Statin therapy is often associated with myalgia. Occasionally however rhabdomyolysis is seen, characterized by an elevated serum creatine kinase, myo-globinuria and acute renal failure.

4 F Long-term treatment with **heparin** may result in osteoporosis; alopecia is also rarely seen.

5 I **Metoclopramide**, a dopamine antagonist, inhibits the dopaminergic neurones that usually prevent prolactin release, thereby causing hyperprolactinaemia.

9 IATROGENIC CAUSES OF GASTROINTESTINAL BLEEDING

1 I   **Alendronate**, in common with other bisphosphonates, can be extremely toxic to the oesophagus. Patients are usually advised to stand for half an hour after taking their medication to prevent oesophageal irritation.

2 J   **Diclofenac** is a commonly used NSAID. These all have the ability to cause gastric erosions and ulceration, and are a common cause of upper gastrointestinal haemorrhage.

3 A   The only medication listed that is likely to be given to a patient with pneumonia is **enoxaparin**. Low-molecular weight heparins are commonly used in hospital practice to prevent deep venous thrombosis.

4 D   **Abciximab**, a platelet glycoprotein IIb/IIIa antagonist, is used to prevent complications in patients undergoing percutaneous coronary intervention. It is only administered by specialists.

5 G   Out of the standard drugs used for secondary prevention of myocardial infarction (**aspirin**, ACE inhibitor, β-blocker, statin), aspirin is associated with gastrointestinal bleeding. Note that clopidogrel is usually only given for one year after a cardiac event.

10 ANTIDOTES 2

1 H   **Vitamin K** can be used to reverse the effects of warfarin if there is minor bleeding, as it usually takes a few hours to work. For more urgent cases prothrombin complex is required.

2 I   **Dimercaprol** is a chelating agent which can be used to aid the elimination of heavy metals such as gold, arsenic, lead and mercury from the body.

3 G   The hyperthermia that can follow ecstasy ingestion resembles neuroleptic malignant syndrome with muscle rigidity, metabolic acidosis and rhabdomyolysis. Treatment is with **dantrolene**, but is often unsuccessful.

4 C   **N-acetylcysteine** increases the liver's supplies of glutathione, which prevents toxicity by binding to the dangerous metabolite of paracetamol.

5 A   Nerve agents such as sarin, VX and tabun irreversibly inactivate acetylcholinesterase and so present with features of parasympathetic overdrive. The drug **pralidoxime** can reactivate this enzyme in cases of severe poisoning, if administered in time.

11 PRESCRIPTION DRUGS

1 A   **Cannabis** is a class C drug and is not available by medical prescription for any purpose. Possession and supply are both criminal offences.

2 B   **Heroin** is the lay name for diamorphine, a controlled substance. All prescriptions must be written by hand; the amount to be supplied must be written in both numbers and words.

3 D   **Temazepam**, due to its potential for addiction, is a controlled substance. However, it is exempt from the prescribing rules that apply to other controlled medication.

4 H   **Co-codamol** 8/500 is available over the counter as a combination of 8 mg of codeine with 500 mg of paracetamol. A prescription is required for the stronger 15/500 and 30/500 preparations.

5 B   The prescription of **heroin** (diamorphine) and cocaine is restricted to doctors specializing in the treatment of addiction.

General surgery

MULTIPLE CHOICE QUESTIONS

1 The following statements are true of testicular cancers:
   a) They are rare in undescended testicles
   b) Early sexual intercourse is a risk factor
   c) Teratomas occur in an older age group than seminomas
   d) Seminomas are radiosensitive
   e) Prognosis is poor

2 Regarding acute appendicitis:
   a) Some cases are best managed conservatively
   b) The risk of developing the disease increases with age
   c) There is no role for antibiotics
   d) Digital rectal examination is useful
   e) Mesenteric adenitis may present in a similar way

3 Features of strangulated bowel obstruction include:
   a) Pyrexia
   b) Troisier's sign
   c) Leucocytosis
   d) Hypercapnia
   e) Peritonism

4 The following statements are true of sigmoid volvulus:
   a) This occurs most commonly in neonates
   b) It is a recognized complication of digital rectal examination
   c) Flexible sigmoidoscopy has no role in the management of this condition
   d) It is usually painless
   e) An abdominal radiograph is of little use

5 The following statements are true of small bowel obstruction:
   a) Strangulated obstruction can usually be managed conservatively
   b) Patients with acute obstruction should be resuscitated with oral fluids
   c) A nasogastric tube is useful in a patient who is vomiting
   d) It can be treated by laparoscopic surgery
   e) Obstruction from adhesions can present years after the original surgical operation

6 Causes of acute pancreatitis include:
   a) Endoscopic retrograde cholangiopancreatography (ERCP)
   b) Diabetes mellitus
   c) Alcohol
   d) Mumps
   e) Coeliac disease

7 Cholecystectomy is an appropriate treatment for the following conditions:
   a) Biliary colic
   b) Cholangitis
   c) Chronic cholecystitis
   d) Acute cholecystitis
   e) Asymptomatic gallstones

8 Regarding haemorrhoids:
   a) First-degree haemorrhoids do not bleed
   b) Second-degree haemorrhoids bleed but do not prolapse
   c) Third-degree haemorrhoids prolapse outside the anus and can be manually replaced
      by the patient
   d) Haemorrhoids are normally painful
   e) Pregnancy is a risk factor

9 The following statements are true of paralytic ileus:
   a) It is treated operatively
   b) It is usually extremely painful
   c) Bowel sounds are hyperactive and tinkling
   d) Vomiting may be a feature
   e) 'Nil by mouth' is not necessary

10 Causes of a lump in the groin include:
   a) Ectopic testis
   b) Diaphragmatic hernia
   c) Bouchard's nodes
   d) Femoral aneurysm
   e) Saphena varix

11 The following factors preclude organ donation:
   a) Diabetes mellitus
   b) Coronary artery disease
   c) Malignancy
   d) Asthma
   e) Human immunodeficiency virus

12 Scrotal swellings that an examiner can 'get above' include:
   a) Epididymitis
   b) Inguinoscrotal hernia
   c) Epididymal cyst
   d) Testicular tumour
   e) Adult hydrocele

13 Regarding scrotal swellings:
   a) Mumps is a cause of orchitis
   b) It is impossible to palpate the cord above an adult hydrocele
   c) Varicoceles usually occur on the right
   d) Epididymal cysts are pre-malignant
   e) 20 per cent of hydroceles cause infertility

14 The following statements are true of testicular torsion:
   a) It is usually bilateral
   b) It is commonest in middle-aged men
   c) An undescended testis is a risk factor
   d) Orchidectomy is always necessary
   e) Testicular malignancy is a complication

15 Causes of a congenital lump in the neck include:
   a) Carotid body tumour
   b) Virchow's node
   c) Branchial cyst
   d) Nodes of Ranvier
   e) Cystic hygroma

16 Triple assessment of breast lumps includes:
   a) Quantification of nipple discharge
   b) Breast computed tomography (CT) scan
   c) Isotope scanning
   d) Mammography
   e) Clinical examination

17 The following increase susceptibility to abdominal hernias:
   a) Pregnancy
   b) Intervertebral disc prolapse
   c) Uraemia
   d) Chronic bronchitis
   e) Constipation

18 Early complications of acute pancreatitis include:
   a) Hypercalcaemia
   b) Erythema nodosum
   c) Adult respiratory distress syndrome
   d) Hyperglycaemia
   e) Acute renal failure

19 The following are risk factors for peritonitis:
   a) Peritoneal dialysis
   b) Irritable bowel syndrome
   c) Prostatic hypertrophy
   d) Ascites
   e) Diverticulitis

20 The following statements are true of inguinal hernias:
  a) They do not occur in children
  b) In women they are rarer than femoral hernias
  c) Laparoscopic repair is possible
  d) An absent cough impulse excludes the diagnosis of hernia
  e) They occur more commonly on the right than the left

21 Causes of paralytic ileus include:
  a) Metoclopramide
  b) Polycythaemia
  c) Generalized peritonitis
  d) Laparotomy
  e) Hypokalaemia

22 The cardinal symptoms of mechanical bowel obstruction are:
  a) Abdominal distension
  b) Melaena
  c) Oliguria
  d) Vomiting
  e) Colicky abdominal pain

23 Late complications of acute pancreatitis include:
  a) Hepatocellular carcinoma
  b) Polyneuropathy
  c) Pancreatic necrosis
  d) Pernicious anaemia
  e) Pseudocyst formation

24 Anal conditions that are usually acutely painful include:
  a) Proctalgia fugax
  b) Anal skin tags
  c) Anal fissure
  d) First-degree haemorrhoids
  e) Perianal haematoma

25 Regarding femoral hernias:
  a) They are more common in females than males
  b) There is a low risk of strangulation
  c) They are usually congenital
  d) The neck lies above and medial to the pubic tubercle
  e) Treatment is usually conservative

26 The following factors predispose to post-operative wound dehiscence:
  a) Obesity
  b) Absorbent dressings
  c) Analgesia
  d) Wound haematoma
  e) Malnutrition

27 Common causes of central abdominal pain include:
   a) Small bowel obstruction
   b) Salpingitis
   c) Leaking abdominal aortic aneurysm
   d) Early appendicitis
   e) Ruptured ovarian cyst

28 Causes of post-operative confusion include:
   a) Urine retention
   b) Compression stockings
   c) Tramadol
   d) Heparin
   e) Myocardial infarction

29 Absorbable sutures include:
   a) Polyglactin (Vicryl)
   b) Silk
   c) Catgut
   d) Prolene
   e) Nylon

30 The following drugs should be routinely stopped pre-operatively before major surgery:
   a) Corticosteroids
   b) Beta-blockers
   c) Warfarin
   d) The oral contraceptive pill
   e) Anti-epileptics

31 Factors preventing spontaneous healing of a post-operative fistula include:
   a) Foreign body
   b) Opioids
   c) Malignant tissue
   d) Antibiotics
   e) Distal obstruction

32 Common causes of left iliac fossa pain include:
   a) Diverticulitis
   b) Gastritis
   c) Cholecystitis
   d) Ectopic pregnancy
   e) Ureteric calculus

33 The following are signs of generalized peritonitis:
   a) Guarding
   b) Fluid thrill
   c) Murphy's sign
   d) Hyperactive bowel sounds
   e) Rigid abdomen

34 Causes of oesophageal rupture include:
a) Foreign body
b) Candidiasis
c) Boerhaave's syndrome
d) Oesophagogastroduodenoscopy (OGD)
e) Nelson's syndrome

35 Consequences of chest trauma include:
a) Cardiac tamponade
b) Pulmonary embolism
c) Flail chest
d) Tension pneumothorax
e) Lung fibrosis

36 Regarding gas gangrene:
a) The offending organism is *Clostridium tetani*
b) It is a Gram-negative infection
c) Necrotic tissue should be excised
d) Gas production is rare
e) Antibiotics are not indicated

37 A painless breast lump may be caused by:
a) Fibroadenoma
b) Carcinoma
c) Acute breast abscess
d) Cyclical nodularity
e) Cyst

38 Recognized complications of cholecystectomy include:
a) Hepatoma
b) Peritonitis
c) Cholestatic jaundice
d) Duodenitis
e) Cholangitis

39 Typical causes of pruritus ani include:
a) Proctalgia fugax
b) Anal candidiasis
c) Pilonidal sinus
d) Fistula-in-ano
e) Poor hygiene

40 Regarding congenital hypertrophic pyloric stenosis:
a) It is inherited in an autosomal recessive manner
b) Males are more commonly affected than females
c) It usually presents at 12–16 weeks of age
d) Vomiting is characteristically bile-stained
e) Treatment is with Heller's myotomy

41 Causes of small bowel obstruction include:
   a) Lymphoma
   b) Crohn's disease
   c) Barrett's oesophagus
   d) Gallstone ileus
   e) Adhesions

42 Regarding indirect and direct inguinal hernias:
   a) Direct hernias are more likely to strangulate
   b) Direct hernias are uncommon in children
   c) Direct hernias are more likely to descend into the scrotum
   d) In females direct inguinal hernias are more common than indirect hernias
   e) An indirect hernia can be controlled by pressure over the internal ring

43 Treatment options for haemorrhoids include:
   a) Injection
   b) Band ligation
   c) Colostomy
   d) Ileo-rectal anastomosis
   e) Surgical ligation

44 Clinical features of acute pancreatitis include:
   a) Left iliac fossa pain
   b) Peritonism
   c) Quincke's sign
   d) Vomiting
   e) Grey Turner's sign

45 Complications of colostomy include:
   a) Parastomal hernia
   b) Stomal stenosis
   c) Peutz–Jeghers' syndrome
   d) Colonic prolapse
   e) Colonic angiodysplasia

46 The following are recognized consequences of severe burns:
   a) Acute renal failure
   b) Peptic ulceration
   c) Pseudomembranous colitis
   d) Limb contractures
   e) Depression

47 Post-operative pain can cause:
   a) Impaired mobility
   b) Confusion
   c) Paralytic ileus
   d) Delayed wound healing
   e) Urine retention

48 Causes of post-operative pyrexia include:
a) Urinary retention
b) Deep vein thrombosis
c) Basal lung atelectasis
d) Epidural analgesia
e) Anastomotic leak

49 Swelling of the parotid gland may be caused by:
a) Staphylococcus
b) Calculus
c) Ramsay–Hunt syndrome
d) Mumps
e) Mikulicz's syndrome

50 Causes of a fistula-in-ano include:
a) Perianal haematoma
b) Anal abscess
c) Rectal prolapse
d) Rectal cancer
e) Crohn's disease

51 Causes of post-operative hypoxia include:
a) Deep vein thrombosis
b) Morphine
c) Basal atelectasis
d) Myocardial infarction
e) Pulmonary embolism

Answers: see pages 284–291

EXTENDED MATCHING QUESTIONS

1 SWELLINGS IN THE INGUINAL REGION

All of the patients below are found to have a lump in the groin. Choose the most likely cause from the options given

A   Saphena varix
B   Femoral artery aneurysm
C   Psoas abscess
D   Hydrocele of the cord
E   Indirect inguinal hernia

F   Ectopic testicle
G   Direct inguinal hernia
H   Femoral hernia
I   Femoral neuroma
J   Inguinal lymphadenopathy

1   A 42-year-old baggage handler goes to see the doctor because he has a lump in his groin. On examination, the lump is reducible but reappears on coughing, even with pressure over the internal ring. The doctor refers the patient to hospital, noting in his letter that the lump is superior and medial to the pubic tubercle.
2   A 26-year-old bartender makes an appointment with his general practitioner (GP). He is embarrassed because he has a yellow urethral discharge. The GP examines him and finds multiple small masses in both groins. A sample of the discharge is sent to the laboratory for further analysis.
3   A 29-year-old Somalian woman comes with her seven children to see the GP. She has noticed a lump in her groin and is having difficulty walking. On examination, there is a soft, fluctuant mass, that the GP cannot reduce, lateral to the femoral artery. He also notices tender discoloured areas on both shins.
4   A 63-year-old head teacher, who has been admitted for coronary angiography, is being examined by some medical students on the ward. One of them becomes quite excited when she finds an expansile and pulsatile mass in the right groin with an associated bruit.
5   The same medical students start to examine the other leg and groin. They find an expansile mass with a cough impulse. One of them shows the others how she can feel a thrill in the groin, just by tapping behind the patient's left knee.

2 ABDOMINAL SCARS

Match the abdominal scars with their descriptions:

A   Kocher's
B   Midline
C   Left paramedian
D   Laparoscopic
E   Gridiron

F   Right paramedian
G   Pfannenstiel
H   Rooftop
I   Mercedes
J   Lanz

1   A low pelvic transverse incision.
2   A vertical incision 3 cm to the right of the linea alba.
3   An 8 cm oblique scar in the right upper quadrant.
4   A small oblique scar passing through McBurney's point.
5   A small transverse scar passing through McBurney's point.

3 ABDOMINAL SCARS 2

Choose the most appropriate incision for each of the patients below

A   Kocher's
B   Midline
C   Left paramedian
D   Laparoscopic
E   Gridiron

F   Right paramedian
G   Pfannenstiel
H   Rooftop
I   Mercedes
J   Lanz

1   A 29-year-old woman is scheduled to have a liver transplant, as she is encephalopathic after a paracetamol overdose.
2   A 27-year-old woman is to have an elective Caesarean section as her baby is in the breech position.
3   A 62-year-old woman is referred to clinic with right upper quadrant pain. She proudly shows the consultant the scar that she was left with after a cholecystectomy 30 years before.
4   A 14-year-old girl is put on the emergency operating list for an open appendicectomy. She is particularly concerned that her scar be as unobtrusive as possible.
5   A 42-year-old woman has an attack of acute cholecystitis. The surgeon arranges for her to have her gallbladder removed 6 weeks later.

4 ABDOMINAL OPERATIONS

Choose the most suitable operation for each of the indications below

A   Left hemicolectomy
B   Right hemicolectomy
C   Sigmoid colectomy
D   Hartmann's procedure
E   Abdominoperineal resection

F   Anterior resection
G   Loop ileostomy
H   End ileostomy
I   Oesophagectomy
J   Gastrectomy

1   A rectal carcinoma 2 cm from the anal verge.
2   An emergency procedure for a perforated diverticulum.
3   A caecal carcinoma.
4   A curative procedure for ulcerative colitis.
5   A rectal carcinoma 9 cm from the anal verge.

5 ABDOMINAL HERNIAS

All the patients below have hernias. Choose the most appropriate hernia from the options given for each of the clinical scenarios

A   Sliding hiatus hernia
B   Littre's hernia
C   Femoral hernia
D   Richter's hernia
E   Para-umbilical hernia

F   Inguinal hernia
G   Maydl's hernia
H   Rolling hiatus hernia
I   Incisional hernia
J   Congenital diaphragmatic hernia

1   A 45-year-old man complains of heartburn to his GP. An upper gastrointestinal endoscopy shows that some of the stomach is in the thorax, but the gastro-oesophageal junction is in the correct place.

2   A 42-year-old woman is taken to theatre with a strangulated hernia. The consultant points out to the house officer, who is assisting, that only part of the bowel wall is involved, which is why the patient was free of the symptoms and signs of obstruction.

3   A 68-year-old man comes back to clinic 6 months after his left hemicolectomy. He has no complaint about the operation, but does note that when he stands up a bulge appears down the middle of his abdomen.

4   A 23-year-old man is having his hernia operation. The registrar becomes quite excited when she finds a Meckel's diverticulum within the hernia sack. The consultant sighs wistfully and says that in his day when he was a registrar, he saw several.

5   A 30-year-old woman complains of a groin lump. She is referred to clinic, where the registrar notes that she has a hernia, the origin of which is above and medial to the pubic tubercle.

6 EPONYMOUS SIGNS IN SURGERY

Each of the patients below demonstrates a clinical sign when their doctor is examining them. Choose the correct sign from the list below

A   Chvostek's sign
B   Cullen's sign
C   Phalen's sign
D   Rovsing's sign
E   Lasègue's sign

F   Troisier's sign
G   Tinel's sign
H   Grey Turner's sign
I   Trousseau's sign
J   Homan's sign

1   A 46-year-old baggage handler complains of back pain. When his GP flexes his right hip and then dorsiflexes the ankle, he screams in pain.

2   A 12-year-old boy is thought to have appendicitis. The surgical registrar demonstrates to some medical students how the boy feels pain in the right iliac fossa when he palpates the left iliac fossa.

3   A 32-year-old alcoholic is admitted to hospital with a fourth attack of severe acute pancreatitis. The night doctor is called to see him some hours later, because the nurses are concerned that the skin around his navel has turned an unusual colour.

4   A 56-year-old policeman goes to see his doctor with tiredness, weight loss and dysphagia. The GP finds a firm hard lump in the left supraclavicular fossa.

5   A 31-year-old pregnant woman makes an appointment to see her GP as she is suffering from pins and needles in her hands. He asks her to flex both wrists while she talks to him. One minute later she finds she can no longer continue as the pins and needles have returned.

7 EPONYMS IN SURGERY

Each of the eponyms below is used to describe an operation, syndrome or sign in surgery. Choose the correct eponym to match the descriptions given

A   Billroth II
B   Heller
C   Murphy
D   Brown–Séquard
E   Rovsing

F   Polya
G   Goodsall
H   Buerger
I   McBurney
J   Boerhaave

1   Surgical division of the lower oesophageal sphincter as a treatment for achalasia.
2   A partial gastrectomy, whereby the remaining stomach is joined to a loop of jejunum.
3   A point two-thirds of the way from the umbilicus to the anterior superior iliac spine.
4   Pressure on the left side of the abdomen in acute appendicitis causes more pain in the right iliac fossa than the left.
5   Oesophageal rupture.

8 POST-OPERATIVE COMPLICATIONS

Choose the most likely post-operative complication for each of the patients below

A   Deep vein thrombosis (DVT)
B   Lower respiratory tract infection
C   Atelectasis
D   Pulmonary embolism
E   Hypoglycaemia

F   Hypovolaemia
G   Wound dehiscence
H   Incisional hernia
I   Wound infection
J   Myocardial infarction

1   A 60-year-old gentleman develops sudden shortness of breath and central chest pain 10 h following a femoral popliteal bypass.
2   An obese 45-year-old woman is seen in the emergency department; she is short of breath and has pleuritic left-sided chest pain. She underwent a laparoscopic cholecystectomy 7 days before. Her chest X-ray shows a small pleural effusion.
3   Two days following an abdominal aortic aneurysm repair, a 62-year-old man is noticed to be breathless. He has a rattling cough, is tachycardic and his saturations are 95 per cent on air. A full blood count is normal.
4   Four days following a hysterectomy, a woman is noticed to be pyrexial and breathless. She has a productive cough and crepitations at the right lung base.
5   The surgical houseman on call is bleeped to the ward. The nurses have just changed a patient's abdominal dressings – he underwent an abdominal aortic aneurysm (AAA) repair 5 days before. They are shocked as it appears that his abdomen has opened up.

9 LEG ULCERS

Choose the most likely cause of lower limb ulceration in each of the patients below

A Malignant melanoma
B Venous ulcer
C Dermatitis artefacta
D Basal cell carcinoma
E Marjolin's ulcer

F Pyoderma gangrenosum
G Neuropathic ulcer
H Arterial ulcer
I Polycythemia rubra vera
J Tabes dorsalis

1 A 78-year-old woman is seen in the outpatients department with a large ulcer over her medial malleolus. The ulcer has sloping edges.
2 A 60-year-old smoker has a deep ulcer on his heel. It is painful and has a punched out appearance.
3 An 85-year-old with a long-standing history of venous ulcers is concerned as the ulcers are changing shape and extending. The ulcers have everted edges, and a biopsy is taken.
4 A 30-year-old develops painful pustular ulcers on his legs. From his notes the GP sees that he has recently been seen by the gastroenterologist for weight loss and diarrhoea.
5 A diabetic man with poor glycaemic control has a large ulcer on the plantar aspect of his right foot. It is non-tender.

10 VASCULAR SURGICAL INTERVENTIONS

Select the most appropriate procedure for each of the patients below

A Endarterectomy
B Sympathectomy
C Embolectomy
D Thrombolysis
E Angioplasty

F Aortic grafting
G Arteriovenous fistula formation
H Amputation
I Endovascular coiling
J Ultrasound scan

1 A 29-year-old lawyer is referred to hospital because of intractable sweating in her armpits. Her clients are complaining that this makes her look extremely nervous in front of juries.
2 A 41-year-old gardener is brought to hospital by ambulance after collapsing in the garden with a sudden cry. He has neck stiffness and rigidity leading to the suspicion of sub-arachnoid haemorrhage. He is wheeled immediately into the CT scanner, and the diagnosis of a still-bleeding ruptured berry aneurysm is confirmed.
3 An 83-year-old man is brought to the emergency department with a cold left leg. On examination, his heartbeat is irregularly irregular, with absent left femoral, popliteal and pedal pulses. The doctor is surprised when she feels good pulses on the other side.
4 A 64-year-old man goes to see his GP with non-specific symptoms of fatigue, lethargy and low mood. Blood tests reveal an elevated urea and creatinine, high phosphate and low calcium. The local nephrologist agrees that the patient would probably benefit from dialysis.
5 An 82-year-old man makes an appointment with his GP to receive the influenza vaccination. The GP decides to examine him and finds a 4 cm pulsatile and expansile mass in the epigastrium.

11 DIAGNOSIS OF BREAST DISEASE

Each of the patients below presents to their GP with problems associated with their breasts. Choose the most likely diagnosis for each of the clinical scenarios below

A   Pregnancy
B   Tietze's syndrome
C   Mastitis
D   Breast carcinoma
E   Cyclical mastalgia

F   Fat necrosis
G   Duct ectasia
H   Lactating abscess
I   Paget's disease of the nipple
J   Phyllodes tumour

1   A 50-year-old woman sees her GP. She complains of pain behind the nipple and a thick, creamy, green nipple discharge over the last few weeks.
2   A middle-aged woman sees her GP complaining of an irregular hard mass in her left breast. She only noticed it 2 weeks ago following a bruise from a seatbelt when she was involved in a road traffic accident.
3   A 55-year-old woman has noticed a hard craggy mass in her left breast. Her left nipple is retracted. She is otherwise well and denies any pain.
4   A 25-year-old complains of monthly breast pain; she is otherwise well.
5   A breast-feeding mother presents to her GP with a red, painful right breast.

12 TREATMENT OF BREAST DISEASE

Each of the patients below seeks medical attention for a breast disorder. Choose the most suitable treatment from the options given

A   Lumpectomy
B   Benzylpenicillin
C   Pamidronate
D   Tamoxifen
E   Mastectomy

F   Trastuzumab
G   Microdochectomy
H   Bilateral mastectomy
I   Anastrozole
J   Flucloxacillin

1   A 43-year-old woman presents with a bloody nipple discharge. There is a small retro-areolar lump, with no associated lymphadenopathy. The GP thinks that the most likely diagnosis is a ductal papilloma.
2   A 61-year-old woman comes to breast clinic with 2 cm left breast lump. A staging CT shows hepatic metastasis. The primary tumour is removed; at the multidisciplinary team meeting the pathologist notes with interest that the tissue is HER2 positive, but negative for oestrogen receptors.
3   A 29-year-old breast-feeding mother presents to her GP with a red, painful breast.
4   A 49-year-old woman with metastatic breast cancer comes to clinic feeling tired and complaining of constipation. A set of blood tests shows a calcium level of 3.2 mmol/L.
5   A 76-year-old woman presents to her GP, complaining of breast discharge. When he examines her, he finds a malodorous fungating mass, with axillary lymphadenopathy. A staging CT scan reveals no further metastasis.

13 SKIN LUMPS

Each of the patients below presents with a skin lesion. Choose the most likely diagnosis from the options given

A   Lipoma
B   Basal cell carcinoma
C   Dermoid cyst
D   Malignant melanoma
E   Campbell de Morgan spots

F   Squamous cell carcinoma
G   Sebaceous cyst
H   Keratoacanthoma
I   Neurofibroma
J   Epidermoid cyst

1 A 78-year-old man has a 3-year history of multiple small red papules on his chest. He is curious to know what they are.
2 A 29-year-old woman gives a 1-week history of a sore lesion on her upper back. It is well circumscribed and has a central punctum.
3 A 63-year-old man goes to see his doctor as he has a lesion on his nose. On examination, it is well circumscribed and has a rolled pearly edge with superficial telangiectasia.
4 A 71-year-old woman seeks medical attention for a lesion on her ear. It started as a small pimple, and has grown rapidly over the past month to about 2 cm in diameter. On examination, there is a central crater surrounded by a well-circumscribed lesion.
5 A 58-year-old gardener presents with a small cystic swelling in the subcutaneous tissue of his right hand. He says it has been there ever since he pricked himself on some rose thorns.

Answers: see pages 291–295

ANSWERS

MCQ ANSWERS

1   a) False. This is a risk factor.
    b) False.
    c) False. The peak age group for teratoma is 20–30 years, and 30–40 years for seminoma.
    d) True.
    e) False. Testicular cancer survival rates have improved significantly.

2   a) True. If an appendix mass has formed, when the patient presents after a few days of abdominal pain, surgery is delayed.
    b) False. Young people are at highest risk.
    c) False. Prophylactic peri-operative antibiotics are indicated.
    d) True. This may reveal tenderness on the right.
    e) True. Inflammation of the mesenteric lymph nodes is an important differential diagnosis in children.

3   a) True. This is part of the systemic inflammatory response.
    b) False. This is a left supraclavicular lymph node (Virchow's node), indicating gastro-intestinal malignancy.
    c) True. It is predominantly a neutrophilia.
    d) False.
    e) True. If perforation occurs, the localized peritonitis will progress to generalized peritonitis.

4   a) False. It occurs in the elderly.
    b) False.
    c) False. Flatus tubes and/or sigmoidoscopy are useful non-operative interventions.
    d) False. It causes colicky pain and large bowel obstruction.
    e) False. Abdominal X-ray reveals a grossly dilated loop of large bowel.

5   a) False. This is a surgical emergency and requires an operation.
    b) False. Fluids must be given intravenously.
    c) True. This helps to decompress the bowel.
    d) True. Bands and adhesions can be relieved laparoscopically.
    e) True.

6   a) True. This is a recognized complication of the procedure.
    b) False.
    c) True. Alcohol and gallstones are the commonest causes in the Western world.
    d) True.
    e) False.

7 a) True. This is a common indication for the operation.
  b) False.
  c) True. Patients troubled by a chronically inflamed gallbladder benefit from chole-cystectomy.
  d) True. Cholecystectomy may be carried out during the same admission, usually after a few days.
  e) False.

8 a) False. They bleed but remain within the anal canal.
  b) False. They prolapse during defecation, and spontaneously return to their normal position.
  c) True.
  d) False. They become painful when they strangulate.
  e) True. This is due to compression of the rectal venous system.

9 a) False. Management is conservative.
  b) False. The bowel is paralysed, so colicky abdominal pain is absent.
  c) False. Bowel sounds are silent.
  d) True. This is due to functional bowel obstruction.
  e) False. Oral intake will exacerbate the functional obstruction.

10 a) True. This may be present in the femoral triangle.
   b) False.
   c) False. These are osteoarthritic swellings of the proximal interphalangeal joints.
   d) True.
   e) True. This is a dilatation of the saphenous vein at its junction with the femoral vein.

11 a) False.
   b) False.
   c) True. Some exceptions exist for donors with localized tumours.
   d) False.
   e) True.

12 a) True.
   b) False. This extends into the abdomen.
   c) True.
   d) True.
   e) True.

13 a) True. It may, rarely, cause infertility.
   b) False. If the cord is not palpable above the swelling, it is an inguinoscrotal hernia or an infantile hydrocele.
   c) False. They are usually left-sided.
   d) False.
   e) False. Hydroceles do not affect fertility.

14 a) False.
  b) False. It occurs most commonly in teenagers and young men.
  c) True.
  d) False. It is only necessary if there is testicular infarction.
  e) False.

15 a) False. This occurs in adulthood.
  b) False. This is a supraclavicular lymph node associated with gastrointestinal malignancy.
  c) True. Although congenital, it usually presents in adolescence or early adulthood. A branchial cyst is a remnant of the branchial arch.
  d) False. These are the unmyelinated sections of neuronal axons.
  e) True. This commonly occurs at the base of the posterior triangle, transilluminates and consists of lymphatic cysts.

16 a) False.
  b) False.
  c) False.
  d) True.
  e) True. Triple assessment comprises clinical examination, imaging (mammography or ultrasound) and fine needle aspiration cytology.

17 a) True. Pregnancy increases intra-abdominal pressure.
  b) False.
  c) False.
  d) True. Chronic coughing increases intra-abdominal pressure.
  e) True. Constipation leads to raised intra-abdominal pressure.

18 a) False. Hypocalcaemia is a complication.
  b) False. This is a cutaneous manifestation of streptococcal infection, sarcoidosis, inflammatory bowel disease etc.
  c) True. An arterial blood gas is an important investigation to detect the possibility of this complication arising.
  d) True.
  e) True.

19 a) True. Bacteria, often staphylococci, can enter the peritoneal space via the peritoneal catheter.
  b) False.
  c) False.
  d) True. Spontaneous bacterial peritonitis is a recognized complication of ascites.
  e) True. Perforation of a diverticulum, if untreated, would lead to peritonitis.

20 a) False. They may occur at any age.
  b) False.
  c) True. This is a very common operation.
  d) False. Cough impulse may be absent due to a tight neck, or the presence of adhesions between the sac and its contents.
  e) True.

21 a) False. This may be helpful in the treatment of the condition.
    b) False.
    c) True. Hence the absence of bowel sounds in peritonitis.
    d) True. It occurs to some extent after every abdominal operation.
    e) True.

22 a) True. This is due to bowel distension proximal to the obstruction.
    b) False. This is a sign of upper gastrointestinal bleeding.
    c) False.
    d) True. This occurs earlier in a high obstruction.
    e) True. The pain becomes continuous if the obstruction becomes strangulated.

23 a) False.
    b) False.
    c) True.
    d) False. This is a lack of intrinsic factor causing vitamin B_{12} deficiency.
    e) True. There is fluid collection in the lesser sac.

24 a) True. There is deep-seated cramp-like rectal pain. This is a benign condition.
    b) False. These are not usually painful.
    c) True. This is a tear in the skin of the anal canal. Pain is worse on defecation.
    d) False. Bleeding is the main symptom; they do not normally cause pain.
    e) True. This often occurs while straining to pass a stool.

25 a) True.
    b) False. The narrow femoral canal makes strangulation a high risk.
    c) False. They normally occur in middle-aged and elderly females.
    d) False. It lies below and lateral to the tubercle. The neck of an inguinal hernia is above
        and medial to the pubic tubercle.
    e) False. Operative repair is recommended due to the high risk of strangulation.

26 a) True. This increases tension across the wound.
    b) False.
    c) False.
    d) True. This weakens the suture line.
    e) True. This impairs wound healing.

27 a) True. This causes colicky, central abdominal pain.
    b) False. This causes iliac fossa pain.
    c) True.
    d) True. The pain classically starts vaguely in the central abdominal area, and then
        localizes to the right iliac fossa.
    e) False. This causes iliac fossa pain.

28 a) True. This can be intensely painful.
    b) False.
    c) True. A commonly used opioid analgesic, it is a frequent cause of confusion.
    d) False.
    e) True.

29　a) True.
　　b) False.
　　c) True.
　　d) False.
　　e) False.

30　a) False. These should be continued, and are given as hydrocortisone i.v. (intravenous) peri-operatively.
　　b) False. Abrupt cessation can precipitate unpredictable haemodynamic effects.
　　c) True. Anticoagulation can be managed with subcutaneous enoxaparin or with a heparin infusion peri-operatively.
　　d) True. This should be stopped due to its prothrombotic effect.
　　e) False.

31　a) True.
　　b) False.
　　c) True.
　　d) False.
　　e) True. Other factors include epithelialization of the fistula and chronic inflammation (e.g. Crohn's disease).

32　a) True.
　　b) False. This causes upper abdominal pain.
　　c) False. This typically causes right upper quadrant pain.
　　d) True.
　　e) True.

33　a) True.
　　b) False. This is a sign of ascites.
　　c) False. This is a sign of acute cholecystitis – there is pain as the patient breathes in with the examiner resting two fingers on the right upper quadrant.
　　d) False. Bowel sounds are absent.
　　e) True.

34　a) True.
　　b) False.
　　c) True. Rare, this is a spontaneous oesophageal rupture, often after profound vomiting, for example after heavy alcohol intake.
　　d) True. This is a recognized complication of the procedure.
　　e) False. This is browning of the skin after bilateral adrenalectomy, due to excess adrenocorticotrophic hormone (ACTH).

35　a) True. Blood accumulates in the pericardium and restricts ventricular filling, causing cardiogenic shock.
　　b) False.
　　c) True. This is a result of several rib fractures; the affected area moves out in expiration and inwards in inspiration.
　　d) True. This is perforation of the pleura, where air is drawn into the pleural space in inspiration, but is unable to escape in expiration.
　　e) False.

36 a) False. *Clostridium perfringens* is responsible.
    b) False. Clostridium is Gram-positive.
    c) True.
    d) False. It is a common feature of the infection.
    e) False. Penicillin is effective.

37 a) True.
    b) True.
    c) False. This causes a painful lump.
    d) True.
    e) True. This may be painful or painless.

38 a) False. Cirrhosis and viral hepatitis are the commonest causes of a hepatocellular carcinoma.
    b) True. Leakage of bile into the peritoneal cavity can cause biliary peritonitis.
    c) True. Stones may be retained in the common bile duct.
    d) False.
    e) True.

39 a) False. This causes intense pain.
    b) True. In the same way that vaginal candidiasis causes pruritus vulvae.
    c) False. This is painful but not normally pruritic.
    d) True. The discharge from the fistula keeps the skin moist, predisposing to pruritus.
    e) True.

40 a) False. It is a familial condition but inheritance is multifactorial.
    b) True.
    c) False. Typical presentation is at 3–6 weeks of age.
    d) False. Vomiting is not bilious as the obstruction is proximal to the duodenum.
    e) False. Ramstedt's pyloromyotomy is the treatment. Heller's myotomy is a treatment for achalasia.

41 a) True. This is a rare cause.
    b) True. The disease has a predilection for the terminal ileum.
    c) False.
    d) True. This occurs when a gallstone perforates from the gallbladder into the small bowel.
    e) True. Adhesions and hernias are the commonest causes.

42 a) False. The narrow opening of the internal ring renders indirect hernias more likely to strangulate.
    b) True. Direct hernias are usually acquired defects.
    c) False. They rarely descend into the scrotum, unlike indirect inguinal hernias, which commonly do so.
    d) False. Direct hernias are uncommon in females.
    e) True. Indirect hernias protrude through the internal ring, whereas direct hernias do not.

43 a) True. Phenol mixed in oil is injected in order to sclerose the haemorrhoid.
   b) True. This strangulates the relevant area.
   c) False.
   d) False.
   e) True. Haemorrhage is an important complication of haemorrhoidectomy.

44 a) False. Classically the pain is epigastric, radiating to the back.
   b) True. Features may include guarding, tenderness, rigid abdomen.
   c) False. This is nail-bed capillary pulsation in aortic regurgitation.
   d) True.
   e) True. This is flank bruising indicating necrotizing pancreatitis.

45 a) True. The colostomy site is an area of weakness within the abdominal wall, pre-
      disposing to hernias.
   b) True. The opening of the stoma site becomes narrower.
   c) False. This is an autosomal dominant condition involving mucocutaneous
      pigmentation and gastrointestinal hamartomas.
   d) True. The bowel prolapses out of the stoma.
   e) False. This is a vascular malformation in the bowel, that can present with bleeding.

46 a) True. This is due to hypovolaemia, and possible rhabdomyolysis.
   b) True. This is Curling's ulcer, occurring as a reaction to stress.
   c) False. This is a complication of broad-spectrum antibiotic therapy.
   d) True. Full-thickness burns heal with scarring, causing contracture.
   e) True.

47 a) True.
   b) True.
   c) False.
   d) True. The sympathetic response stimulated by pain causes reduced wound perfusion,
      thereby impairing healing.
   e) True. Pain, as well as opioid analgesia, can cause urinary retention.

48 a) False.
   b) True. There is mild pyrexia.
   c) True. Again, there is mild pyrexia.
   d) False.
   e) True. Contents of the bowel may spill out, causing peritonitis.

49 a) True. This is the usual cause of bacterial parotitis.
   b) True. Calculi affect the parotid gland less commonly than the submandibular gland.
   c) False. This is herpes zoster infection of the geniculate ganglion, producing a facial
      nerve palsy and vesicles in the external auditory meatus.
   d) True. This is the commonest parotid infection.
   e) True. This is an autoimmune condition involving enlargement of the salivary and
      lacrimal glands and a dry mouth.

50 a) False.
    b) True. This is the usual cause.
    c) False.
    d) True. Infiltration of a tumour can occasionally result in a fistula.
    e) True. Rectal inflammation leads to fistula formation.

51 a) False. This does not cause hypoxia by itself.
    b) True. Opioid overdose can cause respiratory depression.
    c) True. Basal lung collapse is common post-operatively; deep breathing exercises should be encouraged.
    d) True. This can cause left ventricular failure and pulmonary oedema.
    e) True. This typically occurs 5 days post-operatively.

EMQ ANSWERS

1 SWELLINGS IN THE INGUINAL REGION

1 **G** Inguinal hernias originate superior and medial to the pubic tubercle. Indirect hernias pass through the internal ring whereas direct hernias enter the canal through a posterior defect. A hernia that reappears while pressure is applied over the internal ring suggests a **direct inguinal hernia**.

2 **J** Bilateral **inguinal lymphadenopathy** can sometimes be found in association with sexually transmitted infections.

3 **C** Fluid collections or abscesses produce fluctuant masses: in this case an abscess is associated with discoloration of the shins in a Somalian immigrant. The underlying diagnosis is likely to be tuberculosis manifested by erythema nodosum and a **psoas abscess** tracking into the groin. The abscess also explains the difficulty walking, as hip flexion would be painful

4 **B** Pulsatile and expansile masses are signs of aneurysmal dilatation of blood vessels, in this case indicating a **femoral artery aneurysm**. Pseudoaneurysms are a common complication of femoral artery puncture during angiography.

5 **A** The sign being demonstrated here is a fluid thrill being transmitted through a column of fluid, which can be elicited in patients with varicose veins. The mass in the groin with a positive cough impulse is a **saphena varix**, a localized dilatation of the proximal end of the long saphenous vein.

2 ABDOMINAL SCARS 1

1 **G** The **Pfannenstiel** incision is used when access to the contents of the pelvis is required, most commonly when performing a Caesarean section.

2 **F** A **right paramedian** incision can be used to gain access to right-sided structures such as the ascending colon.

3 **A** **Kocher's** incision was the traditional method of opening the abdomen to perform a cholecystectomy, and is still seen in patients who had their surgery before the advent of laparoscopy.

4 **E** A **gridiron** incision is used during an appendicectomy; it passes obliquely through McBurney's point.

5 **J** The **Lanz** incision is similar to the gridiron and passes transverse rather than oblique. It has the advantage that the scar may be hidden within a skin crease, and so is less noticeable.

3 ABDOMINAL SCARS 2

1 I As the liver is such a large organ, a substantial incision is required to gain access to the entire upper abdomen. A **Mercedes** scar, bilateral Kocher's incisions with a central vertical extension, offers excellent exposure of this area.

2 G A **Pfannenstiel** incision, a low transverse pelvic scar, is used in most Caesarean sections as it permits good access to the pelvic contents and may be hidden underneath a bikini.

3 A **Kocher's** incision is a subcostal oblique scar, formerly used when performing open cholecystectomy.

4 J The **Lanz** incision is a small transverse scar that passes through McBurney's point. It may be hidden within a skin crease to render it as unobtrusive as possible. Increasingly, appendicectomies are being carried out laparoscopically.

5 D The vast majority of cholecystectomies are carried out laparoscopically nowadays. **Laparoscopic** scars are extremely small incisions found at three or four different positions in the abdomen.

4 ABDOMINAL OPERATIONS

1 E This carcinoma is too close to the anus for a successful anastomosis between the proximal end of the colon and the anal canal. An **abdominoperineal resection** – excision of the tumour and anus with the colon brought out as a permanent end colostomy – is the only option that permits adequate resection margins of the carcinoma.

2 D **Hartmann's procedure**, leaving a closed distal colonic segment in the abdomen while bringing the proximal colon to the surface as an end colostomy, is commonly performed when there is abdominal contamination and the surgeon cannot risk a primary anastomosis failure.

3 B A **right hemicolectomy** is the treatment of choice for caecal carcinoma.

4 H Ulcerative colitis, by definition, is confined to the colon. A panproctocolectomy with **end ileostomy** formation is therefore curative.

5 F Nine cm is an adequate distance to allow both clear resection margins and enough tissue for primary anastomosis between the rectal stump and distal colon – an **anterior resection**.

5 ABDOMINAL HERNIAS

1 H This gentleman has a hiatus hernia, where part of the stomach is found within the thorax. A **rolling hiatus hernia** occurs with a correctly positioned gastro-oesophageal junction, whereas displacement indicates a sliding hiatus hernia.

2 D **Richter's hernia** occurs when only part of the bowel wall is involved in the hernia. This leaves the lumen patent, allowing the normal passage of luminal contents. Therefore even if the hernia is strangulated, there are no signs of bowel obstruction.

3 I **Incisional hernias** are common after abdominal operations. Bowel prolapses through the defects created in muscle and fascia by the surgeon's knife. As the neck of these hernias is very wide, they have an extremely low risk of strangulation.

4 B **Littre's hernia** is a rare variant where a Meckel's diverticulum is found within the hernial sack.

5 F **Inguinal hernias** have their origins above and medial to the pubic tubercle; femoral hernias arise inferior and lateral to this structure.

6 EPONYMOUS SIGNS IN SURGERY

1 E **Lasègue's sign** is used to assess irritation of the lower lumbosacral nerve roots. It is alternatively known as the straight leg raise test, whereby the patient experiences severe pain when the leg is passively elevated. The pain can be exacerbated by stretching the sciatic nerve by dorsiflexing the foot.

2 D **Rovsing's sign** is said to be positive when palpation in the left iliac fossa elicits greater pain in the right iliac fossa than the left. When pressure is applied to the left side of the abdomen, some peritoneum on the right side is stretched, and if this is inflamed due to underlying appendicitis then the patient experiences pain.

3 B **Cullen's sign**, peri-umbilical discoloration in acute pancreatitis, is caused by retro-peritoneal blood tracking through to the subcutaneous umbilical tissues via the falciform ligament.

4 F **Troisier's sign**, the finding of a palpable left supraclavicular lymph node (Virchow's node), is a sign of gastric carcinoma and indicates a poor prognosis as the cancer has metastasized.

5 C The underlying diagnosis in this pregnant woman is carpal tunnel syndrome. **Phalen's sign**, where the wrists are flexed to cause compression of the median nerve, can reproduce the symptoms of this condition. Tinel's sign, in which the nerve is tapped with a finger to cause paraesthesiae, may also be positive.

7 EPONYMS IN SURGERY

1 B **Heller's** operation, or cardiomyotomy, is the surgical treatment for achalasia and is used in patients who have failed to respond to endoscopic pneumatic dilatation.

2 A A **Billroth II** gastrectomy involves removing part of the stomach and attaching it to the jejunum. The duodenum is closed and left as a blind passage from this new opening.

3 I Pain at McBurney's point indicates that the peritoneum overlying the usual position of the appendix is inflamed. However the position of the appendix may be highly variable and so a high index of suspicion is often needed to diagnosis acute appendicitis.

4 E **Rovsing's** sign occurs because pressure on the left side of the abdomen still stretches the peritoneum on the right. If the peritoneum overlying the appendix is inflamed, and therefore painful, even this small degree of stretching will cause pain.

5 J **Boerhaave's** syndrome typically occurs as a side-effect of forceful vomiting. Gastric contents may escape through the oesophageal perforation, causing mediastinitis.

8 POST-OPERATIVE COMPLICATIONS

1 J This patient is an arteriopath and therefore probably has coronary disease. The timing is too early for pneumonia or pulmonary embolus. It is most likely that he is having a **myocardial infarction**.

2 D This woman may have suffered a **pulmonary embolism**; this post-operative timescale is appropriate. The chest X-ray is also suggestive, with a small pleural effusion; the characteristic wedge-shaped infarct is rarely seen. Obesity, hormonal treatment and periods of immobility are all risk factors.

3 C Post-operative **atelectasis** generally occurs within 48 h. It is an extremely common post-operative complication with some degree of pulmonary collapse occurring after almost every abdominal or transthoracic procedure. The collapsed lung may become secondarily infected by inhaled organisms.

4 B The history is similar to question 3 but this woman has pyrexia and crepitations suggesting a **lower respiratory tract infection** secondary to atelectasis.

5 G **Wound dehiscence** is an uncommon early post-operative complication affecting about 1 per cent of abdominal wounds. It usually occurs about 1 week after an operation and may be preceded by a pink serous discharge. Though alarming, the patient often experiences little pain.

9 LEG ULCERS

1 B **Venous ulcer.** The site of the ulcer gives a clue to the aetiology. Venous stasis tends to occur over the medial aspect of the lower third of the leg, the gaiter area. There may also be a history of varicose veins or DVT.

2 H **Arterial ulcers** occur at pressure points over the metatarsal heads, toe tips, heel or between the toes. There may be a history of atheromatous disease. This punched out ulcer is typical of arterial disease.

3 E The presence of long-standing venous ulcers with a change in shape suggests the development of squamous cell carcinoma (**Marjolin's ulcer**). There is sometimes regional lymphadenopathy.

4 F This man may have inflammatory bowel disease suggesting **pyoderma gangrenosum**. These ulcers are usually multiple and pustular; treatment is often difficult.

5 G Lack of pain suggests that the ulcer is **neuropathic**, and therefore due to diabetes or tabes dorsalis. These ulcers usually occur at pressure points such as the heels.

10 VASCULAR SURGICAL INTERVENTIONS

1 B Hyperhidrosis is an often debilitating and embarrassing condition which can lead to permanently sweaty armpits, palms and face. Some patients gain benefit from bilateral endoscopic transthoracic **sympathectomy** (ETS).

2 I The treatment of bleeding cerebral aneurysms can be via craniotomy or by **endovascular coiling**, in which small coils are introduced into the brain through the femoral artery in an effort to block off the bleeding vessels.

3 C This patient is in atrial fibrillation and has no signs of long-standing peripheral vascular disease (with good pulses in the right leg). The most likely cause of his arterial occlusion is therefore embolus derived from the heart: removal of this with an **embolectomy** is the treatment of choice.

4 G The formation of an **arteriovenous fistula** greatly facilitates the regular access needed for haemodialysis.

5 J Small aortic aneurysms (less than 5.5 cm) are managed by a watch and see approach. Regular **ultrasound** scans allow evaluation of any change in size and whether an operation is indicated.

11 DIAGNOSIS OF BREAST DISEASE

1 G **Duct ectasia** usually presents in the 5th decade with a tender retro-areolar area, erythema and nipple retraction. There is a typical thick, creamy nipple discharge. It is unusual for malignancy to cause pain.

2 F **Fat necrosis** presents as a hard, irregular swelling. There may be overlying skin bruising, or occasionally teeth-marks. Sometimes the lesion is tethered and is difficult to differentiate from carcinoma.

3 D A history of **breast carcinoma** is suggested by nulliparity, early menarche, late menopause and positive family history. In 85 per cent of cases, the lump is painless.

4 E **Cyclical mastalgia** causes tenderness of the breasts in the week preceding a period. It is a common problem in women aged 25–40 years. On examination, the breasts are tender and may feel lumpy.

5 H **Lactating abscess** is the most likely diagnosis in this woman. This condition is usually associated with constitutional upset.

12 TREATMENT OF BREAST DISEASE

1 G Ductal papillomas are benign lesions. A single duct can be surgically removed by **microdochectomy**, resulting in permanent cure.

2 F **Trastuzumab** is a monoclonal antibody which causes destruction of cancerous cells expressing the HER2 receptor. These cancers are generally not responsive to hormonal manipulation. It is increasingly being used in the adjuvant treatment of early breast cancer.

3 J The diagnosis here is probably a lactating breast abscess, usually caused by *Staphylococcus aureus*. Treatment with oral **flucloxacillin** is usually successful.

4 C This patient has symptoms of hypercalcaemia, **Pamidronate**, a bisphosphonate, is used to treat the hypercalcaemia of malignancy. Adequate rehydration is also mandatory.

5 E The clinical scenario being described is a locally advanced breast carcinoma with regional spread, but not distant metastasis. Breast-conserving surgery is not an option when the tumour has infiltrated the skin, and so **mastectomy** is indicated in the first instance.

13 SKIN LUMPS

1 E These small papules are **Campbell de Morgan spots**, alternatively known as angio-keratomas. These benign lesions are extremely common in the elderly population and are of no significance.

2 G The history of a rapidly growing tender lesion with a central punctum in an area of the body rich in sebaceous glands is highly suggestive of a **sebaceous cyst**.

3 B These features are typical of a **basal cell carcinoma**. This is an extremely low grade malignancy which seldom metastasizes, but may erode underlying tissue to form an ulcer.

4 H The rapid growth of this lesion in a sun-exposed area, combined with the central crater, makes **keratoacanthoma** most likely. Histologically, these lesions are very similar to squamous cell carcinomas, but they often resolve spontaneously.

5 C If cells from the epidermis are relocated into the dermis by a penetrating injury, they can continue to grow and form implantation **dermoid cysts**. In this case, this patient's occupation is responsible for his hand lesion.

Ophthalmology

MULTIPLE CHOICE QUESTIONS

1   The following drugs are known to impair vision:
   a) Chloroquine
   b) Gentamicin
   c) Ethambutol
   d) Metformin
   e) Atorvastatin

2   State whether the extraocular muscles are correctly paired with the cranial nerves that innervate them:
   a) Superior rectus; III nerve
   b) Inferior oblique; IV nerve
   c) Lateral rectus; IV nerve
   d) Medial rectus; VI nerve
   e) Superior oblique; III nerve

3   The following statements are true of refractive errors:
   a) Myopia is treated with convex lenses
   b) Astigmatism is not correctable with lenses
   c) In hypermetropia, long-distance vision is better than near-vision
   d) Presbyopia is the progressive development of short-sightedness with age
   e) Hypermetropia is a cause of childhood squint

4   The following are risk factors for open-angle glaucoma:
   a) African-Caribbean origin
   b) Cataract
   c) Hypermetropia
   d) Diabetes mellitus
   e) Myopia

5   Causes of gradual visual loss include:
   a) Retinal artery embolism
   b) Conjunctivitis
   c) Cataract
   d) Open-angle glaucoma
   e) Macular degeneration

6   Medical treatment for primary open-angle glaucoma includes:
    a) Steroid eye drops
    b) Tropicamide eye drops
    c) Beta-blocker eye drops
    d) Pilocarpine eye drops
    e) Prostaglandin analogue eye drops

7   State whether the following visual field defects are paired correctly with the anatomical site of the lesion:
    a) Left optic tract; left monocular blindness
    b) Optic chiasm; homonymous hemianopia
    c) Macula central scotoma
    d) Left occipital cortex; right monocular blindness
    e) Left optic nerve; right homonymous hemianopia

8   Fundoscopy findings in malignant hypertension include:
    a) Cotton wool spots
    b) Silver wiring
    c) Flame haemorrhages
    d) Papilloedema
    e) Arteriovenous nipping

9   Myopia (short-sightedness) is a risk factor for the following:
    a) Retinal detachment
    b) Closed angle glaucoma
    c) Macular degeneration
    d) Episcleritis
    e) Corneal ulceration

10   The following predispose to cataract formation:
    a) Steroid administration
    b) Trauma
    c) Hypertension
    d) Diabetes mellitus
    e) Papilloedema

11   The following are causes of dilated pupils:
    a) Opioid overdose
    b) Brain death
    c) Cocaine
    d) Pontine haemorrhage
    e) Pilocarpine

12   Causes of acute visual loss include:
    a) Keratoconjunctivitis sicca
    b) Retinal vein occlusion
    c) Age-related macular degeneration
    d) Vitreous haemorrhage
    e) Giant cell arteritis

13 The following are recognized ocular complications of diabetes mellitus:
    a) Blepharitis
    b) VI cranial nerve palsy
    c) Chronic simple glaucoma
    d) Retinal detachment
    e) Vitreous haemorrhage

14 Causes of papilloedema include:
    a) Cavernous sinus thrombosis
    b) Raised intracranial pressure
    c) Age-related macular degeneration
    d) Optic neuritis
    e) Retinal vein occlusion

15 Causes of the acute red eye include:
    a) Diabetic maculopathy
    b) Episcleritis
    c) Closed-angle glaucoma
    d) Optic neuritis
    e) Iritis

16 The following are causes of ptosis:
    a) Botulism
    b) Myasthenia gravis
    c) Sjögren's syndrome
    d) Presbyopia
    e) Horner's syndrome

17 Features of diabetic background retinopathy include:
    a) Vitreous haemorrhage
    b) Blot haemorrhages
    c) Cotton wool spots
    d) Retinal neovascularization
    e) Dot haemorrhages

Answers: see pages 303–305

EXTENDED MATCHING QUESTIONS

1 TERMS IN OPHTHALMOLOGY

Choose the appropriate ophthalmological diagnosis for each stem below

A Hyphema
B Myopia
C Chalazion
D Hypopyon
E Presbyopia

F Hypermetropia
G Blepharitis
H Astigmatism
I Keratitis
J Nystagmus

1 A 59-year-old man finds reading increasingly difficult and buys a pair of reading glasses from the supermarket.
2 A fluid level of pus cells in the anterior chamber of the eye.
3 A cyst on the eyelid originating from the Meibomian glands.
4 A fluid level of red blood cells in the anterior chamber of the eye.
5 Inflammation of the lid margins.

2 RED EYE

Each of the patients below presents with a red eye. Choose the most likely diagnosis from the options given

A Subconjunctival haemorrhage
B Acute angle-closure glaucoma
C Corneal ulcer
D Foreign body
E Bacterial conjunctivitis

F Blepharitis
G Anterior uveitis
H Episcleritis
I Scleritis
J Herpes simplex conjunctivitis

1 A 29-year-old woman with sarcoidosis goes to see her doctor, complaining of photophobia, blurred vision, and eye pain. He examines her and finds redness around the cornea, cells in the anterior chamber and parts of the pupil stuck to the lens. The pupil is small.
2 A 41-year-old man goes to the emergency department complaining that both his eyes are uncomfortable and red. In the morning, he notices that there is a yellow crust on his eyelids. On examination, both eyes are red, with a sticky discharge. Visual acuity is normal.
3 A 63-year-old man, with a past medical history of long-sightedness, presents to the emergency department with nausea, vomiting, headache, blurred vision and a painful eye. On examination, he has a red eye, a mid-dilated fixed oval pupil, and decreased visual acuity in the affected eye.
4 A 26-year-old man seeks medical attention for a red eye. He wears contact lenses, and apart from the redness is entirely asymptomatic. Examination reveals a localized area of redness between the iris and the external canthus.
5 A 21-year-old woman goes to see her general practitioner (GP) as she has had a cough for 2 days. Her chest is clear, but she notices a bright red patch in one eye. Visual acuity is normal.

3 LOSS OF VISION

Each of the patients below seeks medical attention for visual loss. Choose the most likely cause of their symptoms from the options given

A Cataract	F Giant cell arteritis
B Retinal detachment	G Optic neuritis
C Age-related macular degeneration	H Amaurosis fugax
D Retinal artery occlusion	I Acute angle-closure glaucoma
E Vitreous haemorrhage	J Tobacco amblyopia

1   A 63-year-old woman goes to see her GP complaining of progressive poor vision. She has reduced acuity in the right eye. Eye movements are normal, but when the GP attempts to elicit the red reflex, all he can see is white.

2   A 71-year-old man is brought to hospital by his wife. He says that he could see normally that morning, and now cannot see out of his right eye. He is unable to read a Snellen chart, and can just about count fingers. The optic disc appears normal, but the retina is pale. The pupil reacts poorly to light; the consensual light reflex is normal.

3   A 69-year-old man goes to hospital as he says he cannot see in one eye. When he is seen, after a 2 h wait, he tells the doctor that his symptoms have resolved, but it was as if a curtain had come down over his eye. Ophthalmic examination is unremarkable. The doctor also feels his pulse and finds him to be in atrial fibrillation.

4   A 34-year-old woman presents with a 4-day history of deteriorating visual loss. She says that colours do not appear as bright as they used to be, and that it is painful to move her eyes.

5   An 83-year-old man presents to hospital with nausea, vomiting, abdominal pain and a red left eye. His abdomen is soft and he has not eaten any unusual foods. His GP treated him with hyoscine 2 days ago for similar abdominal pain. Examination reveals an injected conjunctiva and reduced visual acuity with a fixed pupil in the mid-dilated position.

4 DRUGS USED IN OPHTHALMOLOGY

For each of the patients below, choose the most appropriate drug from the options given

A Ganciclovir	F Pilocarpine
B Fluorescein	G Latanoprost
C Aciclovir	H Chloramphenicol
D Timolol	I Hypromellose
E Tropicamide	J Prednisolone

1   A 41-year-old woman with Sjögren's syndrome complains of dry eyes.

2   A 21-year-old man presents to the emergency department with a headache. The doctor wants to perform fundoscopy.

3   A 29-year-old woman presents with suspected herpes simplex conjunctivitis. The doctor wants to see if there is an associated corneal ulcer.

4   A 31-year-old man with AIDS and a CD4 count of 150/mm^3 presents with visual loss. He has multiple flame-shaped haemorrhages and retinal spots. The medical team suspects cytomegalovirus (CMV) retinitis.

5   A 19-year-old man goes to see his doctor with bilateral red, sticky eyes. He says that there is a yellow crust on his eyelashes in the mornings.

5 EXTERNAL EYE DISEASE

Each of the patients below presents with an eye problem. Choose the best diagnosis for each scenario from the options given

A   Entropion
B   Orbital cellulitis
C   Chalazion
D   Pinguecula
E   Basal cell carcinoma

F   Ptosis
G   Blepharitis
H   Ectropion
I   Stye
J   Lid retraction

1   A 28-year-old man complains of a lump on his eye. On examination, he has a small red swelling originating from an eyelash follicle.
2   A 66-year-old woman goes to see her GP complaining of yellow lumps in her eye. She says she has had them for 9 months. On examination, there are small yellow conjunctival nodules near her nose.
3   An 86-year-old woman goes to see her GP complaining that her eyelashes are always bothering her right eye. On examination, the lower lid is turned inwards, with the lashes pointing into a reddened eye.
4   A 41-year-old man goes to see his doctor as he thinks he has an eye infection. He feels entirely well. On examination, the eyelid is red and swollen.
5   A 43-year-old woman with Graves' disease complains that her eyes are particularly sore, especially when she wakes up in the morning.

6 VISUAL FIELD DEFECTS

Choose the visual field defect most likely to be caused by each of the lesions below

A   Complete blindness
B   Bitemporal hemianopia
C   Left homonymous hemianopia
D   Left superior quadrantanopia
E   Left inferior quadrantanopia

F   Left central scotoma
G   Right homonymous hemianopia
H   Right superior quadrantanopia
I   Right inferior quadrantanopia
J   Right central scotoma

1   Left temporal lobe lesion.
2   Right macular degeneration.
3   Right optic tract lesion.
4   Pituitary tumour.
5   Bilateral occipital lobe lesion.

7 EXAMINATION OF THE EYE

Select the examination feature most likely to be seen in association with each of the conditions below

A   Cotton wool spots
B   Arteriovenous nipping
C   Papilloedema
D   Kayser–Fleischer rings
E   Microaneurysms

F   Flame haemorrhages
G   Pale optic disc
H   Retinal detachment
I   Lisch nodules
J   Lens dislocation

1   Idiopathic intracranial hypertension.
2   Background diabetic retinopathy.
3   Marfan's syndrome.
4   Early hypertensive retinopathy.
5   Advanced diabetic retinopathy.

Answers: see pages 305–307

ANSWERS

MCQ ANSWERS

1 a) True. Screening for visual defects is recommended while taking chloroquine for long periods.
  b) False.
  c) True. Visual acuity must be tested before starting antituberculous therapy with ethambutol; any visual symptoms should be reported immediately.
  d) False.
  e) False.

2 a) True. This muscle, innervated by the oculomotor nerve (III) moves the eye up.
  b) False. The oculomotor nerve (III) innervates the inferior oblique muscle; it moves the eye up in adduction.
  c) False. The abducens nerve (VI) innervates the lateral rectus muscle; it moves the eye laterally i.e. abduction.
  d) False. The oculomotor nerve (III) innervates the medial rectus; it moves the eye medially i.e. adduction.
  e) False. The trochlear nerve (IV) innervates the superior oblique muscle; it moves the eye down in adduction.

3 a) False. Concave lenses bring the image of distant objects further back, onto the retina.
  b) False.
  c) True. This is long-sightedness.
  d) False. Near vision deteriorates with age.
  e) True. It causes a convergent squint.

4 a) True.
  b) False.
  c) False. This is a risk factor for closed-angle glaucoma.
  d) True.
  e) True.

5 a) False. Visual loss is sudden.
  b) False. This is usually self-limiting, and does not affect acuity.
  c) True. There is opacification of the lens.
  d) True. High intraocular pressure causes optic nerve damage.
  e) True. This is loss of central vision occurring in the elderly. Macular drusen may be evident on fundoscopy.

6 a) False. These are used for inflammatory conditions.
  b) False. This is a short-acting mydriatic used for fundoscopy.
  c) True. They reduce intraocular pressure by decreasing aqueous humour production. An example is timolol.
  d) True. This is a miotic drug that reduces aqueous outflow resistance.
  e) True. These increase uveoscleral outflow, for example, latanoprost.

7 a) False. This results in homonymous hemianopia.
   b) False. This results in bitemporal hemianopia.
   c) True. There is loss of vision in the centre of the visual field, e.g. in age-related macular degeneration.
   d) False. This results in right homonymous hemianopia with macular sparing.
   e) False. This results in left monocular blindness.

8 a) True. These occur in grade 3 retinopathy.
   b) False. This describes the shiny walls of retinal arteries found in grade 1 retinopathy.
   c) True. These occur in grade 3 retinopathy.
   d) True. This is a sign of grade 4 retinopathy. Grades 3 and 4 are features of malignant hypertension.
   e) False. This is compression of the retinal veins where they are crossed by retinal arteries; it occurs in grade 2 retinopathy.

9 a) True.
   b) False. Hypermetropia is a risk factor for closed-angle glaucoma.
   c) True.
   d) False.
   e) False.

10 a) True.
   b) True.
   c) False.
   d) True.
   e) False.

11 a) False. This produces pupil constriction.
   b) True. The pupils are fixed and dilated.
   c) True. This is a sympathomimetic.
   d) False. Pontine damage gives rise to pinpoint pupils.
   e) False. This is a miotic drug, in the form of eye drops, used in glaucoma.

12 a) False. This is reduced tear formation causing dry eyes, found in Sjögren's syndrome.
   b) True.
   c) False. The visual loss occurs gradually.
   d) True. Floaters and loss of the red reflex are features of this condition. Diabetes mellitus is a risk factor.
   e) True. This may cause central retinal artery occlusion, causing sudden severe visual loss.

13 a) False.
   b) True. Cranial nerves III and VI are more prone to mononeuropathy.
   c) True. Diabetes is a risk factor for chronic glaucoma.
   d) True. This occurs in advanced retinopathy.
   e) True. This is a feature of proliferative retinopathy.

14 a) True.
   b) True.
   c) False.
   d) True.
   e) True.

15 a) False.
    b) True. This requires steroid eye drops.
    c) True. This must be treated urgently, with pilocarpine and acetazolamide.
    d) False.
    e) True. Features include photophobia and reduced acuity.

16 a) True. This is a severe type of food poisoning caused by *Clostridium botulinum*. Gastrointestinal and visual paralytic symptoms occur.
    b) True. This causes weakness of ocular muscles.
    c) False. Features include keratoconjunctivitis sicca (reduced lacrimation) and xerostomia (decreased salivation).
    d) False. This is the long-sightedness that occurs with age.
    e) True. There is interruption of the sympathetic pathway to the eye.

17 a) False. This occurs in proliferative retinopathy.
    b) True. These represent ruptured microaneurysms.
    c) False. These occur in pre-proliferative retinopathy; they are due to oedema from areas of retinal infarction.
    d) False. New vessel formation is a feature of proliferative retinopathy.
    e) True. These are microaneurysms.

EMQ ANSWERS

1 TERMS IN OPHTHALMOLOGY

1 E **Presbyopia** is the diminished capacity of the eye to accommodate with age as a result of the lens becoming less elastic. Correction is with slightly convex lenses to help focus near objects.

2 D A **hypopyon** is usually caused by an infectious or inflammatory process within the eye. An urgent ophthalmological referral is indicated for further management.

3 C A **chalazion** is a small mass occurring at the lid margin due to blockage of a Meibomian gland duct. They often resolve spontaneously.

4 A A **hyphema** usually occurs secondary to trauma, and can predispose to sudden acute glaucoma and visual loss. If severe, the blood can be drained by an ophthalmologist.

5 G **Blepharitis** is an inflammation of the eyelash follicles, and can cause swollen, crusted eyelids. Treatment is with good hygiene and cleansing of the lid margins.

2 RED EYE

1 G **Anterior uveitis** (or iritis) is most commonly idiopathic but may be associated with systemic diseases, such as sarcoidosis, ankylosing spondylitis, and human leucocyte antigen (HLA)-B27 arthritides. Cells in the anterior chamber are frequently seen in this condition.

2 E **Bacterial conjunctivitis** is the most likely diagnosis, given the history of red, sticky eyes with discharge. Note that visual acuity is not affected and that the eyes are uncomfortable but not painful.

3 B The presentation here is typical of **acute angle-closure glaucoma**. This patient also has risk factors: he is over 50 years old and is known to be long-sighted. Urgent treatment is needed with drugs aimed at lowering intraocular pressure.

4 H The localized inflammation without symptoms suggests **episcleritis**, possibly secondary to contact lens wear. Occasionally rheumatoid arthritis is aetiologically implicated.

5 A A **subconjunctival haemorrhage** results from a ruptured small blood vessel, and may occur after trauma or coughing. It generally resolves spontaneously without adverse effects.

3 LOSS OF VISION

1 A **Cataracts** are common in the elderly, and result from opacification of the lens. The slow, progressive loss of vision with the inability to elicit the red reflex makes the diagnosis.

2 D Central **retinal artery occlusion** causes a sudden painless loss of vision, often with a relative afferent pupillary defect, as in this case. The pale retina is caused by widespread ischaemia.

3 H **Amaurosis fugax** is due to a temporary interruption to the retinal blood supply, often due to an embolus. In this case, this is most likely to be secondary to atrial fibrillation.

4 G **Optic neuritis** causes visual loss in a younger population than most other ophthalmic conditions. Painful eye movements and the loss of colour vision are highly suggestive; there may also be a relative afferent pupillary defect or a central scotoma.

5 I Sometimes extra-ocular symptoms can be the presenting complaint of **acute angle-closure glaucoma**. The fixed dilated pupil and red eye suggest this diagnosis, perhaps precipitated by the administration of an anticholinergic agent (hyoscine).

4 DRUGS USED IN OPHTHALMOLOGY

1 I **Hypromellose** is commonly used as an artificial tear replacement solution.

2 E **Tropicamide** is a short-acting weak mydriatic that is used to dilate the pupil so that the fundus can be accurately seen. Care should be taken in patients with glaucoma as it may precipitate acute angle-closure.

3 B **Fluorescein** is used to stain the eyes before slit-lamp examination, thereby allowing corneal ulcers to be visualized.

4 A CMV retinitis is an important condition as it may rapidly threaten sight in the immunocompromised. **Ganciclovir** is the treatment of choice.

5 H This patient has conjunctivitis. First-line therapy is with **chloramphenicol**, a broad-spectrum antibiotic.

5 EXTERNAL EYE DISEASE

1 I   A **stye** is an infected eyelash follicle. It is common in the general population and can be effectively treated with topical antibiotics.

2 D   **Pinguecula** are small yellow conjunctival nodules, which may be related to sun damage. They are harmless and do not require treatment unless they become infected.

3 A   **Entropion**, or inturning of the lid, is seen most frequently in the elderly population. The eyelashes cause local trauma to the eye, resulting in watering and inflammation. Taping the lid into the correct position may help.

4 B   **Orbital cellulitis** is a soft tissue infection around the eye, most commonly caused by *Staphylococcus* and *Streptococcus*. Intravenous antibiotics are usually administered to decrease the chances of the infection spreading and causing meningitis.

5 J   **Lid retraction** occurs with exophthalmos, so that the eyelids do not fully cover the eyes when closed. The exposed eyes are not lubricated with tears, and become dry and inflamed.

6 VISUAL FIELD DEFECTS

1 H   Temporal lobe lesions cause a **homonymous superior quadrantanopia**, whereas parietal lobe lesions cause a homonymous inferior quadrantanopia. Remember PITS – parietal inferior/temporal superior.

2 J   Right-sided macular degeneration – the loss of the central part of the retina – results in a **right central scotoma**. Local lesions affecting the eye and optic nerve before the chiasm cause unilateral visual loss.

3 C   A **left homonymous hemianopia** results from lesions of the right optic tract, whereas lesions of the optic radiation cause quadrantanopias.

4 B   Pressure on the optic chiasm by a pituitary tumour causes **bitemporal hemianopia** due to pressure on the nasal fibres from both optic nerves.

5 A   If both occipital lobes are severely damaged, the patient suffers **complete blindness**, known as cortical blindness. The characteristic features associated with this condition are called Anton's syndrome: the patient typically lacks insight into their inability to see, and may deny their blindness.

7 EXAMINATION OF THE EYE

1 C   **Papilloedema** is seen in all cases of raised intracranial pressure. On fundoscopy the margins of the optic discs appear indistinct and merge into the surrounding retina.

2 E   **Microaneurysms**, small capillary outpouchings, and dot and blot haemorrhages are seen in background diabetic retinopathy. New vessel formation and exudates signify more advanced disease.

3 J   Superior **lens dislocation** is a feature of Marfan's syndrome. Patients also usually have poor eyesight due to myopia and astigmatism.

4 B   **Arteriovenous nipping** is one of the early changes of hypertensive retinopathy, corresponding to grade 2 on the Keith–Wagener–Barker grading. Haemorrhages, cotton wool spots and papilloedema are seen in more severe disease.

5 H   Patients with advanced diabetic eye disease suffer from **retinal detachment**, vitreous haemorrhage and scarring of the retina. There is a high chance of progression to significant visual loss.

Oncology

MULTIPLE CHOICE QUESTIONS

1 Side-effects of chemotherapy include:
   a) Bone marrow suppression
   b) Polymyositis
   c) Wegener's granulomatosis
   d) Alopecia
   e) Cystic fibrosis

2 Regarding the treatment of breast cancer:
   a) Mastectomy is only offered to women with metastatic cancer
   b) Oophorectomy is an option for postmenopausal women
   c) Radiotherapy is useful after wide local excision and axillary surgery
   d) Tamoxifen is only used in premenopausal women
   e) Monoclonal antibodies are a useful therapeutic option

3 Complications of axillary lymph node clearance for breast malignancy include:
   a) Sensory loss
   b) Breast discharge
   c) Lymphoedema
   d) Biceps tendonitis
   e) Reduced shoulder movement

4 Smoking is implicated in the aetiology of the following cancers:
   a) Bladder
   b) Prostate
   c) Oesophagus
   d) Larynx
   e) Liver

5 Risk factors for breast cancer include:
   a) Multiparity
   b) Early first pregnancy
   c) Oral contraceptive pill
   d) Smoking
   e) Early menopause

6   Match the following tumour markers with the cancer they are most commonly associated with:
   a) Prostate-specific antigen (PSA); rectum
   b) Alpha-fetoprotein; prostate
   c) CA 125; lung
   d) CA 19.9; pancreas
   e) CA 15.3; brain

7   Side-effects of radiotherapy include:
   a) Pneumonitis
   b) Scurvy
   c) Spinal cord compression
   d) Proctitis
   e) Antiphospholipid syndrome

8   Regarding breast cancer:
   a) Some breast cancers are hereditary
   b) It is the third largest cause of cancer deaths among women in the UK
   c) It does not affect males
   d) Mammography screening is offered every 5 years to women over the age of 45 years
   e) It metastasizes to bone

9   The following are associated with breast malignancy:
   a) Peau d'orange
   b) Fibroadenoma
   c) Periductal mastitis
   d) Paget's disease of the nipple
   e) Gynaecomastia

10   Radiotherapy may be useful for the following oncological problems:
   a) Spinal cord compression
   b) Bone pain
   c) Superior vena cava obstruction
   d) Neutropenic sepsis
   e) Raised intracranial pressure

11   The following statements are true of tamoxifen:
   a) It is given as 3-monthly intramuscular injections
   b) It reduces mortality from breast cancer
   c) Hot flushes are a side-effect
   d) Its use is associated with an increased risk of endometrial cancer
   e) It is offered to all patients with breast cancer

12   Regarding breast cancer:
   a) The inferior medial quadrant of the breast is affected most commonly
   b) Ultrasound provides better imaging than mammography in under-35-year-olds
   c) Nipple discharge usually reflects a malignant cause
   d) It is usually a sarcoma
   e) The breast lump is usually painful

13 The following are oncological emergencies:
   a) Weight loss
   b) Spinal cord compression
   c) Constipation
   d) Jaundice
   e) Superior vena cava obstruction

14 Treatment options for metastatic prostatic cancer include:
   a) Bilateral orchidectomy
   b) Cyproterone
   c) Octreotide
   d) Goserelin
   e) Whipple's procedure

Answers: see pages 315–317

EXTENDED MATCHING QUESTIONS

1 THE AETIOLOGY OF CANCER

Choose the malignancy most associated with each of the carcinogens below

A Gastric carcinoma
B Melanoma
C Bronchial carcinoma
D Nasopharyngeal carcinoma
E Bladder carcinoma
F Oesophageal carcinoma
G Mesothelioma
H Oral cancer
I Hepatocellular carcinoma
J Anal carcinoma

1 Betel nut.
2 Aflatoxin.
3 Asbestos.
4 Human papillomavirus.
5 Epstein–Barr virus.

2 INVESTIGATIONS USED IN ONCOLOGY

Choose the most helpful investigation from the options given for each of the patients below

A Computed tomography (CT) of the abdomen
B X-ray of the spine
C Full blood count
D Urea and electrolytes
E Clotting
F Chest X-ray
G Magnetic resonance imaging (MRI) of the spine
H CT of the thorax
I CT of the brain
J Myelogram

1 A 41-year-old woman, who last received a dose of chemotherapy for non-Hodgkin's lymphoma 10 days ago, presents to the emergency department with a sore throat and pyrexia of 39°C.
2 A 78-year-old man with known chronic obstructive pulmonary disease (COPD) and bronchial carcinoma is seen in oncology clinic. He complains of increasing shortness of breath, headache, and a feeling of fullness in his head. On examination, his jugular venous pressure is raised and he is plethoric with dilated veins across his thorax.
3 A 68-year-old woman with multiple myeloma goes to see her doctor with malaise, nausea, vomiting and constipation. She says that she feels thirsty all the time, and has recently noticed that she has to get up at night-time to pass urine at least twice.
4 A 69-year-old woman with bronchial carcinoma is brought to hospital by her husband. She complains of new-onset urinary retention and faecal incontinence. The registrar detects lax anal tone.
5 A 17-year-old boy is diagnosed with acute myeloid leukaemia. The on-call doctor is asked to see him as he has developed epistaxis and rectal bleeding.

3 DRUGS USED TO TREAT COMPLICATIONS OF CANCER

For each of the patients below, choose the most appropriate drug from the options given

A   Paracetamol
B   Loperamide
C   Dexamethasone
D   Oramorph
E   Co-danthramer

F   Ondansetron
G   Filgrastim
H   Pamidronate
I   Subcutaneous morphine pump
J   Ceftazidime/gentamicin

1   An 87-year-old man with known metastatic prostate cancer presents with a spastic paraparesis.
2   A 72-year-old man, who last received a dose of chemotherapy for lymphoma about a week ago, presents to the emergency department with a pyrexia of 39°C. He says he feels well.
3   A 28-year-old woman, with metastatic adenocarcinoma of unknown origin, becomes febrile overnight on the ward. The doctor suspects neutropenic sepsis, which is confirmed by a full blood count. The consultant says that he would like to give her some medication to increase her white cell count.
4   A 63-year-old woman with metastatic ovarian carcinoma is receiving palliative treatment only. She calls her GP out to see her at home because she says she is extremely constipated and has not opened her bowels for the last 5 days.
5   A 72-year-old woman is diagnosed with ovarian carcinoma. Her oncologist wants to treat her with cisplatin. The patient is concerned as she has read on the internet that cisplatin causes severe vomiting. The oncologist pats her on the shoulder and says he will do his best to make sure that this does not affect her.

4 DRUGS USED TO TREAT MALIGNANT DISEASE

From the options given, choose the drug that best fits each of the descriptions

A   Irinotecan
B   Trastuzumab
C   Vincristine
D   Doxorubicin
E   All trans-retinoic acid

F   Rituximab
G   Methotrexate
H   Chlorambucil
I   Anastrozole
J   Thalidomide

1   An alkylating agent.
2   An antitumour antibiotic.
3   An antimetabolite.
4   A plant-derived alkaloid.
5   A monoclonal antibody used in breast cancer.

5 THE ORIGIN OF MALIGNANCY

Choose the malignancy associated with each tissue below

A   Astrocytoma
B   Ependymoma
C   Cholangiocarcinoma
D   Ewing's sarcoma
E   Rhabdomyosarcoma

F   Wilms' tumour
G   Leiomyosarcoma
H   Mesothelioma
I   Myxoma
J   Chondrosarcoma

1 Striated muscle.
2 Bile duct.
3 Bone marrow.
4 Pleura.
5 Cartilage.

6 TUMOUR MARKERS

Choose the tumour marker most associated with each of the malignancies below

A   Alpha-fetoprotein
B   β-human chorionic gonadotrophin (HCG)
C   CA 19-9
D   CA 125
E   CA 15-3

F   Carcinoembryonic antigen
G   Prostate-specific antigen
H   Calcitonin
I   Thyroglobulin
J   Adrenocorticotrophic hormone (ACTH)

1 Pancreatic carcinoma.
2 Colonic carcinoma.
3 Hepatocellular carcinoma.
4 Ovarian carcinoma.
5 Choriocarcinoma.

Answers: see pages 317–319

X-RAY QUESTIONS

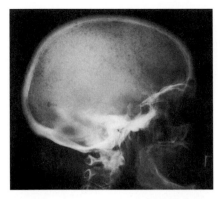

1

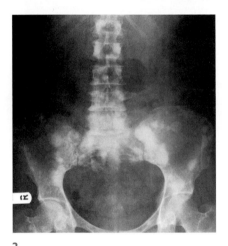

2

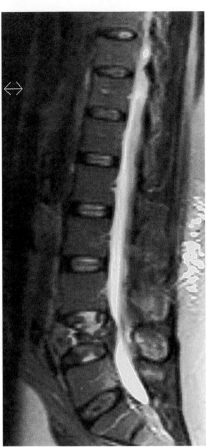

3

To answer the questions below, please refer to the corresponding numbered X-ray images above.

1 A 69-year-old man goes to see his GP saying that he feels tired all the time. The GP performs some blood tests, and asks for an X-ray of his skull.

   a) What is the cause of these appearances?

   b) Which blood tests are typically used to diagnose this condition?

2 An 83-year-old man sees his GP, complaining of weight loss of 8 kg in the past 3 months. He has also noticed some pain around his pelvis. The GP requests an X-ray.

   a) What is the diagnosis?

   b) What is the likely underlying cause of these appearances?

3 A 62-year-old woman, with a history of breast carcinoma, presents to the emergency department with leg weakness. The doctor finds that lower limb tone is decreased, and the plantars are downgoing.

   a) Which type of imaging has been performed?

   b) What is the cause of this patient's symptoms?

Answers: see page 319

ANSWERS

MCQ ANSWERS

1 a) True. Anaemia and thrombocytopenia can be managed with transfusions. Neutropenia must be monitored closely, with a low threshold for starting antibiotics.
   b) False. This is an inflammatory myopathy.
   c) False. This is a granulomatous vasculitis, often affecting the kidneys and respiratory tract.
   d) True.
   e) False. This is an autosomal recessive respiratory disorder, predisposing to bronchiectasis.

2 a) False. A mastectomy is performed if adequate margins cannot be gained with a lumpectomy or if a poor cosmetic result is expected.
   b) False. It is only indicated in premenopausal women.
   c) True.
   d) False. It is used in women of all ages.
   e) True. Trastuzumab (Herceptin), a monoclonal antibody, is used in breast cancers that express the Her-2 receptor.

3 a) True.
   b) False.
   c) True.
   d) False.
   e) True.

4 a) True. Transitional cell carcinoma is linked with smoking.
   b) False.
   c) True. Smoking is a risk factor for both adenocarcinoma and squamous cell carcinoma.
   d) True. The disease is uncommon in non-smokers.
   e) False.

5 a) False. Nulliparity is a risk factor.
   b) False. A late first pregnancy is a risk factor.
   c) True.
   d) False.
   e) False. This is protective.

6 a) False. It is linked to prostate cancer.
   b) False. It is associated with hepatocellular carcinoma or teratomas.
   c) False. It is linked to ovarian carcinoma.
   d) True.
   e) False. It is associated with breast cancer.

7 a) True.
   b) False. This is caused by vitamin C deficiency.
   c) False.
   d) True. This causes diarrhoea.
   e) False.

8 a) True. The *BRCA1* and *BRCA2* genes predispose to familial breast cancer.
   b) False. It is second, behind lung cancer.
   c) False. Male breast cancer does occur, but accounts for less than 1 per cent of breast cancers in the UK.
   d) False. It is available every 3 years over the age of 50.
   e) True.

9 a) True. This is an orange-peel appearance of the skin, caused by lymphatic blockage by a breast carcinoma.
   b) False. This is a benign cause of a breast lump.
   c) False. This is inflammation around dilated milk ducts, causing pain and discharge.
   d) True. This is caused by an intraduct carcinoma spreading within the epidermis of the skin of the nipple.
   e) False. This is a benign condition of breast enlargement in males.

10 a) True.
   b) True.
   c) True.
   d) False. It is treated with antibiotics.
   e) True.

11 a) False. It is administered orally.
   b) True.
   c) True.
   d) True. Patients must be vigilant about abnormal vaginal bleeding.
   e) False. The cancer must be oestrogen-sensitive.

12 a) False. The superior lateral quadrant is most affected.
   b) True.
   c) False. Most cases of discharge are due to benign disease.
   d) False. It is an adenocarcinoma.
   e) False. Typically the lump is painless.

13 a) False.
   b) True. This may be treated with steroids and/or radiotherapy.
   c) False.
   d) False.
   e) True. This may be treated with steroids, anticoagulation, and radiotherapy or chemotherapy.

14 a) True. This reduces testosterone production.
   b) True. This is an anti-androgen.
   c) False.
   d) True. This is a gonadotrophin-releasing hormone (GnRH) analogue that reduces testicular testosterone production.
   e) False. This is a pancreatoduodenectomy.

EMQ ANSWERS

1 THE AETIOLOGY OF CANCER

1 H **Oral cancer** is widespread in Asia where betel nut consumption is common; malignancy is particularly prone to develop in the areas of the mouth where the quid is held.

2 I Ingestion of aflatoxin, a carcinogenic metabolic product of *Aspergillus flavus*, predisposes to **hepatocellular carcinoma**. Aflatoxin can be found in stored foods, especially grains, in tropical areas.

3 G **Mesothelioma**, malignancy of the pleura, is extremely rare without a history of direct or indirect asbestos exposure.

4 J Both **anal carcinoma** and cervical carcinoma are associated with HPV infection, especially types 16 and 18.

5 D **Nasopharyngeal carcinoma** is linked to infection with the Epstein–Barr virus. Other aetiological factors are also likely, as this malignancy is particularly prevalent in Asia, despite Epstein–Barr virus infection occurring worldwide.

2 INVESTIGATIONS USED IN ONCOLOGY

1 C This is a typical history for neutropenic sepsis, which is commonly seen about 10 days after the last dose of chemotherapy. An urgent **full blood count** would show an extremely low neutrophil count, though the administration of antibiotics should not wait until the results of this are available.

2 H Extrinsic compression of the superior vena cava by a bronchial carcinoma causes venous congestion in the head and thorax giving rise to these signs. A **CT of the thorax** will show the lesion impinging on the superior vena cava.

3 D This patient is complaining of constitutional symptoms with nausea, vomiting, constipation, polyuria and polydipsia: all hallmarks of hypercalcaemia, which is associated with multiple myeloma. Measurement of the **urea and electrolytes** would show an elevated serum calcium.

4 G Sphincter disturbance is extremely suggestive of spinal cord compression. An urgent **MRI of the spine** is most helpful, as it clearly shows the level and nature of the lesion pressing on the cord. Plain X-rays are seldom helpful, and myelography (injection of contrast into the spinal canal) is obsolete.

5 E A subtype of acute myeloid leukaemia is associated with disseminated intravascular coagulation, in which there is consumption of clotting factors because of deposition of fibrin within the vascular tree. This may manifest itself as bleeding, in this case from the nose and rectum. A blood sample for **clotting** studies would reveal prolonged prothrombin time (PT)/activated partial thromboplastin time (APTT) with low fibrinogen.

3 DRUGS USED TO TREAT COMPLICATIONS OF CANCER

1 C The onset of spastic paraparesis in a patient with known metastatic cancer (especially prostate cancer which has a predilection for bone) is most probably due to spinal cord compression. Urgent radiotherapy is indicated, but in the interim **dexamethasone** can decrease swelling.

2 J This gentleman is at high risk for neutropenic sepsis, having recently received chemotherapy. Urgent broad-spectrum antibiotics are indicated after blood cultures are taken. Local policies vary, but a reasonable choice would be **ceftazidime/gentamicin.**

3 G **Filgrastim**, recombinant human granulocyte colony-stimulating factor (G-CSF), can be used by specialists to reduce the duration of neutropenia in patients undergoing chemotherapy for cancer.

4 E Patients receiving high doses of opioids may become extremely constipated. **Co-danthramer** is a powerful laxative, but due to the theoretical risk of carcinogenesis, is only used in the terminally ill.

5 F Drugs such as cisplatin, dacarbazine and cyclophosphamide are highly emetogenic. Prophylactic administration of 5-HT$_3$ antagonists, such as **ondansetron**, is highly effective at reducing nausea and vomiting suffered by patients.

4 DRUGS USED TO TREAT MALIGNANT DISEASE

1 H **Chlorambucil** binds to the DNA of rapidly dividing cells and alters it sufficiently that the cell cannot continue with its cell cycle. Other agents in this group include cyclophosphamide and busulfan.

2 D **Doxorubicin**, an anthracycline antibiotic, disrupts DNA synthesis by activating topo-isomerase II, which causes breaks in DNA. An important side-effect of doxorubicin is cardiotoxicity.

3 G **Methotrexate**, an inhibitor of dihydrofolate reductase, is used widely both in oncology and rheumatology. Antimetabolites prevent cellular division by inhibiting essential enzymes. Other drugs in this class include 5-fluorouracil and cytarabine, which interferes with pyrimidine synthesis.

4 C **Vincristine**, a vinca alkaloid, inhibits formation of the mitotic spindle in dividing cells. Neurotoxicity is common, and can manifest itself as paraesthesiae. Other agents in this class include vinblastine and vinorelbine.

5 B **Trastuzumab** is used to treat HER-2 positive breast cancer, which is often a more aggressive form than oestrogen receptor-positive disease.

5 THE ORIGIN OF MALIGNANCY

1 E **Rhabdomyosarcoma** is a rare tumour of striated muscle that usually affects children. The commonest affected areas are the head, neck and bladder, although sometimes tumours affecting the limbs are seen. If possible, treatment is by surgical resection.

2 C **Cholangiocarcinoma** is a malignancy of the bile ducts, and may be intrahepatic or extrahepatic. Patients present with obstructive jaundice, weight loss and abdominal pain. It is unusual for the lesion to be resectable, and consequently the prognosis is generally poor.

3 D **Ewing's sarcoma** is a primary bone tumour affecting children, thought to originate from the red bone marrow. It is highly aggressive and can metastasize to the lung, other bones and to lymph nodes. The characteristic appearance on X-ray is that of an 'onion skin' periosteal reaction.

4 H **Mesothelioma** is strongly associated with asbestos exposure. At the time of presentation, the disease is usually widespread, and curative treatment is never possible. The interval between the primary exposure and the development of mesothelioma may be up to 40 years.

5 J **Chondrosarcoma** is an unusual malignancy of cartilage. The mainstay of treatment is surgical excision: chemotherapy and radiotherapy are usually largely ineffective.

6 TUMOUR MARKERS

1 C Elevated **CA 19-9** levels are seen in 80–90 per cent of pancreatic carcinomas and a lower proportion of biliary tract cancers.

2 F **Carcinoembryonic antigen** is used as a marker to follow up patients who have had their colonic carcinomas resected. A rise in the level often signifies a return of the disease. Note that smokers have higher normal baseline levels of carcinoembryonic antigen than non-smokers.

3 A **Alpha-fetoprotein** is elevated in hepatocellular carcinoma and non-seminomatous germ cell testicular tumours.

4 D Levels of **CA 125** are elevated in most patients with ovarian carcinoma; however, levels also rise in the presence of ascites, fibroids, cirrhosis and pregnancy.

5 B Levels of **β-HCG** are usually markedly elevated in choriocarcinoma and are used to monitor the response to treatment.

X-RAY ANSWERS

1 a) The X-ray shows widespread small lytic lesions in the cranial vault, an appearance that is characteristic of multiple myeloma.

   b) Serum protein electrophoresis usually shows an abnormal immunoglobulin para-protein in myeloma. Other abnormalities of blood may include anaemia, an elevated erythrocyte sedimentation rate (ESR), hyperuricaemia, hypercalcaemia and an elevated alkaline phosphatase.

2 a) There are diffuse sclerotic bone lesions, most likely to be metastatic in origin.

   b) In men, prostate carcinoma is the most likely cause of sclerosing metastases. In a patient presenting with metastatic disease such as this, a hunt should be undertaken to find the primary tumour to guide treatment.

3 a) An MRI scan of the spine is shown. MRI is excellent at visualizing soft tissues, such as spinal cord.

   b) The L4 vertebra has been replaced by bony metastasis, thereby causing compression of the spinal cord. Malignant cord compression is a medical emergency necessitating urgent imaging and radiotherapy.

Ear, nose and throat

MULTIPLE CHOICE QUESTIONS

1   Regarding hearing tests:
    a) The optimum tuning fork to use is 128 Hz in frequency
    b) Weber's test involves placing the tuning fork on the mastoid process
    c) A normal ear should be Rinne negative
    d) The Rinne and Weber tests do not differentiate between conductive and sensori-neural deafness
    e) In Weber's test, sound is heard louder in an ear with conductive deafness

2   Causes of conductive deafness include:
    a) Otosclerosis
    b) Loud noise
    c) Acoustic neuroma
    d) Glue ear
    e) Cholesteatoma

3   Causes of sensorineural deafness include:
    a) Presbyacusis
    b) Otosclerosis
    c) Gentamicin
    d) Warfarin
    e) Ménière's disease

4   Causes of ear discharge include:
    a) Ménière's disease
    b) Presbyacusis
    c) Otitis media
    d) Cholesteatoma
    e) Basal skull fracture

5   Causes of sensorineural deafness include:
    a) Furosemide
    b) Otitis media
    c) Paget's disease
    d) Acoustic neuroma
    e) Bell's palsy

6 Causes of ear pain include:
   a) Barotrauma
   b) Glue ear
   c) Tinnitus
   d) Otitis externa
   e) Benign positional vertigo

7 The following measures can be used to treat epistaxis:
   a) Nasal packing
   b) Arterial ligation
   c) Foley catheter
   d) Cautery
   e) Sengstaken–Blakemore tube

8 Causes of chronic nasal obstruction include:
   a) Deviated nasal septum
   b) Choanal atresia
   c) Kallmann's syndrome
   d) Enlarged adenoids
   e) Sinusitis

9 Causes of a hoarse voice include:
   a) Singer's nodules
   b) Bronchial carcinoma
   c) Oesophagitis
   d) Choanal atresia
   e) Laryngeal carcinoma

10 Ménière's disease:
   a) Is inherited as autosomal recessive
   b) Causes tinnitus
   c) Causes deafness
   d) Is treated with gabapentin
   e) May have nystagmus as a feature

Answers: see pages 324–325

EXTENDED MATCHING QUESTIONS

1 EAR DISEASE

Each of the patients below seeks medical attention for an ear problem. Choose the best diagnosis from the options given for each of the clinical scenarios

A   Acute otitis media
B   Chronic otitis media
C   Cholesteatoma
D   Ménière's disease
E   Mastoiditis

F   Barotrauma
G   Ramsay–Hunt syndrome
H   Otitis externa
I   Pinna haematoma
J   Labyrinthitis

1   A 31-year-old boxer goes to see his doctor the morning after a prize fight, which he proudly states that he won. He asks the doctor to look at his right ear, which is swollen and painful.

2   A 9-year-old boy goes to see his doctor with fever and ear pain. On examination, the area just behind the ear is slightly red and tender, and the tympanic membrane is erythematous and bulging.

3   A 6-year-old boy goes to see his general practitioner (GP) with his mother. He has had a fever for the last 2 days and says he has ear pain. When the GP looks in his ear, there is a red, bulging tympanic membrane.

4   A 55-year-old man goes to see his GP complaining of a foul-smelling discharge from his right ear, and hearing loss. On examination, there is a pearly white mass within the auditory canal.

5   A 32-year-old man is referred to hospital by his GP with a left VIIth nerve palsy. On examination, the registrar finds a vesicular eruption in the external auditory meatus.

2 NECK LUMPS

Each of the patients below seeks medical attention for a neck lump. Choose the best diagnosis from the options given for each of the clinical scenarios

A   Torticollis
B   Thyroglossal cyst
C   Cystic hygroma
D   Tonsillitis
E   Pharyngeal pouch

F   Branchial cyst
G   Carotid body tumour
H   Cervical rib
I   Lymphadenopathy
J   Goitre

1   A 21-year-old man presents with a soft discrete 3 cm mass just anterior to the sternocleidomastoid, at the junction of the upper and middle thirds. It does not move on swallowing and does not transilluminate.

2   A 6-month-old boy, who was born with the assistance of forceps, is brought in to his GP by his mother. She is worried as his head is permanently tilted to the left. The GP feels a lump in the sternocleidomastoid.

3   A 67-year-old man is referred to hospital with a lump in his neck and dysphagia. He has a smooth 5 cm swelling, which he says he has noticed gurgling at night. The consultant notes that the patient has been admitted three times in the past year with aspiration pneumonia.

4   A 71-year-old woman is found to have a pulsatile left-sided neck mass. She says that it has been there for some time, but has been slowly enlarging.

5   A 24-year-old man seeks medical attention as he has noticed a lump in his neck. On examination, there is a painless 1 cm swelling in the midline. It moves superiorly when the patient sticks out his tongue.

Answers: see pages 325–326

ANSWERS

MCQ ANSWERS

1 a) False. A 512 Hz tuning fork is ideal.
   b) False. It is placed on the forehead or upper incisors.
   c) False. Air conduction is better than bone conduction in normal ears; this is known as Rinne positive.
   d) False. By combining the tests, the side and the nature of the deafness can be determined.
   e) True.

2 a) True. The stapes becomes fixed to the oval window, preventing sound conduction to the inner ear.
   b) False. This causes sensorineural deafness.
   c) False. This is a cause of sensorineural deafness.
   d) True. Chronic secretory otitis media produces a middle ear effusion, causing deafness.
   e) True. This is proliferation of skin in the middle ear cleft, causing discharge and deafness.

3 a) True. This is the deafness of old age – primarily to high-frequency sounds.
   b) False. This is a degenerative cause of conductive deafness.
   c) True. This is a well-known ototoxic drug.
   d) False. This is not a recognized side-effect.
   e) True. Deafness, vertigo and tinnitus are features.

4 a) False.
   b) False. This is sensorineural deafness of old age.
   c) True. This causes a purulent discharge.
   d) True. This produces an offensive discharge.
   e) True. This can give rise to cerebrospinal fluid otorrhoea.

5 a) True. This is a rare side-effect.
   b) False. This has a conductive cause.
   c) True. Excessive new bone formation can cause compression of the eighth cranial nerve.
   d) True. This is an eighth nerve sheath neurofibroma at the cerebellopontine angle.
   e) False. This is an idiopathic facial nerve palsy.

6 a) True. When atmospheric pressure increases, a patent Eustachian tube allows pressure equalization of the middle ear. A blocked Eustachian tube can predispose to damage to the middle or inner ear as external pressure increases, for example while diving.
   b) True. This is chronic secretory otitis media.
   c) False.
   d) True. This is inflammation of the external ear.
   e) False.

7 a) True. Ribbon gauze is inserted into the nose to stop bleeding.
   b) True. This can be done endoscopically.
   c) True. The balloon can be inflated in the pharynx and pulled upwards to provide pressure posteriorly.
   d) True. Topical silver nitrate is effective.
   e) False. This is used for oesophageal variceal bleeds.

8 a) True.
   b) True. This is a rare cause of nasal obstruction in children.
   c) False. This is a genetic disorder causing anosmia.
   d) True.
   e) True.

9 a) True. These are keratinous nodules that may appear on the vocal cords due to overuse of the voice.
   b) True. Extension of the carcinoma can involve the recurrent laryngeal nerve, giving rise to hoarseness.
   c) False.
   d) False. This is a cause of nasal obstruction in children.
   e) True. This is a squamous cell carcinoma. Glottic tumours produce hoarseness earlier and therefore present more quickly, giving a better prognosis.

10 a) False. It is not an inheritable disease.
    b) True.
    c) True. Tinnitus, deafness and vertigo are all symptoms of the disease.
    d) False. Betahistine, diuretics, antihistamines and phenothiazines are all used in the treatment of the condition.
    e) True.

EMQ ANSWERS

1 EAR DISEASE

1 I A **pinna haematoma** is a collection of blood between the cartilage and the perichondrium, and is secondary to trauma. Drainage of the haematoma is needed to prevent the permanent deformity of cauliflower ear.

2 E **Mastoiditis** is an important complication of otitis media. There is spread of infection to the mastoid process. Treatment with intravenous antibiotics is urgently indicated to prevent infection spreading into the cranial vault.

3 A **Acute otitis media** is common in children, and is usually caused by *Streptococcus pneumoniae*, *Haemophilus influenzae* or *Moraxella catarrhalis*. Treatment is with oral antibiotics and analgesics.

4 C A **cholesteatoma** is an overgrowth of squamous epithelial cells within the middle ear. This typically appears as a pearly white mass on otoscopy. Surgery is required to prevent destruction of local tissues.

5 G Involvement of the geniculate ganglion of the facial nerve by herpes zoster, the **Ramsay–Hunt syndrome**, leads to a lower motor neurone VIIth nerve palsy, loss of taste in the anterior two-thirds of the tongue, and vesicles within the ear.

2 NECK LUMPS

1 F A **branchial cyst** is a congenital lesion that may not present until adulthood, and is usually derived from the embryological second branchial cleft. The location of the neck lump is characteristic. Treatment is by surgical excision.

2 A Trauma to the sternocleidomastoid during delivery can cause **torticollis** in children. Presentation is usually with a tilted head and a thickening or a lump within the sterno-cleidomastoid muscle.

3 E A **pharyngeal pouch** is an extrusion of the pharynx through the neck muscles, and typically causes dysphagia with a neck mass. It predisposes to aspiration pneumonia, as regurgitated food may be inhaled.

4 G Pulsatile masses imply vascular involvement: in this case, the best answer is **carotid body tumour**. These usually grow slowly, but may metastasize in the later stages of the disease.

5 B **Thyroglossal cysts** are embryological remnants of the thyroid gland. They are attached to the base of the tongue and therefore characteristically move upwards on tongue protrusion.

CHAPTER 16

Public health and statistics

MULTIPLE CHOICE QUESTIONS

1   The following types of study require follow-up:
   a) Cohort study
   b) Case–control study
   c) Randomized controlled trial
   d) Meta-analysis
   e) Ecological study

2   The following are notifiable diseases in England:
   a) Tuberculosis
   b) Gonorrhoea
   c) Hepatitis A
   d) Chickenpox
   e) Rabies

3   There are nationalized screening programmes for the following diseases in the UK:
   a) Hepatitis C
   b) Colon cancer
   c) Prostate cancer
   d) Phenylketonuria
   e) Abdominal aortic aneurysm

4   Immunization is available for the following infections:
   a) Influenza
   b) Hepatitis C
   c) Typhoid
   d) Malaria
   e) Chickenpox

5   The following are acceptable entries in section 1a of a death certificate, unqualified by any other entry:
   a) Myocardial infarction
   b) Exhaustion
   c) Bronchopneumonia
   d) Heart failure
   e) Diabetes mellitus

6   The following routine steps are essential when certifying death:
   a) Checking pupil reflexes
   b) Auscultating for breath sounds
   c) Testing capillary refill
   d) Measuring body temperature
   e) Checking blood pressure

7   State whether the following terms are correctly matched with their definitions:
   a) Sensitivity; proportion of subjects who test positive for a disease who actually have that disease
   b) Specificity; proportion of healthy subjects who test negative for a disease
   c) Positive predictive value; proportion of subjects with a disease who test positive for that disease
   d) Negative predictive value; proportion of subjects who test negative for a disease who are clear of the disease
   e) Incidence; the number of people with a disease in a defined population

8   The following are criteria for screening for a disease:
   a) The disease is fatal
   b) The screening programme should reduce mortality or morbidity
   c) The disease prevalence must be greater than 1 per cent
   d) There should be an effective treatment for the disease
   e) Screening should be cost-effective

Answers: see pages 331–332

EXTENDED MATCHING QUESTIONS

1 TERMS USED IN STATISTICS 1

Select the most appropriate statistical term for each of the clinical scenarios below

A   Sensitivity
B   Specificity
C   Positive predictive value
D   Negative predictive value
E   Number needed to treat

F   Relative risk
G   Incidence
H   Prevalence
I   Absolute risk reduction
J   Confidence interval

1 A general practitioner (GP) recommends that his patients go for cervical smear testing. A young executive makes an appointment and asks him the exact proportion of cases of cervical dysplasia picked up by the test.

2 A 31-year-old woman has some blood tests for systemic lupus erythematosus. The anti-nuclear antibody (ANA) is positive. She wants to know how likely she is to have the disease.

3 A GP refers a 28-year-old man to hospital for a renal ultrasound, as he has discovered that his mother has polycystic kidney disease. The patient is extremely worried and returns 1 week later for the results. The GP tells him that his kidneys appear normal, but the young man wants to know, given this information, what his chances are of having polycystic kidneys.

4 A teenager has her contraceptive medication changed by her doctor. She is concerned about the risk of deep venous thrombosis, and wants to know how much more likely she is to have a blood clot while on this medication.

5 A 58 year-old woman is treated for breast cancer with anastrozole, but suffers from debilitating hot flushes. She is considering stopping the treatment, and wants to know how many women have to take the drug for one to gain a benefit.

2 TERMS USED IN STATISTICS 2

Select the statistical term that best fits each of the calculations below

A   Sensitivity
B   Specificity
C   Positive predictive value
D   Negative predictive value
E   Number needed to treat

F   Relative risk
G   Incidence
H   Prevalence
I   Absolute risk reduction
J   Confidence interval

1 $\dfrac{1}{\text{Absolute risk reduction}}$

2 $\dfrac{\text{True positive test result}}{\text{All positive test results}}$

3 $\dfrac{\text{True negative test results}}{\text{All patients without disease}}$

4 The number of new cases of a disease within a specific time period.

5 $\dfrac{\text{Chance of disease in exposed population}}{\text{Chance of disease in unexposed population}}$

3 EVIDENCE-BASED MEDICINE

Select the most appropriate data source for each of the scenarios below

A   Case–control study
B   Randomized controlled trial
C   Cohort study
D   Crossover study
E   Phase 1 trial

F   Phase 2 trial
G   Phase 4 trial
H   Case report
I   Meta-analysis
J   Cross-sectional study

1   A pharmaceutical company wants to test a new substance to see if it works in patients.

2   A professor of medicine wants to see if there is any overall benefit in using statins to prevent stroke, as to his mind, none of the trials to date have been adequately powered.

3   The government wants to find out how common chronic obstructive pulmonary disease (COPD) is in the community.

4   The management of a nuclear power plant wants to find out if workers exposed to plutonium have a higher chance of developing leukaemia.

5   A consultant respiratory physician makes the diagnosis of pulmonary alveolar micro-lithiasis in one of her patients. There have only ever been 300 reported cases in the world in the last century. She wonders how to treat the patient.

Answers: see pages 332–333

ANSWERS

MCQ ANSWERS

1 a) True. A control group and a group of people with risk factors for a disease are followed up, with analysis of the numbers of new cases of the disease.
   b) False. Cases and controls are tested for prior exposure to a risk factor for a particular disease.
   c) True. The efficacy of an intervention is tested in an experimental group and compared with a control group.
   d) False. This is a statistical analysis of several different studies.
   e) False. This is a study comparing the characteristics of different populations.

2 a) True.
   b) False.
   c) True. All forms of viral hepatitis are notifiable.
   d) False.
   e) True.

3 a) False.
   b) False.
   c) False.
   d) True. The Guthrie test in newborns screens for this disease as well as congenital hypothyroidism.
   e) False.

4 a) True. The elderly and other high-risk groups are advised to take a yearly vaccine against seasonal influenza.
   b) False.
   c) True.
   d) False.
   e) True. It is offered to non-immune healthcare workers.

5 a) True.
   b) False. Section 1a requires a disease or condition leading directly to death, not the mechanism of death.
   c) True.
   d) False. Organ failure is not acceptable if the underlying cause is not stated.
   e) False. The immediate, direct cause of death must be given, for example, diabetic ketoacidosis.

6 a) True. The pupils must be fixed and dilated.
   b) True.
   c) False.
   d) False.
   e) False.

7 a) False. It is the proportion of subjects with a disease who test positive.
   b) True.
   c) False. The positive predictive value is the proportion of subjects who test positive for a disease who actually have that disease.
   d) True.
   e) False. Incidence measures the number of new cases in a population per unit time.

8 a) False.
   b) True.
   c) False.
   d) True.
   e) True.

EMQ ANSWERS

1 TERMS USED IN STATISTICS 1

1 A This patient is asking how good a test is at picking up cases of disease. This is known as the **sensitivity**, the proportion of diseased patients identified out of all the diseased patients tested.

2 C The question here is: given a positive test result (ANA), what is the likelihood of having the disease? The **positive predictive value** answers this question.

3 D **Negative predictive value.** This stem asks the opposite of question 2: given a negative test result, what is the likelihood of not having the disease?

4 F The **relative risk** is the patient's risk of developing the condition, compared to a normal population. For example, women on the contraceptive pill are approximately two times more likely to develop deep venous thrombosis than those not taking any medication.

5 E The **number needed to treat** is a useful figure as it is the number of patients who have to take a treatment for one to benefit. For example, eighty healthy people need to take a statin to lower their cholesterol for one myocardial infarction to be prevented.

TERMS USED IN STATISTICS 2

1 E The **number needed to treat** is the absolute number of patients who need to take the treatment for one to derive a benefit. For example, if a new drug decreases the chance of myocardial infarction by 4 per cent, 25 people (1 ÷ 0.04) need to take the drug to prevent one event.

2 C This calculation assesses the proportion of patients with a positive test result who actually have the disease, the **positive predictive value**.

3 B **Specificity.** This calculation assesses what proportion of patients without disease will have an accurate negative result, i.e. how good the test is at correctly identifying healthy people.

4 G The **incidence** describes the number of new cases of a disease in a specific time period; it differs from the prevalence which measures all cases of a disease, not just new ones.

5 F The **relative risk** is the ratio of the risk of disease in the exposed population compared to the unexposed population. For example, the relative risk of smoking causing lung cancer is 15: smokers are 15 times more likely to develop this condition than matched non-smokers.

3 EVIDENCE-BASED MEDICINE

1 F New substances that drug companies want to test on humans first undergo Phase 1 trials on healthy volunteers or patients to test that the drug is safe and to ascertain the correct dose. The first time that the clinical efficacy is assessed is in **Phase 2 trials.**

2 I A **meta-analysis** in this setting would combine the data from the inadequately powered trials to try to produce results that were statistically significant in order to answer the clinical question. An alternative would be a new, large, randomized controlled clinical trial – this however would be time-consuming and extremely expensive in comparison.

3 J A **cross-sectional study** would involve taking a representative sample of the population, measuring the prevalence of COPD, and then extrapolating those data to the entire population.

4 A A **case–control study** is the most efficient use of resources for evaluating rare exposures, such as plutonium. Workers from the plant could be matched with similar workers at, for example, a coal-fired power station to see if there was any difference in the incidence of leukaemia.

5 H Pulmonary alveolar microlithiasis is an exceptionally rare disease. It is extremely unlikely that any clinical trials have been done on such a small patient population. Therefore, the best quality of data available is likely to be from **case reports.**

Index

Note: References for questions are given in the form of the starting page number followed in brackets by the question number(s) which may run over on to the following page. The few references without brackets indicate the page ranges of chapter topics.